Gastroenterology

Editors

AMIR E. SOUMEKH
PHILIP O. KATZ

CLINICS IN GERIATRIC MEDICINE

www.geriatric.theclinics.com

February 2021 • Volume 37 • Number 1

ELSEVIER

1600 John F. Kennedy Boulevard • Suite 1800 • Philadelphia, Pennsylvania, 19103-2899

http://www.theclinics.com

CLINICS IN GERIATRIC MEDICINE Volume 37, Number 1
February 2021 ISSN 0749–0690, ISBN-13: 978-0-323-75634-1

Editor: Katerina Heidhausen
Developmental Editor: Laura Fisher

Clinics in Geriatric Medicine (ISSN 0749-0690) is published quarterly by Elsevier Inc., 360 Park Avenue South, New York, NY 10010-1710. Months of issue are February, May, August, and November. Business and Editorial Offices: 1600 John F. Kennedy Blvd., Suite 1800, Philadelphia, PA 191023-2899. Periodicals postage paid at New York, NY, and additional mailing offices. Subscription prices are $295.00 per year (US individuals), $875.00 per year (US institutions), $100.00 per year (US & Canadian student/resident), $320.00 per year (Canadian individuals), $928.00 per year (Canadian institutions), $418.00 per year (international individuals), $928.00 per year (international institutions), and $195.00 per year (international student/resident). Foreign air speed delivery is included in all *Clinics* subscription prices. All prices are subject to change without notice. POSTMASTER: Send address changes to *Clinics in Geriatric Medicine,* Elsevier Health Sciences Division, Subscription Customer Service, 3251 Riverport Lane, Maryland Heights, MO 63043. **Telephone: 1-800-654-2452 (U.S. and Canada); 314-447-8871 (outside U.S. and Canada). Fax: 314-447-8029. E-mail:** journalscustomerservice-usa@elsevier.com **(for print support)** or journalsonlinesupport-usa@elsevier.com **(for online support).**

Reprints. For copies of 100 or more, of articles in this publication, please contact the Commercial Reprints Department, Elsevier Inc., 360 Park Avenue South, New York, New York 10010-1710. Tel.: 212-633-3874; Fax: 212-633-3820, E-mail: reprints@elsevier.com.

Clinics in Geriatric Medicine is covered in *MEDLINE/PubMed (Index Medicus), EMBASE/Excerpta Medica, Current Contents/Clinical Medicine (CC/CM),* and the *Cumulative Index to Nursing & Allied Health Literature.*

Contributors

EDITORS

AMIR E. SOUMEKH, MD
Assistant Professor of Clinical Medicine, Jay Monahan Center for Gastrointestinal Health, Weill Cornell Medical College, New York, New York

PHILIP O. KATZ, MD
Professor of Medicine, Division of Gastroenterology and Hepatology, Jay Monahan Center for Gastrointestinal Health, Weill Cornell Medical College, New York, New York

AUTHORS

AIYA ABOUBAKR, MD
Department of Medicine, NewYork-Presbyterian Hospital/Weill Cornell Medicine, New York, New York

ANDREA L. BETESH, MD
Assistant Professor of Medicine, Department of Gastroenterology and Hepatology, NewYork-Presbyterian Hospital/Weill Cornell Medicine, New York, New York

ANKIT CHHODA, MD
Chief Resident, Department of Internal Medicine, Bridgeport Hospital, Yale New Haven Hospital System, New Haven, Connecticut

MICHELLE S. COHEN, MD
Assistant Professor of Clinical Medicine, Division of Gastroenterology and Hepatology, Weill Cornell Medicine, New York, New York

SHIRLEY COHEN-MEKELBURG, MD, MS
Assistant Professor, Inflammatory Bowel Disease Program, VA Ann Arbor Healthcare System, VA Center for Clinical Management Research, Clinical Lecturer, Division of Gastroenterology and Hepatology, Department of Internal Medicine, Michigan Medicine, Institute for Healthcare Policy and Innovation, University of Michigan, Ann Arbor, Michigan

NICHOLAS J. COSTABLE, MD
Department of Internal Medicine, Icahn School of Medicine at Mount Sinai, New York

CARL V. CRAWFORD, MD
Assistant Professor of Medicine, Division of Gastroenterology, Weill Cornell Medicine, NewYork-Presbyterian Hospital, New York, New York

GREGORY DAKIN, MD, FACS
Chief, Division of GI, Metabolic, and Bariatric Surgery, Weill Cornell Medical Center, New York, New York

ENAD DAWOD, MD
Resident Physician, Department of Medicine, Weill Cornell Medicine, NewYork-Presbyterian Hospital, New York, New York

DAVID A. GREENWALD, MD, FACG
Director of Clinical Gastroenterology and Endoscopy, Department of Internal Medicine, Division of Gastroenterology, Icahn School of Medicine at Mount Sinai, New York

LUCINDA A. HARRIS, MS, MD
Associate Professor of Medicine, Division of Gastroenterology and Hepatology, Alix School of Medicine, Mayo Clinic, Scottsdale, Arizona

PRASAD G. IYER, MSc
Division of Gastroenterology and Hepatology, Mayo Clinic, Rochester, Minnesota

PHILIP O. KATZ, MD
Professor of Medicine, Division of Gastroenterology and Hepatology, Jay Monahan Center for Gastrointestinal Health, Weill Cornell Medical College, New York, New York

TIBOR KRISKO, MD
Assistant Professor of Medicine, Director of Endoscopy, Associate Site Director, LMH/NYP, Division of Gastroenterology and Hepatology, Joan & Sanford I. Weill Department of Medicine, Weill Cornell Medicine, New York, New York

MINDY WINGHIN LEE, MD
Assistant Professor, Division of Gastroenterology and Hepatology, Weill Cornell Medical College, New York, New York

SUSAN LUCAK, MD
Affiliated Clinical Assistant Professor of Clinical Medicine, Weill Cornell Medicine, Special Lecturer, Columbia University Irving Medical Center, New York, New York

TISHA N. LUNSFORD, MD
Assistant Professor of Medicine, Division of Gastroenterology and Hepatology, Alix School of Medicine, Mayo Clinic, Scottsdale, Arizona

SRIHARI MAHADEV, MD, MS
Assistant Professor of Medicine, Advanced Endoscopy, Division of Gastroenterology and Hepatology, Weill Cornell Medicine, New York, New York

BAHARAK MOSHIREE, MD, MSc
Director of Motility, Professor of Medicine, Atrium Health-Charlotte, UNC School of Medicine, Charlotte, North Carolina

SAURABH S. MUKEWAR, MD
Assistant Professor of Medicine, Advanced Endoscopy, Division of Gastroenterology and Hepatology, Weill Cornell Medicine, New York, New York

CAROLYN NEWBERRY, MD
Co-Director, Innovative Center for Health and Nutrition in Gastroenterology (ICHANGE), Division of Gastroenterology, Weill Cornell Medical Center, New York, New York

FOUAD OTAKI, MD
Assistant Professor of Medicine, Division of Gastroenterology and Hepatology, Oregon Health & Science University, Portland, Oregon

TRISHA PASRICHA, MD
Clinical Research Fellow, Department of Gastroenterology, Massachusetts General Hospital, Boston, Massachusetts

FELICE H. SCHNOLL-SUSSMAN, MD
Professor of Clinical Medicine, Department of Gastroenterology and Hepatology, NewYork-Presbyterian Hospital/Weill Cornell Medicine, New York, New York

MORGAN A. SENDZISCHEW SHANE, MD
Clinical Instructor, Division of Gastroenterology, Department of Medicine, University of Miami Miller School of Medicine, Miami, Florida

KYLE STALLER, MD, MPH
Director, Gastrointestinal Motility Laboratory, Assistant Professor of Medicine, Department of Gastroenterology, Massachusetts General Hospital, Boston, Massachusetts

AKBAR K. WALJEE, MD, MSc
Staff Physician and Research Scientist, Inflammatory Bowel Disease Program, VA Ann Arbor Healthcare System, VA Center for Clinical Management Research, Associate Professor, Division of Gastroenterology and Hepatology, Department of Internal Medicine, Michigan Medicine, Institute for Healthcare Policy and Innovation, University of Michigan, Michigan Integrated Center for Health Analytics and Medical Prediction (MiCHAMP), University of Michigan, Ann Arbor, Michigan

DAVID WAN, MD
Assistant Professor of Medicine, Division of Gastroenterology and Hepatology, Joan & Sanford I. Weill Department of Medicine, Weill Cornell Medicine, New York, New York

Contents

The elderly are particularly prone to developing upper gastrointestinal disturbances. Changes are due to the aging process, diabetes, cardiovascular risk factors, and neurologic issues. Medications used to treat these underlying conditions can cause gastrointestinal symptoms. Dysphagia is common and can be oropharyngeal and/or esophageal. Gastroparesis is due to either medications such as opiates, or due to neurologic sequala of diabetes, cerebrovascular accidents, or neurologic diseases such as Parkinson's disease. Given limitations in many commonly used prokinetics with a wide range of side effect profiles including neurologic and cardiac, the focus of treatment should be on symptom management with dietary changes.

As our population continues to age, the early diagnosis and optimal management of patients with gastroesophageal reflux disease becomes paramount. Maintaining a low threshold for evaluating atypical symptoms in this population is key to improving outcomes. Should patients develop complications including severe esophagitis, peptic stricture, or Barrett esophagus, then a discussion of medical, endoscopic, and surgical treatments that accounts for patient's comorbidities and survival is important. Advances in screening, surveillance, and endoscopic treatment of Barrett esophagus have allowed us to dispel concerns of futility and treat a larger subset of the at-risk population.

Advanced age, history of peptic ulcer disease, Helicobacter pylori, coadministration of nonsteroidal antiinflammatory drugs (NSAIDs), corticosteroids, anticoagulation, and antiplatelets are risk factors for gastrointestinal bleeding in the elderly. Awareness of these risks and appropriate use of NSAIDs, particularly in those needing antiplatelet or anticoagulant therapy, is critical to optimal management. Careful selection of elderly patients requiring antiplatelet, anticoagulation, or chronic NSAID therapy for cotherapy with proton pump inhibitors can significantly reduce morbidity and mortality from gastrointestinal bleeding.

Geriatric patients tend to have subtle presentations of biliary disorders and, if untreated, can decompensate acutely. Each biliary disorder warrants formulation of an individualized treatment plan with a multidisciplinary approach. Acute cholecystitis, a common complication of gallstones, is initially managed by conservative measures and subsequently, among patients with optimal surgical risk, through laparoscopic or open cholecystectomy. High-risk patients undergo temporization, percutaneous or endoscopic, followed by definitive intervention. Acute cholecystitis with complications (ie, perforation, gangrene, or small bowel obstruction) warrants emergent cholecystectomy. Gallstone migration into the biliary system can cause choledocholithiasis, often complicated by biliary pancreatitis or cholangitis if not intervened. Therapy for choledocholithiasis is based on biliary clearance through endoscopic and, infrequently, surgical approaches.

Fecal incontinence can be a challenging and stigmatizing disease with a high prevalence in the elderly population. Despite effective treatment options, most patients do not receive care. Clues in the history and physical examination can assist the provider in establishing the diagnosis. Direct inquiry about the presence of incontinence is key. Bowel disturbances are common triggers for symptoms and represent some of the easiest treatment targets. We review the epidemiology and impact of the disease, delineate a diagnostic and treatment approach for primary care physicians to identify patients with suspected fecal incontinence and describe appropriate treatment options.

Chronic constipation affects one-third of the US population and occurs disproportionately in the elderly and female individuals, increasing in older individuals who are institutionalized. This condition has a significant impact on health care costs and quality of life. Clinicians need to consider primary as well as secondary causes of constipation in elderly individuals because the cause is often multifactorial. Diagnostic algorithms should eliminate red-flag symptoms that may indicate a malignancy but also consider pelvic floor dysfunction, which is more common in this age group. An appropriate treatment plan is tailored to the severity of the patient's symptoms.

Diarrhea is a fairly common problem among the elderly that has a higher morbidity and mortality compared with the general population. There are multiple reasons for diarrhea in the elderly that can be stratified by different mechanisms: infectious, osmotic, secretory, inflammatory, and malabsorptive. Oral hydration and dietary management are the basic management principles for all forms of diarrhea but specific treatment should address the root cause of diarrhea in order to improve outcomes.

Functional bowel disorders refer to disorders of gut-brain interaction that affect the intestinal tract. Irritable bowel syndrome (IBS) is the most common functional bowel disorder and affects individuals regardless of age and gender. It can result in impaired quality of life and significant health care utilization and is therefore important to recognize and manage. The diagnosis of IBS is based on clinical symptoms. IBS is categorized based on predominant bowel habit (constipation, diarrhea, mixed, or unclassified), and the treatment of IBS is individually tailored based on subtype and symptom severity.

Aging alters the way the body digests food, absorbs nutrients, and metabolizes energy. Changes in deglutition, digestion, and metabolism in this population are well described and may lead to alterations in oral intake, body composition, and overall health status. Elderly persons are at high risk for developing sarcopenia as well as sarcopenic obesity characterized by accelerated reduction in lean muscle mass and enhancement of body fat. Nutritional screening is important to identify high-risk individuals and facilitate care management planning. The most common assessment tool in elderly patients is the Mini Nutritional Assessment, which analyzes oral intake, health status, and anthropometrics.

Diverticulosis consists of outpouching of colonic mucosa and submucosa through the muscularis. Although prevalence of diverticulosis increases with age, clinically-relevant diverticular diseases remain rare. This includes diverticulitis, which presents as acute abdominal pain and is traditionally managed with antibiotics, and in complicated cases, surgery. Diverticular hemorrhage, the most-common etiology of lower gastrointestinal bleeding, typically manifests with large volume red blood per rectum. Diverticular diseases place a significant burden on the healthcare system, and recent developments have altered the timing and choice of traditional management decisions. Lifestyle interventions such as high-fiber diet and tobacco cessation are effective at preventing diverticular disease.

Upper gastrointestinal (GI) bleeding is a common reason for hospital admission in older adult patients and carries a high morbidity and mortality if not properly managed. Risk factors include advanced age, Helicobacter pylori infection, medication use, smoking, and history of liver disease. Patients with known or suspected liver disease and suspected variceal bleeding should also receive antibiotics and somatostatin analogues. Risk stratification scores should be used to determine patients at highest risk for further decompensation. Upper endoscopy is both a diagnostic and therapeutic tool used in the management of upper GI bleeding. Endoscopy should be performed within 24 hours of presentation after appropriate resuscitation. Management of anticoagulation in upper GI bleeding largely depends on the indication for anticoagulation, the risk of continued bleeding with continuing the medication, and the risk of thrombosis with discontinuing the medication. A multidisciplinary approach to the decision of anticoagulation continuation is preferred when possible.

Colorectal cancer (CRC) is a common and preventable malignancy, and routine CRC screening is recommended for average risk individuals between the ages of 50 and 75 years. Screening has been shown to decrease CRC incidence and mortality. Once patients are older than 75 years, the risk to benefit ratio of ongoing screening begins to shift. As comorbidities increase and life expectancy decreases, the future potential benefits of CRC prevention become less robust, and risk for screening-related complications grows. However, firm age cutoffs are not sufficient to guide these decisions, as there is substantial physiologic heterogeneity among individuals of the same age.

Although management of inflammatory bowel disease follows a similar approach for all adults, there are certain characteristics making its treatment more challenging in older patients. The advent of novel medical treatments has changed the paradigm of inflammatory bowel disease, with an increasing focus on preventing disease progression in addition to controlling symptoms. The safety of these therapies in the elderly needs to be considered. Management of inflammatory bowel disease in the elderly is confounded by comorbidities that can increase the risk of medication or surgical complications; polypharmacy and altered pharmacokinetics also increase the risk of drug–drug interactions and adverse events.

CLINICS IN GERIATRIC MEDICINE

THE CLINICS ARE AVAILABLE ONLINE!
Access your subscription at:
www.theclinics.com

Preface

Common Gastroenterology Disorders in the Elderly

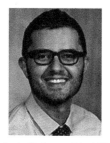
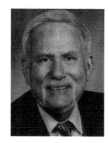

Amir E. Soumekh, MD   Philip O. Katz, MD

Editors

We are not victims of aging, sickness, and death. These are part of scenery, not the seer, who is immune to any form of change. This seer is the spirit, the expression of eternal being.

—Deepak Chopra

The world is aging. With improved access to nutrition, hygiene, vaccinations, preventative care, and medical care for chronic diseases, the global average age continues to rise as does the number of elderly patients. The United Nations estimates approximately 1 in 10 people in the world are over the age of 65 and expects this figure to climb. Furthermore, the proportion of adult life spent beyond age 65 has seen a steady rise. As physicians, we will be challenged by the unique medical needs of this population.

The gastrointestinal (GI) tract presents particular challenges to the aging patient and the clinician. Approximately 30 feet long, the GI tract is the largest immune organ in the body as well as the largest endocrine organ, contains more bacterial cells than there are human cells in the body, has a dedicated nervous system that functions independently of the central nervous system, and has a complex muscular structure. The GI organs are responsible for intake of food, secretion of numerous enzymes and fluids, digestion, extraction and absorption of nutrients, immune protection against infectious agents, immune tolerance of beneficial bacteria, and, finally, excretion of waste products. These functions occur continuously and seamlessly with perfect coordination— except when they don't! As patients age, in addition to normal physiologic changes, numerous factors, including environmental exposures, acquired genetic and cellular changes, medications, and medical procedures, lead to increased disruptions of normal GI function.

Clin Geriatr Med 37 (2021) xiii–xiv
https://doi.org/10.1016/j.cger.2020.10.001
0749-0690/21/© 2020 Published by Elsevier Inc.

Elderly patients experience increased rates of esophageal and gastric disorders, with a higher incidence of motility abnormalities, gastroesophageal reflux, reflux complications (such as Barrett's, dysplasia, and esophageal cancer), gastric ulcers, and GI bleeding. Similarly, lower GI diseases, such as pelvic floor disorders (and fecal incontinence), constipation, diarrheal illness, diverticular disease, inflammatory bowel disease, and colorectal cancer, present with increased frequency and often atypically in the geriatric patient. Older patients also face unique nutritional challenges, with both malnutrition and obesity being common problems.

The authors of this issue delve deep into the unique GI challenges geriatric patients and their physicians face and provide a broad, up-to-date, and clinically useful overview of these common GI diseases. We would like to thank all the authors who made invaluable contributions to this issue, for their time and effort in creating this comprehensive issue. We hope our readers find it a helpful resource.

Amir E. Soumekh, MD
Jay Monahan Center for Gastrointestinal Health
Weill Cornell Medical College
1315 York Avenue, Ground Level
New York, NY 10021, USA

Philip O. Katz, MD
Jay Monahan Center for Gastrointestinal Health
Weill Cornell Medical College
1315 York Avenue, Ground Level
New York, NY 10021, USA

E-mail addresses:
Ams2041@med.cornell.edu (A.E. Soumekh)
Phk9009@med.cornell.edu (P.O. Katz)

Esophageal and Gastric Motility Disorders in the Elderly

Morgan A. Sendzischew Shane, MD[a],*,
Baharak Moshiree, MD, MSc[b]

KEYWORDS

- Oropharyngeal dysphagia • Gastroparesis • Dyspepsia • Nausea and vomiting
- Dysphagia • Parkinson's disease

KEY POINTS

- Gastrointestinal and motility disorders in the elderly are more commonly a sequelae of systemic disease or medication side effects rather than related to age.
- Many medications have unwanted gastrointestinal side effects; polypharmacy is a significant concern in the elderly.
- Dysphagia is common in elderly and can be oropharyngeal and/or esophageal, requiring a dedicated motility workup using barium swallow studies and esophageal motility testing to determine the cause.
- Gastroparesis in the elderly is mostly due to complications of diabetes or some neurologic diseases like Parkinson's disease; its treatment is limited given the cardiac and neurologic side effects of currently available medications.
- Opiates cause several gastrointestinal disturbances, including esophageal dysmotility, gastric emptying delay, and constipation and should be used sparingly and with caution in the elderly population.

INTRODUCTION

Similar to other organ systems, the gastrointestinal (GI) tract experiences age-related physiologic changes. Some disorders are a result of structural and functional changes owing to age, but most upper GI disorders are secondary to age-related disease burden and the medications used to treat those diseases.[1] Older patients report symptoms infrequently, a phenomenon often leading to delayed diagnosis and more severe complications.[2] Clinicians need to not only be aware of the more

[a] Division of Gastroenterology, Department of Medicine, University of Miami Miller School of Medicine, 1120 Northwest 14th Street, CRB 1184, Miami, FL 33136, USA; [b] Atrium Health-Charlotte, UNC School of Medicine, Charlotte Campus, 1025 Morehead Medical Drive, Suite 300, Charlotte, NC 28204, USA
* Corresponding author.
E-mail address: msendz@med.miami.edu

Clin Geriatr Med 37 (2021) 1–16
https://doi.org/10.1016/j.cger.2020.08.002
0749-0690/21/© 2020 Elsevier Inc. All rights reserved.

common GI diseases effecting elderly patients, but keep these conditions in the fore-front when evaluating older patients to ensure prompt diagnosis.

ESOPHAGEAL DISEASE
Physiology of the Aging Esophagus

To diagnose and treat upper GI tract disorders in the elderly, one must first understand how the physiology of the upper GI tract changes with increasing age. The term pres-byesophagus, first coined in 1964, was used to describe a tortuous esophagus more often seen in older individuals.[3] More specifically, this term describes age-related changes, including decreased esophageal contractile amplitudes, polyphasic waves in the esophageal body, incomplete lower or upper sphincter relaxation, and esopha-geal dilation. With endoscopy, and the advent of more sophisticated testing modalities like esophageal high-resolution manometry, we have now come to understand that this term, in its original understanding, is obsolete.

Varied data exist on the change in esophageal physiology with age. Although initial studies showed significant alterations in motility, a subsequent retrospective study failed to show significant age-related changes.[4,5] Healthy subjects over age 75 were found to have lower basal lower esophageal sphincter (LES) tone, a lower percentage of swallows with complete LES relaxation, and an increase in the mean integrated relaxation pressure, which measures relaxation at the esophagogastric junction.[6] The increase in peristaltic velocity when upright seen in the younger patients was not seen in this older cohort. There was also an increase in the time to recovery of LES tone back to baseline after swallow-induced relaxation in the older subjects.

Gastroesophageal Reflux Disease

Gastroesophageal reflux disease (GERD)—defined as symptoms or lesions resulting from the reflux of gastric contents into the distal esophagus—is the most commonly seen upper GI condition by primary care providers. GERD accounts for nearly one-third of visits to primary care in patients over age 65.[7] Roughly 20% of these patients experience symptoms of GERD once weekly, and nearly 60% have symptoms monthly.[8] GERD is more prevalent in the elderly owing to medications that decrease LES tone, the increased prevalence of hiatal hernia, and impaired esophageal motility.[9] Impaired saliva production and decreased salivary bicarbonate concentra-tion impair esophageal acid clearance.[10] Decreased physical activity and more time recumbent increases reflux.[11]

Older adults can also have poor primary and secondary peristalsis, leading to increased acid exposure time. Esophageal manometry and pH impedance data show that both the frequency and duration of esophageal acid exposure increases with age.[12] Despite the increase in the prevalence of GERD in the elderly, symptom reporting is low owing to decreased pain perception in this age group.[13,14] Endo-scopic studies show a worse reflux complications, such as esophagitis and peptic strictures in the elderly.[15–17] Older patients also more frequently present with atypical symptoms of GERD, as well as extraesophageal manifestations like asthma, chronic cough, globus, and laryngitis.[18]

Proton pump inhibitors (PPIs) are the mainstay of acid suppression treatment for GERD; however, more attention has been paid in recent years to potential side effects of long-term use. Although conflicting data exist, PPIs have been linked to increased risk of infections like *Clostridium difficile*,[19] pneumonia,[20] bone fractures,[21] and kidney disease.[22,23] Although dementia was once conjectured to be a side effect of PPIs, newer data suggest no association.[24,25]

Dysphagia

Dysphagia, the subjective sensation of difficulty with swallowing, is common in the elderly. An estimated 14% to 33% of community-dwelling elderly patients experience dysphagia with rates as high as 70% in nursing homes.[26–28] Dysphagia can affect not only quality of life, but also lead to malnutrition, which impacts overall health status leading to frailty.

Oropharyngeal dysphagia is characterized by difficulty initiating a swallow, and is most often due to diseases affecting the structures of the oral cavity, pharynx, and upper esophageal sphincter. Multiple conditions can cause this. Poor dentition can affect mastication. Xerostomia (dry mouth) can affect bolus formation and transfer. Conditions common to the elderly resulting in dry mouth are poorly controlled diabetes, atrophic gastritis, and medications such as anticholinergics and antihistamines, impairing transfer of food bolus into the esophagus.[29] Patients with neurologic disorders like cerebrovascular accidents, amyotrophic lateral sclerosis, and myasthenia gravis may experience dysphagia owing to decreased lingual control, impaired or absent swallowing reflex, or weakened laryngopharyngeal musculature.[30] Dysphagia is also a hallmark of more advanced Parkinson's disease.[31]

Esophageal dysphagia in the elderly may be structural or functional in etiology. Structural causes of dysphagia include malignancies, benign strictures (such as reflux-induced strictures), hernias, rings, webs, cricopharyngeal bars, and esophageal diverticula. Functional causes of esophageal dysphagia include age-related changes in primary motility disorders (with achalasia being the most well-studied), motility disorders that are secondary to another medical disorder or age-related changes in peristaltic function. One study found that, with age, even when overall esophageal function is preserved, a functional reduction in percentage of swallows with complete LES relaxation can be seen.[6] Ineffective esophageal motility, a minor disorder of peristalsis according to Chicago Classification v3.0, is characterized by weak peristalsis in more than 50% of swallows.[32] Ineffective esophageal motility can be due to longstanding GERD, esophageal involvement of connective tissue disorders like scleroderma or Sjogren's syndrome, and idiopathic owing to smooth muscle fibrosis and dysfunction, all of which is more common in older adults.[33,34]

Gastroesophageal hernias, particularly paraesophageal hernias, may cause dysphagia through an esophageal outlet obstruction. Paraesophageal hernias (**Fig. 1**) comprise 5% to 10% of all hiatal hernias, and are more common to the elderly.[35,36] Although some are asymptomatic, many patients present with postprandial pain, dysphagia, and dyspnea. Previously standard management of paraesophageal hernias was prophylactic repair to prevent higher risk emergent surgery owing to gastric volvulus; however, newer data suggest there may be only some indications for repair in asymptomatic patients.[37] Laparoscopic paraesophageal hernias repair is safe in older individuals with good patient satisfaction and limited morbidity.[38,39] In very high-risk surgical patients, gastropexy is the preferred method of treatment.

Cricopharyngeal bars and hypopharyngeal diverticula are both functional and structural abnormalities in the pharynx that can result in dysphagia. Cricopharyngeal bar, a defect in the esophagus at the level of the cricopharyngeus muscle, can lead to decreased compliance and narrowing of the upper esophageal sphincter.[40] Zenker's diverticulum (**Fig. 2**)—an outpouching of the mucosa and submucosa through Killian's triangle, an area of muscular weakness between the cricophayngeus and the thyropharyngeus muscles near the upper esophageal sphincter—is more common in older males, usually in the seventh or eighth decades of life.[41] Zenker's diverticulum is

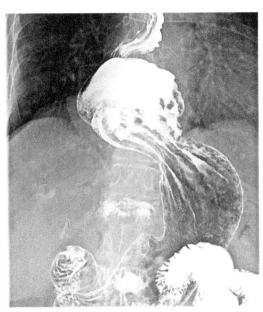

Fig. 1. Barium radiograph of a paraesophageal hernia in an elderly patients with dysphagia.

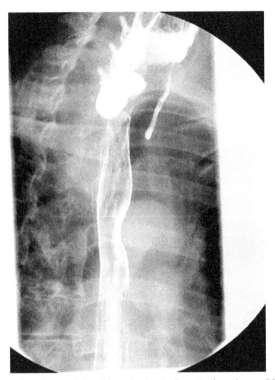

Fig. 2. Esophagram showing a right-sided Zenker's diverticulum in an 80-year-old patient with oropharyngeal dysphagia and halitosis. Patient had a myotomy performed at the level of the upper esophageal sphincter with complete symptom resolution.

caused by increased intraluminal pressure in the oropharynx during swallowing against inadequate relaxation of the cricopharyngeal muscle.[42] Symptoms include dysphagia, regurgitation, chronic cough, aspiration, halitosis, and weight loss.[43] Given the increased prevalence in the elderly, if a Zenker's diverticulum or cricopharyngeal bar is suspected, dedicated imaging with a modified barium swallow is performed initially to make a diagnosis. Rarely, a condition called distal idiopathic hyperskeletal hyperostosis causes direct compression of esophagus by cervical osteophytes is also seen more commonly in the elderly.

Achalasia

Achalasia is a rare esophageal motor disorder defined by the functional loss of myenteric plexus ganglion cells in the distal esophagus, causing lack of swallow-induced LES relaxation with abnormal motility of the esophageal body, leading to impaired esophageal clearance.[44,45] Patients present with dysphagia and even regurgitation of undigested food. The true etiology of achalasia is unknown. Although more common between the ages of 20 and 40 years, achalasia has a secondary peak in those above the age of 65[46] (**Fig. 3**). Sequelae are cumulative, and complications of the disease are more often seen in older individuals. Without treatment, achalasia can lead to irreversible structural changes in the esophagus. End-stage achalasia is characterized by severe dilation (>6 cm diameter) and tortuosity of the esophagus resembling what is termed sigmoid esophagus.[47] Other complications include epiphrenic diverticula, candida esophagitis, malnutrition, aspiration pneumonia, and squamous esophageal cancer. Treatment of achalasia depends on multiple disease and patient factors, but treatment options include per oral endoscopic myotomy, laparoscopic Heller myotomy, pneumatic dilation, botulinum toxin injection, and medications like nitrates and calcium channel blockers.[48] Typically, treatment should be targeted toward the type of achalasia.[49,50] For older individuals, pneumatic dilation is preferred, although per oral endoscopic myotomy has also been found to be safe.[51,52] In poor surgical or endoscopic candidates, botulinum toxin injection can also be considered.[53]

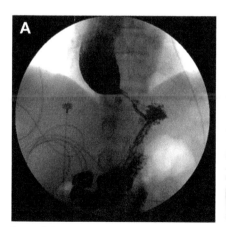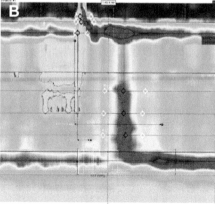

Fig. 3. (*A*) Barium swallow image of a patient with suspected achalasia showing a narrowing at the esophagogastric junction. (*B*) High-resolution manometry image shows a hypertensive LES with pan-pressurization and a high integrated relaxation pressure consistent with type II achalasia. (*B*) Failed relaxation of the LES with elevated integrated relaxation pressure median of 34 mm Hg (upper limit of normal, <15).

Medications for LES relaxation in poor surgical candidates like nitrates and calcium channel blockers can be considered, but are only moderately effective and carry cardiovascular side effects.

GASTRIC DISEASES IN ELDERLY
Physiology of the Aging Stomach

Physiologic changes in the stomach are subtle, and data are conflicting. Gastric motility is regulated by the interaction of smooth muscle cells and the interstitial cells of Cajal. An age-related decline in the number of interstitial cells of Cajal may account for early satiety and decreased food intake in the elderly.[54,55] Age-associated changes in the migratory motor complexes of the eighth and ninth decades of life occurs; however, other investigators have not demonstrated an age-related change in antral motility either in the fasting or postprandial state.[56,57] Other data may suggest that gastric emptying of liquids and mixed meals may be impaired in the elderly owing to changes in fundic accommodation and activity.[58]

Gastroparesis

Gastroparesis, defined as delayed gastric emptying in the absence of a mechanical obstruction, is most commonly caused by type 1 and type 2 diabetes, although idiopathic causes, rarely systemic diseases such as amyloidosis and neurologic diseases, and medication side effects can also contribute.[59] Over 10% of the US population has diabetes in 2020.[60] The resultant chronic peripheral neuropathy is the most common extrinsic neurologic disorder that leads to GI motor dysfunction.[61] Symptoms include nausea, vomiting, postprandial fullness, early satiety, and bloating or epigastric pain, and can lead to weight loss, malnutrition, and impaired glycemic control. As many as 12% of patients with diabetes have reported symptoms attributable to gastroparesis.[62] The incidence of gastroparesis increases with age.[63] Unfortunately, once present, despite subsequent adequate glucose control, symptoms of gastroparesis tend to persist and can significantly impact quality of life.

Diabetes decreases gastric emptying owing to less frequent antral contractions during phase 3 of the interdigestive motor complex and postprandial period. Histopathology of the vagus nerve of patients with diabetes has shown a significant decrease in the density of unmyelinated axons, and smaller caliber of the surviving axons, indicating an overall decrease in the innervation.[64] Loss or dysfunction of the interstitial cells of Cajal plays a major role in disordered gastric emptying in diabetes.[65] Diabetes causes antroduodenal dyscoordination and pylorospasm, preventing gastric contents from emptying into the small bowel for further digestion.[66] Diabetes and gastroparesis can also predispose patients to development of small intestinal bacterial overgrowth from small bowel stasis or rapid transit from uncoordinated small bowel activity.[61]

Gastroparesis may also result from commonly used medications. PPIs, taken by approximately 10% of elderly patients, may delay gastric emptying.[67] Opiates and anitcholinergics lead to delayed gastric emptying.[68,69] Ironically, although elevated blood glucose can delay gastric emptying, some antihyperglycemic medications like the exenatides as glucagon-like peptide receptor agonist impair gastric emptying by inhibiting glucagon secretion to promote satiety.[69–71] It is critical to review the medication lists of older patients to not only evaluate for polypharmacy and drug interactions, but also to monitor side effects of medications used commonly in the treatment of diseases more prevalent in the elderly.

Treatment of Gastroparesis

Treatment of gastroparesis can be complicated. First and foremost, control of glucose is critical, because gastric emptying is delayed with elevated blood sugar.[70] Although there are an increasing number of medications becoming available for the treatment of gastroparesis, in older adults many medications carry undesired side effects. Cisapride, a 5-HT$_4$ receptor agonist, was initially used for the treatment of gastroparesis, but later removed from the market owing to an increased risk of arrhythmia.[72] Bethanechol, a muscarinic receptor agonist, decreases fundic contractions allowing for improved gastric accommodation, as well as increasing pyloric contractility to improve gastric emptying.[73] Metoclopramide, a dopamine D2 receptor antagonist, is the only medication approved by the US Food and Drug Administration (FDA)for the treatment of gastroparesis.[74] Side effects of parkinsonism and tardive dyskinesia ultimately led to an FDA black box warning in 2009.[75,76] As a result, there is maximum duration of use of 3 months, and use is heavily cautioned in patients older than 65 years of age. Metoclopramide, cisapride, and bethanechol all have side effects of tardive dyskinesia, confusion, and drowsiness, which are more likely in an elderly population.[77,78] Domperidone—which is only available in the United States via an Investigational New Drug program—is a more selective peripheral dopamine antagonist with less central penetration, but side effects can include QT prolongation and with significant cardiac disease in older adults, and this agent must be used with extreme caution.[79] Tegaserod, used for constipation-predominant irritable bowel syndrome, significantly improves gastric emptying; however, it is only approved for female patients under 65 years of age, and therefore not applicable to our elderly population.[80] Prucalopride, a selective 5-HT$_4$ receptor agonist, is FDA approved for the treatment of chronic idiopathic constipation and has also shown efficacy for the treatment of gastroparesis in Europe, but is not yet FDA approved for this purpose.[81] Unlike cisapride and tegaserod, prucalopride does not interact with the cardiac hERG potassium channels or serotonergic receptors in blood vessels responsible for the major cardiovascular events seen with the former drugs.[82] Relamorelin, a potent investigational synthetic ghrelin analog, accelerates gastric emptying, and has been shown to decrease gastric retention of solids in patients with diabetes, and may be a viable option for nondiabetic gastroparesis with few side effects.[83,84]

Motilin agonists, azithromycin and erythromycin are potent prokinetics used for gastroparesis; however, tachyphylaxis development limits their use.[85] Erythromycin can have significant drug interactions with medications metabolized by CYP3A4, and can cause QT prolongation, so it should only be used with caution in an older population with an increased prevalence of cardiac disease. Approved in 2000 for the management of diabetic and idiopathic gastroparesis, gastric electrical stimulation delivers high-frequency, lower energy electrical stimulation. Gastric stimulators may be an option in few patients if operable candidates.[86]

Small Intestinal Bacterial Overgrowth

Small intestinal bacterial overgrowth, is defined by an increased proliferation of enteric flora within the small bowel. Patients can present with bloating, abdominal pain, bowel disturbance, and weight loss.[87] Polypharmacy may be a contributing factor, with the use of PPIs, narcotics, steroids, and anticholinergic medications associated with positive xylose breath testing diagnostic of small intestinal bacterial overgrowth.[88] Although this study only found an increase in small intestinal bacterial overgrowth in older women, there may be an age-associated change in microbiota leading to small intestinal bacterial overgrowth in elderly.

CONDITIONS PREDISPOSING THE ELDERLY TO GASTROINTESTINAL MOTILITY DISTURBANCES

Cardiovascular Disease

Heart disease is the leading cause of death for both men and women in the United States.[89] Rampant obesity, hypertension, dyslipidemia, and inactivity are contributing to a worsening epidemic. Cardiovascular issues can affect GI motility. Cardiomyopathy from hypertension, inherited structural abnormalities, valvulopathies, or infiltrative disease can lead to an enlarged heart and dilated aortic root. The aortic arch crosses in front of the esophagus in the superior mediastinum, and the lower esophagus lies anteriorly to the left atrium. Enlargement in either of these structures can lead to exterior compression on the esophagus that is otherwise collapsed when no food is present in the lumen. These points of compression can lead to intermittent obstruction and symptoms of dysphagia.

Stroke

Globally, stroke is the second leading cause of death behind ischemic heart disease.[90] Risk of stroke increases with age, and more than 60% of patients hospitalized for stroke are over the age of 65.[91] Dysphagia after a stroke owing to damage to the cortex and subcortical structures is a common and early complication and is an independent predictor of poor outcome and institutionalization.[92,93] As many as 50% of patients have persistent dysphagia at 6 months.[94] Stroke patients with dysphagia have a higher mortality, primarily related to the increase in risk of aspiration pneumonia.[95]

Neuromuscular Diseases

Neuromuscular disorders are more prevalent in the elderly, and can affect GI motility. The myenteric and submucosal plexi control smooth muscle activity of the GI tract, and depend on neurotransmitters like dopamine, serotonin, and acetylcholine, all of which impact GI function. Diseases and medications that affect the production or degradation of these neurotransmitters can have a significant effect on GI motility, making GI side effects common and critical in multiple disorders.

Parkinson's Disease and Parkinsonism

Enteric neurons produce dopamine, which regulates GI motility. Parkinson's disease, a disorder of dopamine production, results in significant GI disturbances, and may originate in the gut.[96] PD affects 1% of the population over the age of 60.[97] GI symptoms are present in nearly 60% to 80% of these patients, with some symptoms present up to 5 years before the development of the typical motor symptoms—a phenomenon called Braak's hypothesis.[98] GI complications are among the most common reasons for patients with PD to present for emergency evaluation, and older age in PD is associated with more GI complications. Although constipation is most prevalent, upper GI motility disorders including dysphagia, gastroparesis, small intestinal bacterial overgrowth, and malnutrition are also common.[99]

Dysphagia is a key feature of Parkinson's pathology. Xerostomia and drooling are common.[96] Dysphagia in PD can result from dyscoordination of muscular contraction at any phase of deglutition. Disorder of the oropharyngeal phase is most common, affecting nearly one-third of patients, is due to decreased motor control of the tongue, delayed swallowing reflex, and laryngeal movement deficits.[100] Esophageal dysphagia can result from aperistalsis, esophageal spasm, and slower esophageal transit. Incomplete bolus clearance is worsened by impaired LES relaxation leading to an increased risk of aspiration.[101] PD patients with dysphagia are at risk for aspiration with a nearly 70% mortality rate.[102]

Nearly 20% of patients with PD experience nausea and vomiting, felt to be a side effect of the antiparkinsonian medications rather than the disease itself.[103] Carbidopa, often coadministered with levodopa, can worsen nausea.[104] Nausea can be present in untreated patients, likely secondary to gastroparesis, which is present in up to 90% of Parkinson's patients.[105] Delayed gastric emptying is due to decrease stomach motility, leading to nausea, early satiety, weight loss, abdominal pain, and bloating.[106] Although dysphagia can improve with medication optimization, gastroparesis symptoms maybe worsened by levodopa, a medication most commonly used to treat the disorder.[61] Delayed gastric emptying effects absorption of PD medications, impairing improvement in motor symptoms, but continuous delivery formulations of these medications per enteral tubes can help.[107]

Other treatments of gastroparesis in PD are mostly focused on symptom management.[108] Metoclopramide and other dopaminergic antagonists often used in gastroparesis treatment are contraindicated in PD because they worsen motor symptoms.[109] Domperidone, a peripheral dopamine antagonist, does not mostly cross the blood–brain barrier and has shown 100% efficacy in treating nausea and vomiting in PD, but is only available by an Investigational New Drug program owing to cardiac risk.[110]

OPIATES AND THE UPPER GASTROINTESTINAL TRACT

Nearly one-half of older adults report pain that interferes with normal function, and more than 50% of nursing home patients report daily pain.[111,112] Persons over age 65 comprise 25% of chronic opiate users.[113] Opioid pain medications lead to dyspepsia, nausea and vomiting, esophageal dysmotility, and the well-known opiate-induced constipation–narcotic bowel syndrome.[114] In the esophagus, opiates can lead to esophagogastric junction outlet obstruction, wherein esophageal peristalsis is otherwise normal, but there is impaired LES relaxation. Although this phenomenon can be seen in early or evolving achalasia, it can also be a result of mechanical obstruction, or a side effect seen in opiate use. The frequency of type III (spastic) achalasia is much higher in patients using opiates, and may in fact be the predominating cause.[115] Opiate medications also lead to delayed gastric emptying, but have been paradoxically used to treat abdominal pain but should be avoided.[116,117] Opiates in older adults can lead to changes in cognition and, therefore, neuromodulators may be more beneficial instead.

SUMMARY

There are expected to be more than 80 million patients aged 65 and older in the United States in 2040.[118] Although there are some age-related physiologic changes, the majority of GI motility disorders in the elderly result from effects of systemic diseases. Oropharyngeal dysphagia can result from stroke, Parkinson's disease, and other neuromuscular disease. Esophageal dysphagia can be due to structural changes such as hernias, motility disorders like achalasia, or severe or complicated GERD. Gastroparesis is also a significant concern for the elderly, but the majority of treatment medications have undesired and even dangerous side effects in this demographic. Perhaps most important, polypharmacy and medication side effects can create or exacerbate many upper GI motility disorders in the elderly. It is important to investigate GI symptoms in the elderly to diagnose their underlying pathology, but particular care needs to be taken in choosing a treatment regimen in these patients.

DISCLOSURE

B. Moshiree reports grant support from Takeda (Japan), Ironwood (USA), Abbvie now owns Allergan (Ireland) Cairn Diagnostics, Medtronic, and Salix; is on the speakers bureau for Salix and Takeda Pharmaceuticals; and is on the advisory board of Takeda, Cairn Diagnostics, and Salix. M.A. Sendzischew Shane has nothing to disclose.

CLINICS CARE POINTS

- A multidisciplinary approach in caring for the geriatric population is paramount.
- Careful attention to polypharmacy and the side effect profiles of many medications such as commonly misused opiates in the elderly should be provided and their use should be minimized if possible.
- An important part of every care plan for the elderly should include a careful history of their medications and their interactions and possible GI and CNS side effects.
- Several noninvasive diagnostic tests are now available to enhance our physiologic workup of GI symptoms in the elderly and guide treatments with measurable positive outcomes.
- These tests include esophageal manometry and pH testing, barium swallow studies both for upper and lower esophageal disorders, gastric emptying scintigraphy for gastroparesis, Anorectal manometry and balloon expulsion testing to evaluate constipation and fecal incontinence and several breath tests used to evaluate for small bowel bacterial overgrowth.
- Age is not necessarily a precursor to GI distress or dysmotility, but systemic illnesses seen more commonly in geriatrics can lead to GI dysmotility.

REFERENCES

1. Gidwaney NG, Bajpai M, Chokhavatia SS. Gastrointestinal dysmotility in the elderly. J Clin Gastroenterol 2016;50(10):819–27.
2. Maekawa T, Kinoshita Y, Okada A, et al. Relationship between severity and symptoms of reflux oesophagitis in elderly patients in Japan. J Gastroenterol Hepatol 1998;13:927–30.
3. Soergel KH, Zboralske FF, Amberg JR. Presbyesophagus: esophageal motility in nonagenarians. J Clin Invest 1964;43(7):1472–9.
4. Ferriolli E, Dantas RO, Oliveira RB, et al. The influence of ageing on oesophageal motility after ingestion of liquids with different viscosities. Eur J Gastroenterol Hepatol 1996;8(8):793–8.
5. Robson KM, Glick ME. Dysphagia and advancing age: are manometric abnormalities more common in older patients? Dig Dis Sci 2003;48(9):1709–12.
6. Besanko LK, Burgstad CM, Cock C, et al. Changes in esophageal and lower esophageal sphincter motility with healthy aging. J Gastrointest Liver Dis 2014;23(3):243–8.
7. Crane SJ, Talley NJ. Chronic gastrointestinal symptoms in the elderly. Clin Geriatr Med 2007;23(4):721–34.
8. Locke GR III, Talley NJ, Fett SL, et al. Prevalence and clinical spectrum of gastroesophageal reflux: a population based study in Olmsted County, Minnesota. Gastroenterology 1997;112:1448–56.
9. Achem AC, Achem SR, Stark MR, et al. Failure of esophageal peristalsis in older patients: association with esophageal acid exposure. Am J Gastroenterol 2003; 98(1):35–9.

10. Sonnenberg A, Steinkamp U, Weise A, et al. Salivary secretion in reflux esophagitis. Gastroenterology 1982;83:889–95.
11. Pilotto A, Maggi S, Noale M, et al. Association of upper gastrointestinal symptoms with functional and clinical characteristics in elderly. World J Gastroenterol 2011;17(25):3020–6.
12. Lee J, Anggiansah A, Anggiansah R, et al. Effects of age on the gastroesophageal junction, esophageal motility, and reflux disease. Clin Gastroenterol Hepatol 2007;5(12):1392–8.
13. Pilotto A, Franceschi M, Leandro G, et al. Clinical features of reflux esophagitis in older people: a study of 840 consecutive patients. J Am Geriatr Soc 2006; 54(10):1537–42.
14. Mold JW, Rankin RA. Symptomatic gastroesophageal reflux in the elderly. J Am Geriatr Soc 1987;35(7):649–59.
15. Johnson DA, Fennerty MB. Heartburn severity underestimates erosive esophagitis severity in elderly patients with gastroesophageal reflux disease. Gastroenterology 2004;126(3):660–4.
16. Collen MJ, Abdulian JD, Chen YK. Gastroesophageal reflux disease in the elderly: more severe disease that requires aggressive therapy. Am J Gastroenterol 1995;90:1053–7.
17. El-Serag HB, Sonnenberg A. Associations between different forms of gastro-oesophageal reflux disease. Gut 1997;41:594–9.
18. Soumekh A, Schnoll-Sussman FH, Katz PO. Reflux and acid peptic diseases in the elderly. Clin Geriatr Med 2014;30:29–41.
19. McDonald EG, Milligan J, Frenette C, et al. Continuous proton pump inhibitor therapy and the associated risk of recurrent Clostridium difficile infection. JAMA Intern Med 2015;175:784–91.
20. Gulmez SE, Holm A, Frederiksen H, et al. Use of proton pump inhibitors and the risk of community-acquired pneumonia: a population-based case-control study. Arch Intern Med 2007;167:950–5.
21. Ngamruengphong S, Leontiadis GI, Radhi S, et al. Proton pump inhibitors and risk of fracture: a systematic review and meta-analysis of observational studies. Am J Gastroenterol 2011;106:1209–18.
22. Nochaiwong S, Ruengorn C, Awiphan R, et al. The association between proton pump inhibitor use and the risk of adverse kidney outcomes: a systematic review and meta-analysis. Nephrol Dial Transplant 2018;33:331–42.
23. Haastrup PF, Thompson W, Søndergaard J, et al. Side effects of long-term proton pump inhibitor use: a review. Basic Clin Pharmacol Toxicol 2018;123(2): 114–21.
24. Gomm W, von Holt K, Thome F, et al. Association of proton pump inhibitors with risk of dementia: a pharmacoepidemiological claims data analysis. JAMA Neurol 2016;73:410–6.
25. Wod M, Hallas J, Andersen K, et al. Lack of association between proton pump inhibitor use and cognitive decline. Clin Gastroenterol Hepatol 2018;16(5): 681–9.
26. Roy N, Stemple J, Merrill RM, et al. Dysphagia in the elderly: preliminary evidence of prevalence, risk factors, and socioemotional effects. Ann Otol Rhinol Laryngol 2007;116:858.
27. Kawashima K, Motohashi Y, Fujishima I. Prevalence of dysphagia among community-dwelling elderly individuals as estimated using a questionnaire for dysphagia screening. Dysphagia 2004;19:266.

28. Steele CM, Greenwood C, Ens I, et al. Mealtime difficulties in a home for the aged: not just dysphagia. Dysphagia 1997;12:43.
29. Tiisanoja A, Syrjälä AM, Komulainen K, et al. Anticholinergic burden and dry mouth among Finnish, community-dwelling older adults. Gerodontology 2018; 35(1):3–10.
30. Altman KW, Richards A, Goldberg L, et al. Dysphagia in stroke, neurodegenerative disease, and advanced dementia. Otolaryngol Clin North Am 2013;46(6): 1137–49.
31. Suttrup I, Warnecke T. Dysphagia in Parkinson's disease. Dysphagia 2016; 31(1):24–32.
32. Kahrilas PJ, Bredenoord AJ, Fox M, et al. The Chicago Classification of esophageal motility disorders, v3.0. Neurogastroenterol Motil 2015;27(2):160–74.
33. Roman S, Lin Z, Kwiatek MA, et al. Weak peristalsis in esophageal pressure topography: classification and association with Dysphagia. Am J Gastroenterol 2011;106:349–56.
34. Gyawali CP, Bredenoord AJ, Conkli JL, et al. Evaluation of esophageal motor function in clinical practice. Neurogastroenterol Motil 2013l;25(2):99–133.
35. Lal D, Pelligrini C, Oelschalager B. Laparoscopic repair of paraesophageal hernia. Surg Clin North Am 2005;85:105–18.
36. Gangopadhyay N, Perrone JM, Soper NJ, et al. Outcomes of laparoscopic paraesophageal hernia repair in elderly and high risk patients. Surgery 2006;140(4): 491–8.
37. Stylopoulos N, Gazelle GS, Rattner DW. Paraesophageal hernias: operation or observation? Ann Surg 2002;236(4):492–501.
38. Newton AD, Clanahan J, Herbst DA, et al. Laparoscopic gastropexy for large paraesphpageal hernia in the elderly. Gastroenterology 2019;156(6):S-1–388.
39. Parker DM, Rambhajan AA, Horsley RD, et al. Laparoscopic paraesophageal hernia repair is safe in elderly patients. Surg Endosc 2017;31:1186–91.
40. Dantas RO, Cook IJ, Dodds WJ, et al. Biomechanics of cricopharyngeal bars. Gastroenterology 1990;99(5):1269–74.
41. Bizzotto A, Iacopini F, Landi R, et al. Zenker's diverticulum: exploring treatment options. Acta Otorhinolaryngol Ital 2013;33(4):219–29.
42. Sen P, Lowe DA, Farnan T. Surgical interventions for pharyngeal pouch. Cochrane Database Syst Rev 2005;3:CD004459.
43. Siddiq MA, Sood S, Strachan D. Pharyngeal pouch (Zenker's diverticulum). Postgrad Med J 2001;77(910):506–11.
44. Pandolfino JE, Gawron AJ. Achalasia: a systematic review. JAMA 2015;313(18): 1841–52.
45. Zaninotto G, Bennett C, Boexckxstaens G, et al. The 2018 ISDE achalasia guidelines. Dis Esophagus 2018;31(9). https://doi.org/10.1093/dote/doy071.
46. Castell DO. Esophageal disorders in the elderly. Gastroenterol Clin North Am 1990;19:235–54.
47. Eckardt VF, Hoischen T, Bernhard G. Life expectancy, complications, and causes of death in patients with achalasia: results of a 33-year follow-up investigation. Eur J Gastroenterol Hepatol 2008;20(10):956–60.
48. Pandolfino JE, Kwiatek MA, Nealis T, et al. Achalasia: a new clinically relevant classification by high-resolution manometry. Gastroenterology 2008;135: 1526–33.
49. Moonen A, Annese V, Belmans A, et al. Long-term results of the European achalasia trial: a multicenter randomized control trial comparing pneumatic dilation vs laparoscopic heller myotomy. Gut 2016;65(5):732–9.

50. Kahrilas PJ, Katzka D, Richter JE. Clinical practice update: the use of per-oral endoscopic myotomy in achalasia: expert review and best practice advice from the American Gastroenterological Association. Gastroenterology 2017, 153(5):1205–11.
51. Richter JE, Boeckxstaens GE. Management of achalasia: surgery or pneumatic dilation. Gut 2011;60(6):869–76.
52. Kahrilas PJ, Katzka D, Richter JE. Clinical practice update: the use of per-oral endoscopic myotomy in achalasia: expert review and best practice advice from the AGA Institute. Gastroenterology 2017;153(5):1205–11.
53. Boeckxstaens GE, Zaninotto G, Richter JE. Achalasia. Lancet 2014;383(9911): 83–93.
54. Gomez-Pinilla PJ, Gibbons SJ, Sarr MG, et al. Changes in interstitial cells of Cajal with age in the human stomach and colon. Neurogastroenterol Motil 2011;23:36–44.
55. Parker BA, Chapman IM. Food intake and ageing—the role of the gut. Mech Ageing Dev 2004;125:859–66.
56. Bortolotti M, Frada GJR, Barbagallo-Sangiogi G, et al. Interdigestive gastroduodenal motor activity in the elderly (Abstract). Gut 1984;25:A1320.
57. Fich A, Camilleri M, Phillips SF. Effect of age on human gastric and small bowel motility. J Clin Gastroenterol 1989;11(4):416–20.
58. Evans MA, Triggs EJ, Cheung M, et al. Gastric emptying rates in the elderly: implication for drug therapy. J Am Geriatr Soc 1981;29:201–5.
59. Camilleri M, Bharucha AE, Farrugia G. Epidemiology, Mechanisms and management of diabetic gastroparesis. Clin Gastroenterol Hepatol 2011;9(1):5–e7.
60. Centers for Disease Control and Prevention. National Diabetes Statistics Report, 2020. Atlanta, GA: Centers for Disease Control and Prevention, US. Department of Health and Human Services; 2020.
61. Camilleri M. Disorders of gastrointestinal motility in neurologic diseases. Mayo Clin Proc 1990;65:825–46.
62. Maleki D, Locke GR III, Camilleri M, et al. Gastrointestinal tract symptoms among persons with diabetes mellitus in the community. Arch Intern Med 2000;160:2808–16.
63. Jung HK, Choung RS, Locke GR 3rd, et al. The incidence, prevalence, and outcomes of patients with gastroparesis in Olmsted County, Minnesota, from 1996 to 2006. Gastroenterology 2009;136:1225–33.
64. Guy RJ, Dawson JL, Garrett JR, et al. Diabetic gastroparesis from autonomic neuropathy: surgical considerations and changes in vagus nerve morphology. J Neurol Neurosurg Psychiatr 1984;47:686–91.
65. Mihai BM, Mihai C, Cijevschi-Prelipcean C, et al. Bidirectional relationship between gastric emptying and plasma glucose control in normoglycemic individuals and diabetic patients. J Diabetes Res 2018;2018:1736959.
66. Houghton LA, Read NW, Heddle R, et al. Relationship of the motor activity of the antrum, pylorus, and duodenum to gastric emptying of a solid-liquid mixed meal. Gastroenterology 1988;94:1285–91.
67. Sanaka M, Yamamoto T, Kuyama Y. Effects of proton pump inhibitors on gastric emptying: a systematic re- view. Dig Dis Sci 2010;55(9):2431–40.
68. Jeong ID, Camilleri M, Shin A, et al. A randomised, placebo-controlled trial comparing the effects of tapentadol and oxycodone on gastrointestinal and colonic transit in healthy humans. Aliment Pharmacol Ther 2012;35(9):1088–96.
69. Camilleri M, Parkman HP, Shafi MA, et al. Clinical guideline: management of gastroparesis. Am J Gastroenterol 2013;108(1):18–38.

70. Phillips LK, Deane AM, Jones KL, et al. Gastric emptying and glycaemia in health and diabetes mellitus. Nat Rev Endocrinol 2015;11(2):112–28.
71. Drucker DJ. Mechanisms of action and therapeutic application of glucagon-like peptide-1. Cell Metab 2018;27(4):740–56.
72. Shaffer D, Butterfield M, Pamer C, et al. Tardive dyskinesia risks and metoclopramide use before and after U.S. market withdrawal of cisapride. J Am Pharm Assoc (2003) 2004;44(6):661–5.
73. James AN, Ryan JP, Crowell MD, et al. Regional gastric contractility alterations in diabetic gastroparesis mouse model: effects of cholinergic and serotonergic stimulation. Am J Physiol Gastrointest Liver Physiol 2004;287(3):G612–9.
74. Gudsoorkar V, Quigley EM. Choosing a prokinetic for your patient beyond Metoclopramide. Am J Gastroenterol 2020;115(1):5–8.
75. Ehrenpreis ED, Deepak P, Sifuentes H, et al. The metoclopramide black box warning for tardive dyskinesia: effect on clinical practice, adverse event reporting, and prescription drug lawsuits. Am J Gastroenterol 2013;108(6):866–72.
76. Rao AS, Camilleri M. Review article: metoclopramide and tardive dyskinesia. Aliment Pharmacol Ther 2010;31(1):11–9.
77. Rowland LP, Bede P, Elamin M, et al. Medical mimics of neurodegenerative diseases. In: Hardiman O, Doherty C, Elamin M, et al, editors. Neurodegenerative disorders. Cham (Switzerland): Springer; 2016. p. 199–212.
78. Patterson D, Abell T, Rothstein R, et al. A double-blind multicenter comparison of domperidone and metoclopramide in the treatment of diabetic patients with symptoms of gastroparesis. Am J Gastroenterol 1999;94:1230–4.
79. Drolet B, Rousseau G, Daleau P, et al. Domperidone should not be considered a no-risk alternative to cisapride in the treatment of gastrointestinal motility disorders. Circulation 2000;102:1883–5.
80. Camilleri M. Tegaserod. Aliment Pharmacol Ther 2001;15:277–89.
81. Carbone F, Van den Houte K, Clevers E, et al. Prucalopride in gastroparesis: a randomized placebo-controlled crossover study. Am J Gastroenterol 2019;114: 1265–74.
82. Vijayvargiya P, Camilleri M. Use of prucalopride in adults with chronic idiopathic constipation. Expert Rev Clin Pharmacol 2019;12(7):579–89.
83. Lembo A, Camilleri M, McCallum R, et al. Relamorelin reduces vomiting frequency and severity and accelerates gastric emptying in adults with diabetic gastroparesis. Gastroenterology 2016;151(1):87–96.
84. Camilleri M, Acosta A. Relamorelin: a novel gastrocolokinetic synthetic ghrelin agonist. Neurogastroenterol Motil 2015;27(3):324–32.
85. Richards RD, Davenport K, McCallum RW. The treatment of idiopathic and diabetic gastroparesis with acute intravenous and chronic oral erythromycin. Am J Gastroenterol 1993;88:203–7.
86. Abell T, McCallum R, Hocking M, et al. Gastric electrical stimulation for medically refractory gastroparesis. Gastroenterology 2003;125(2):421–8.
87. Dukowicz AC, Lacy BE, Levine GM. Small intestinal bacterial overgrowth: a comprehensive review. Gastroenterol Hepatol 2007;3:112–22.
88. Schatz RA, Zhang Q, Lodhia N, et al. Predisposing factors for positive D-Xylose breath test for evaluation of small intestinal bacterial overgrowth: a retrospective study of 932 patients. World J Gastroenterol 2015;21(15):4575–82.
89. Heron M. Deaths: leading causes for 2017. National Vital Statistics reports; 68(6). Available at: https://www.cdc.gov/heartdisease/facts.htm. Accessed January 20, 2020.

90. Benjamin EJ, Blaha MJ, Chiuve SE, et al. Heart disease and stroke statistics-2017 update: a report from the American Heart Association [published correction appears in Circulation. 2017;135(10):c646] [published correction appears in Circulation. 2017 Sep 5;136(10):e196]. Circulation 2017;135(10):e146–603.

91. Hall MJ, Levant S, DeFrances CJ. Hospitalization for stroke in U.S. hospitals, 1989-2009. NCHS data brief, No. 95. Hyattsville (MD): National Center for Health Statistics; 2012.

92. Cohen DL, Roffe C, Beavan J, et al. Post-stroke dysphagia: a review and design considerations for future trials. Int J Stroke 2016;11(4):399–411.

93. Smithard D, Smeeton N, Wolfe C. Long-term outcome after stroke: does dysphagia matter? Age Ageing 2007;36:90–4.

94. Mann G, Hankey GJ, Cameron D. Swallowing disorders following acute stroke: prevalence and diagnostic accuracy. Cerebrovasc Dis 2000;10:380–6.

95. Wilson RD. Mortality and cost of pneumonia after stroke for different risk groups. J Stroke Cerebrovasc Dis 2012;21:61–7.

96. Fasano A, Visanji NP, Liu LWC, et al. Gastrointestinal dysfunction in Parkinson's disease. Lancet Neurol 2015;14(6):625–39.

97. Tynes OB, Storstein A. Epidemiology of Parkinson's disease. J Neural Transm (Vienna) 2017;124(8):901–5.

98. Cerspsimo MG, Raina GB, Pecci C, et al. Gastrointestinal manifestations in Parkinson's disease: prevalence and occurrence before motor symptoms. J Neurol 2013;260:1332–8.

99. Ramprasad C, Douglas JY, Moshiree B. Parkinson's disease and current treatments for its gastrointestinal neurogastromotility effects. Curr Treat Options Gastroenterol 2018;16(4):489–510.

100. Kalf JG, de Swart BJ, Bloem BR, et al. Prevalence of oropharyngeal dysphagia in Parkinson's disease: a meta-analysis. Parkinsonism Relat Disord 2012;18: 311–5.

101. Pfeiffer RF. Gastrointestinal dysfunction in Parkinson's disease. Lancet Neurol 2003;2(2):107–16.

102. Martinez-Ramirez D, Almeida L, Giugni JC, et al. Rate of aspiration pneumonia in hospitalized Parkinson's disease patients: a cross-sectional study. BMC Neurol 2015;15:104.

103. Postuma R, Romenets SR, Rakheja R. Physician Guide: non-motor symptoms of Parkinson's disease. Montreal (Canada): McGill University Health Centre; 2012.

104. Poirier AA, Aubé B, Côté M, et al. Gastrointestinal dysfunctions in Parkinson's disease: symptoms and treatments. Parkinsons Dis 2016;2016:6762528.

105. Goetze O, Nikodem AB, Wiezcorek J, et al. Predictors of gastric emptying in Parkinson's disease. Neurogastroenterol Motil 2006;18(5):369–75.

106. Hardoff R, Sula M, Tamir A, et al. Gastric emptying time and gastric motility in patients with Parkinson's disease. Mov Disord 2001;16(6):1041–7.

107. Postuma R, Romenets SR, Rakheja R. Physician Guide: non-motor symptoms of Parkinson's disease. Montreal (Canada): McGill University Health Centre; 2012.

108. Heetun ZS, Quigley EM. Gastroparesis and Parkinson's disease: a systematic review. Parkinsonism Relat Disord 2012;18(5):433–40.

109. Cloud LJ, Greene JG. Gastrointestinal features of Parkinson's disease. Curr Neurol Neurosci Rep 2011;11(4):379–84.

110. Soykan I, Sarosiek I, Shifflett J, et al. Effect of chronic oral domperidone therapy on gastrointestinal symptoms and gastric emptying in patients with Parkinson's disease. Mov Disord 1997;12(6):952–7.

111. AGS Panel on Persistent Pain in Older Persons. The management of persistent pain in older persons. J Am Geriatr Soc 2002;50(6 Suppl):S205–24.
112. Patel KV, Guralnik JM, Dansie EJ, et al. Prevalence and impact of pain among older adults in the United States: findings from the 2011 National Health and Aging Trends Study. Pain 2013;154(12):2649–57.
113. Mojtabai R. National trends in long-term use of prescription opioids. Pharmacoepidemiol Drug Saf 2018;27(5):526–34.
114. Jehangir A, Parkman HP. Chronic opioids in gastroparesis: relationship with gastrointestinal symptoms, healthcare utilization and employment. World J Gastroenterol 2017;23(40):7310–20.
115. Ravi K, Murray JA, Geno DM, et al. Achalasia and chronic opiate use: innocent bystanders or associated conditions? Dis Esophagus 2016;29(1):15–21.
116. Tuteja AK, Biskupiak J, Stoddard GJ, et al. Opioid-induced bowel disorders and narcotic bowel syndrome in patients with chronic non-cancer pain. Neurogastroenterol Motil 2010;22:424–30.
117. Lee AA, Hasler WL. Opioids and GI motility-friend or foe? Curr Treat Options Gastroenterol 2016;14:478–94.
118. 2017 National population Projection tables. Available at: https://www.census.gov/data/tables/2017/demo/popproj/2017-summary-tables.html. Accessed January 15, 2020.

Gastroesophageal Reflux Disease and Barrett Esophagus in the Elderly

Fouad Otaki, MD[a],*, Prasad G. Iyer, MSc[b]

KEYWORDS

- Gastroesophageal reflux disease • GERD • Barrett esophagus
- Esophageal adenocarcinoma • Elderly

KEY POINTS

- The early diagnosis and optimal management of elderly patients is vital to the delivery of high quality care in an aging patient population.
- Maintaining a low threshold is essential given atypical presentations and increased repercussions of a delayed or missed diagnosis.
- Contextualizing a discussion regarding management of complications and treatments in the elderly should be personalized and account for patient comorbidities.
- Novel minimally invasive screening, surveillance and treatments of GERD and Barrett's esophagus have allowed us to manage a larger at-risk elderly patient population.

INTRODUCTION

An aging population is a global phenomenon, with minor regional variations in the demographic transition. Average life expectancy continues to increase and many countries are experiencing population contraction and decreasing fertility. Nine percent of the world's population was older than 65 years in 2015, and that proportion is projected to increase to 17% by 2050.[1] This pattern is evident in North America, which is second only to Europe as the oldest region, with 21.4% of population being 65 years or older. In fact, 20 million individuals will be older than 85 years in 2050.[2]

This demographic change is also affecting the way we diagnose and manage the most common upper gastrointestinal indication for primary care physician clinic visits, gastroesophageal reflux disease (GERD). GERD is defined as reflux of gastric contents

Funding: Supported in part by NIH, USA R01 grant CA 241064 (to P.G. Iyer).
[a] Division of Gastroenterology and Hepatology, Oregon Health and Science University, L461, 3181 SouthWest Sam Jackson Park Road, Portland, OR 97229, USA; [b] Barrett's Esophagus Unit, Division of Gastroenterology and Hepatology, Mayo Clinic, 200 First Street SouthWest, Rochester, MN 55905, USA
* Corresponding author.
E-mail address: otaki@ohsu.edu

into the esophagus, oropharynx, nasopharynx, larynx, or lungs with resultant symptoms and complications.[3] Heartburn, manifest as epigastric burning with radiation to the chest or neck, is a common typical symptom.[3] It is estimated that one-fifth of the adult Americans population experiences heartburn at least once a week, with 15 million suffering from symptoms on a daily basis.[4] Original studies indicated increasing incidence of GERD with age, with 6% to 17% of the elderly US population reporting these symptoms.[5] GERD also accounts for nearly a quarter of primary care physician visits for patients 65 years or older,[6] and it is the sixth most common disorder in nursing home residents.[7]

Various studies have attempted to identify the frequency of esophageal mucosal injury in GERD, and overall incidence for esophagitis varied from 6.4% to 15.5% in population studies.[8] Severe reflux esophagitis was more prevalent (37%) in patients 70 years or older in a population study of 12,000 patients compared with 12% in patients 21 year old or younger.[9] This likely underrepresents the at-risk cohort, given impaired sensory function with age. Patients 65 years or older have shown to have decreased and delayed reporting of balloon esophageal distention[10] and sensitivity to esophageal acid perfusion.[11]

Not only is GERD more common, but the presentation is often atypical and more severe in the elderly. Atypical symptoms include dyspepsia, epigastric pain, anorexia, dysphagia, odynophagia, weight loss, anemia, and belching.[3] In fact, only 40% of patient 65 years or older reported typical symptoms in an evaluation of 600 patients with erosive esophagitis.[12] In another study, older patients with Barrett esophagus had symptom scores that were comparable with that of control patients without reflux.[12] Hence there are significant clinical implications to a delay in diagnosis. A systemic review and meta-analysis identified more severe patterns of reflux and esophagitis in the elderly despite no change in GERD symptoms.[13]

Beyond esophageal injury, elderly patients are also prone to GERD-associated aspiration, which carries a significant risk of morbidity and mortality.[14] Manometric changes in the upper esophageal sphincter (UES) have included lower baseline pressure, decreased relaxation, and increased pharyngeal contractility.[15] Moreover, the UES response to reflux is reduced.[16] Laryngopharyngeal reflux (LPR), with or without classic GERD, is associated with a significantly higher economic burden, with 5438$ per person compared with 971$ for GERD.[17] Although it is likely that LPR is more common in the elderly, the absence of classical symptoms and limited objective testing in the population makes it difficult to ascertain true incidence. Associated symptoms include reactive airway disease, chronic cough, laryngitis, hoarseness, and voice change.[18]

PATHOPHYSIOLOGY

The pathophysiology of GERD in the elderly is multifaceted. Changes include structural and dynamic changes at the level of the lower esophageal sphincter (LES), increased incidence of hiatal hernias that are often larger than younger cohorts, increased gastric refluxate, ineffective esophageal clearance, and luminal stasis in the setting of esophageal dysmotility.[4] Other factors include limitation in activities of daily living and musculoskeletal postural changes.[6]

Larger hiatal hernias and lower LES pressures have also been reported more frequently in an elderly population.[19] Frequent transient lower esophageal sphincter relaxation (TLESRs) are part of pathophysiological underpinnings for the increased frequency of GERD. There is no clear association between age and TLESRs,[20] but the polypharmacy commonly seen in the elderly includes many medications that have been associated with more frequent TLESRs. These include nitrates, calcium channel blockers, benzodiazepines, anticholinergics, antidepressants, and lidocaine.[21] Broadly combined into presbyesophagus, the subtle changes in the esophageal body are less clear. Retrospective reviews of various institutional experiences associate aging with major motility disorders.[22–25] Elderly patients with endoscopic or impedance evidence of GERD are more likely to have an esophageal motility disorder on manometry (44% 70 years or older vs 13% 17–39 years old)[26] and lower rates of swallow-induced peristalsis on impedance study. Increasing age was also associated with more frequent reflux but less severe reflux episodes.[20,27] The clinical implications of cellular changes in autopsy studies indicating decrease in ganglionic cells and increased lymphocytic infiltration in esophageal biopsies when compared with young individuals are uncertain.[28] Yet similar changes have been noted in major esophageal motility disorders.[29]

In additional to mechanical stasis the reflexive ability to increase salivary bicarbonate is diminished in the elderly despite the absence of change in volume and baseline bicarbonate levels.[25] This weakened neutralizing salivary secretion is paired with increased gastric refluxate in the setting of a growing epidemic of obesity, which has not spared the elderly and makes reflux worse via multifactorial pathways.[30]

TESTING

The low risk of complications from esophagogastroduodenoscopy (EGD) are often pitted against the odds of an endoscopic finding that would validate the diagnosis or ideally change medical management. Many would favor of an empirical proton pump inhibitor (PPI) trial instead of an EGD in many scenarios. This is most applicable to a primary care setting and young otherwise healthy patient population. PPI trial is an acceptable option, as it is available, noninvasive, and inexpensive, with sensitivity ranging from 68% to 83%.[4,11,31] Typically, EGDs are recommended to assess refractory symptoms or to patients who are unable to wean off medical therapy or patients who are unable to wean off medical therapy or to assess complications.

Given atypical symptoms or absence of symptoms in the elderly and a higher prevalence of severe disease and complications, EGD is encouraged earlier in the elderly, as it helps complete a thorough workup and avoids delay in diagnostic care. Although there is no guideline recommendation to support EGD in this group yet, visual evaluation has the added advantage of assessing the presence of and degree of esophagitis and identifying and treating GERD complications including strictures and Barrett esophagus (with or without malignancy).[3]

Esophageal functional testing with pH and impedance is the most informative test in GERD. Metrics of disease continue to be defined and validated, with esophageal acid exposure time being the most reliable thus far. Impedance monitors allow for a detailed functional analysis of distal and proximal esophageal reflux events.[32] These results should be interpreted with caution, as normative values may not apply to a geriatric population.[33,34]

Radiographically, a well-performed double contrast esophagram complements an endoscopy and can identify a subtle stricture that would have otherwise been missed. Esophagrams may identify changes associated with esophagitis yet they lack the necessary sensitivity for a screening test.[3] Although they are financially disincentivized and being performed less frequently, esophagrams continue to play a role in tailoring antireflux surgery and improving outcomes via the careful assessment of gastroesophageal junction (GEJ) anatomy relative to the diaphragm and other anatomic details. They can also add informative data on patients with postoperative symptoms. Additional predictive metrics include barium tablets, where a delay in the 13-mm tablet may suggest a tight fundoplication.[35]

Evaluating LPR is challenging. Beyond the field of view of a standard EGD, structural evaluation with laryngoscopy is essential but findings typically associated with GERD are nonspecific. Functional testing such as esophageal pH/impedance has poor sensitivity. Oropharyngeal pH testing and salivary pepsin evaluation are not as widely adopted due to unclear utility. More accurate sensors and indices that are objective and validated are needed to help guide some of the more targeted chemical and pH testing of proximal pharyngeal reflux.[36]

TREATMENT
Lifestyle Modifications

The efficacy of lifestyle modifications is not limited to young patients. Elderly patients can benefit a great deal from minor changes in their dietary and sleeping habits. The latter includes head of bed elevation, ideally by using wedge mattress inserts.[37–39] Moreover, appropriate utilization of positive ventilation in patients with obstructive sleep apnea has been shown to help reduce nocturnal reflux.[40] Effective dietary changes include avoiding late evening meals and meals with a high fat content.[41] Finally, weight gain increases frequency and severity of GERD. Hence, weight loss is a recommended and effective measure to reduce reflux.[30]

Medical Therapy

Antacids are very effective in the rapid treatment of pyrosis symptoms (typically 30–60 minutes) but their long-term efficacy is limited. They are readily available over the counter in various formulations that have comparable efficacy. Uniquely a few formulations have the added benefit of an antireflux barrier in the form of an alginate raft.[42] Although antacids are typically considered safe, there are some side effects that are more concerning in elderly patients. Antacids can interfere with absorption of other essential medications, have undesirable effects on bowel habits (aluminum and calcium containing agents worsening constipation), and may increase overall salt intake (with preparations containing sodium bicarbonate). Milk alkali syndrome can occur, albeit rarely, with increased dosing. This is often exacerbated by concomitant use of angiotensin-converting enzyme inhibitors, thiazides, and nonsteroidal anti-inflammatory medications. Finally, there are some reports associating aluminum containing antacids with Alzheimer disease.[43]

Antihistamines (H2 receptor antagonists [H2RAs]) are a step-up therapy. They are commonly used for reflux and are effective over an extended period of time, yet they are less potent than PPI and have a shorter duration of action. In a meta-analysis of 7000 patients, erosive esophagitis was healed 84% versus 52% on PPI versus H2RAs.[44] Although there is some concern over tachyphylaxis, the effective use of H2RA as solo therapy or additive therapy for nocturnal symptoms is common. Beyond recent concerns for impurities in ranitidine formulations, there are some concerns of mental status changes associated with H2RAs. These are most relevant to patients with renal and hepatic impairment. Cimetidine is less commonly used than other H2 receptor antagoniists in part because of its effect on cytochrome enzymes, and this can have significant downstream consequences for elderly patients with polypharmacy, particularly in combination with medication with narrow therapeutic windows.[45]

Potent suppression of gastric acid production with PPI is the most effective medical treatment of GERD regardless of age. Although plasma clearance decreases with age, no dose deescalation is necessary in elderly patients.[46] Pantoprazole and esomeprazole pharmacokinetics seem to be relatively unaffected by age.[47] Direct comparison between various PPI has indicated slight superiority for esomeprazole in healing of mucosal erosion,[48] and omeprazole-sodium bicarbonate in achieving prolonged intragastric suppression,[49] but there are no substantial clinical differences.[3]

Management of GERD in the elderly predicates on the principle of the least invasive intervention with the greatest potential benefit. Common side effects of PPI are mild and include headaches, nausea, abdominal pain, change bowel habits, rash, and dizziness. Typically considered a mainstay of treatment of GERD, PPIs were widely prescribed and likely overutilized. There is momentum to move away from a standardized approach, given growing literature on potential long-term side effects.[50] This literature includes retrospective cross-sectional studies, randomized control trials, and metanalysis with conflicting data. Side effects can be grouped into malabsorptive, infectious, and other rare complications.

Gastric acid suppression theoretically leads to vitamin B12 deficiency through an inability to liberate intrinsic factor. This is more profound in elderly who are at a greater risk of pernicious anemia. Associations between vitamin B12 deficiency and PPI use have been limited to case series and retrospective reviews.[51–53] Current guidelines and expert opinion do not advocate for serum vitamin B12 measurements.[4] Other concerns include decreased absorption of divalent minerals such as calcium and magnesium. The concern with calcium pertains to the risk of poor bone health, which is particularly concerning in postmenopausal women who are at risk of osteoporotic fractures.[54] There are also some retrospective studies associating PPIs with increased cardiovascular and renal events. Beyond checking vitamin D levels, there are no data to support additional testing.

In the absence of gastric acid barrier there is a theoretic increased risk of infection. Community-acquired pneumonia and *Clostridium difficile* infections have been most widely studied. Respiratory infections are postulated to be related to increased bacterial colonization in the upper gastrointestinal tract.[55] Despite the publication of randomized control trials and meta-analysis the results continue to be mixed.[54] The risk with enteric infections, particularly *C difficile* is more pathophysiologically plausible and data supported.[56]

Dementia and altered mental status have been suggested in retrospective cohort studies but not validated in prospective case control studies.[57–59] Autoimmune interstitial nephritis is a well-categorized entity that represents a very rare complication of PPI use.[60]

An 8-week course of any PPI once a day achieves healing of esophagitis in 73% to 91% of patients.[61] Elderly patients may require greater acid suppression for esophagitis healing,[62] and relapse in the elderly can be as high as 90% on stopping PPI therapy.[63] Nonetheless, overprescribing PPIs and the failure to discontinue them affects 66% of hospital admissions. It likely represents a significant proportion of the huge health care cost associated with reflux. Early appropriate discontinuation of PPI and H2A has now become a quality metric with several societal and institutional initiatives.[64]

Several prokinetics have been considered and evaluated in the treatment of GERD, with the purported mechanism of increasing gastric acid secretion and improving LES tone. Until recently the only FDA-approved prokinetic agents were erythromycin and metoclopramide. The dopamine antagonist, metaclopramide, has been shown to increase LES pressure and improve gastric emptying.[65] There is a black box warning for idiosyncratic reaction of irreversible tardive dyskinesia. Moreover, it has been associated with muscles tremors, spasms, agitation, anxiety, insomnia, and drowsiness in up to one-third of patients.[66] Domperidone is not available in the United States and shares many prokinetic properties with metoclopramide but has a higher safety profile given limited central nervous system interaction.[67]

Surgical Therapy

In patients who forego medical therapy (in part due to polypharmacy) or are refractory to medical therapy, surgical repair of the hiatal defect and the creation of a more efficient antireflux barrier is possible. A laparoscopic fundoplication is the standard of care. In addition to decades in refinement of surgical technique, personalized surgical planning with a presurgical evaluation is widely adopted. Structural examination includes esophagram and endoscopy, whereas preoperative functional testing includes pH/impedance testing, manometry, and a gastric emptying study. Randomized control trials have identified comparable efficacy between PPI therapy and laparoscopic fundoplication.[68] Results have been durable over 5 years[69] with only a minority requiring reinitiation of PPI.[70] Durability beyond the first decade and need for redo fundoplication are less applicable in an elderly population.[19,71–73] Although some data suggest that elderly are more susceptible to earlier complications,[74–76] studies with open and laparoscopic fundoplication show no increase in mortality or morbidity in this age group,[77–79] which further supports the need for careful patient selection and a complete and through presurgical evaluation.

Endoscopic Therapy

Endoscopic antireflux therapy provides a middle ground between surgical and medical therapies and has been a target of extensive biomedical advancement. Many devices with promising early data have gone out of stock due to a lack of durable benefit and unacceptable complications. Available options include augmentation of the GEJ through submucosal radio frequency ablation scarring (Stretta) and endoscopically placed gastroesophageal junction t-fasteners (transoral incisionless fundoplication).[4] These minimally invasive interventions have varying degrees of evidence and societal support. At present insurance coverage and careful selection of patients will allow us to best identify a subset of elderly patients who would benefit from such interventions and avoid some of the risks associated with surgical or medical therapy.

BARRETT ESOPHAGUS

In addition to esophagitis, strictures, Barrett esophagus, and esophageal adenocarcinoma (EAC) are potential complications of long-term GERD.[80] Incidence of all seems to increase with age.[81–85]

Barrett esophagus is defined as metaplastic growth of specialized intestinal epithelium that appears as columnar mucosa in the distal esophagus on an endoscopic evaluation. The incidence of Barrett esophagus seems to increase with age,[86] in part due to pathophysiological barrier breakdown at the level of the esophagogastric junction and progression in size of the hiatal hernia. This validates epidemiologic data indicating peak incidence of EAC in the sixth and seventh decade of life.[87] The sensitivity of symptoms to suggest Barrett esophagus is low; in fact almost one-third of elderly patients are asymptomatic.[88]

Various societies have adopted an age threshold (commonly 50 years) as a risk factor that is incorporated into determining patients who should undergo screening. These guidelines also advocated for an age limit on screening.[89–91] This is partly due to increasing comorbidities and nonesophageal cancer-related mortality in the elderly. A discussion regarding likelihood of survival over the next 5 years is recommended. There is limited literature on the life expectancy of elderly men with Barrett esophagus. In a recent cross-sectional study of 4252 veterans, a quarter of patients were 80 years old or older. One-third of them had limited life expectancy at the time of their Barrett esophagus diagnosis and a quarter of them died within 4 years of diagnosis.[92]

Dysplasia remains the only readily available and reliable predictor of progression to adenocarcinoma.[93] Misattribution of inflammation to dysplasia is common[94] and might be more challenging in the elderly given concomitant esophagitis. In addition to less frequently causing symptoms, esophagitis is typically more severe in the elderly.[9] It is therefore strongly encouraged that histologic risk assessment is delayed until esophagitis is healed. On medical optimization the interval for surveillance depends on degree of dysplasia: 3 to 5 years for nondysplastic Barrett esophagus and 6 to 12 months for Barrett esophagus with low-grade dysplasia (LGD). Endoscopic ablation is an acceptable alternative in patients with LGD with reasonable life expectancy. Patients with high-grade dysplasia are uniformly recommended to undergo endoscopy therapy. The guidelines do not recommend different intervals based on age.[89–91]

Esophagectomy remains a treatment of high-grade dysplasia and for endoscopically untreatable adenocarcinoma. There is significant increased morbidity and mortality associated with an esophagectomy in the elderly despite advances in technique and postsurgical care.[95,96] Because of the advent of effective and durable endoscopic esophageal sparing procedures, there are arguments to extend the age limit of screening and testing.[90] In fact studies have suggested a preferentially improved 2-year survival rate for elderly patients treated endoscopically.[97] The outcomes of endoscopic and surgical therapies are significantly improved in high volume centers.[98] This is most applicable in elderly patients in whom early detection of complications and management of comorbidities play a significant part.

Identifying a potent chemoprophylactic agent that can reduce the progression to advanced dysplasia and cancer has been actively sought. Many medications with antiinflammatory or antineoplastic potential have been evaluated. Aspirin (ASA) has chemoprophylactic properties against various gastrointestinal cancers.[99,100] A recent prospective multicenter trial, AspECT, found the greatest benefit was for a combination of high-dose PPI and ASA. It should be noted that although ASA toxicity is low, there is a risk for bleeding, intestinal ulceration, and strictures.[101] Several randomized trials have recently found nearly double the risk of bleeding with no to little cardiovascular benefit in patient receiving ASA chemoprophylaxis.[102] USPSTF now recommends a more tailored role for ASA that accounts for the weight of various bleeding risk factors.[103] Although chronic PPI use for chemoprophylaxis use in Barrett esophagus has more evidence behind it, the use of ASA solely for chemoprevention in Barrett esophagus remains controversial.

SUMMARY

As our population continues to age, the early diagnosis and optimal management of patients with GERD becomes paramount. Maintaining a low threshold for evaluating atypical symptoms in this population is key to improving outcomes. Should patients develop complications including severe esophagitis, peptic stricture, or Barrett esophagus then a discussion of medical, endoscopic, and surgical treatments that accounts for patient's comorbidities and survival is important. Advances in screening, surveillance, and endoscopic treatment of Barrett esophagus have allowed us to dispel concerns of futility and treat a larger subset of the at-risk population. Given that GERD persistently accounts for high per patient and health care costs, it is essential we continue to improve the quality of our health care delivery.

DISCLOSURE

P.G. Iyer: Research funding from C2 Therapeutics, Nine Point Medical, Exact Sciences, Consultant: Medtronic, CSA Medical, Symple Surgical; F. Otaki has nothing to disclose.

REFERENCES

1. UC B. An aging world: 2015. 2015. Available at: https://www.census.gov/library/%20publications/2016/demo/P95-16-1.html. Accessed March 3, 2020.
2. US Department of Health and Human Services A Profile of Older Americans: 2017. 2017. Available at: https://acl.gov/sites/default/files/Aging%20and%20Disability%20in%20America/2017OlderAmericansProfile.pdf. Accessed March 3, 2020.
3. Katz PO, Gerson LB, Vela MF. Guidelines for the diagnosis and management of gastroesophageal reflux disease. Am J Gastroenterol 2013;108(3):308–28 [quiz: 29].
4. Soumekh A, Schnoll-Sussman FH, Katz PO. Reflux and acid peptic diseases in the elderly. Clin Geriatr Med 2014;30(1):29–41.
5. Locke GR 3rd, Talley NJ, Fett SL, et al. Prevalence and clinical spectrum of gastroesophageal reflux: a population-based study in Olmsted County, Minnesota. Gastroenterology 1997;112(5):1448–56.
6. Pilotto A, Maggi S, Noale M, et al. Association of upper gastrointestinal symptoms with functional and clinical charateristics in elderly. World J Gastroenterol 2011;17(25):3020–6.
7. Moore KL, Boscardin WJ, Steinman MA, et al. Age and sex variation in prevalence of chronic medical conditions in older residents of U.S. nursing homes. J Am Geriatr Soc 2012;60(4):756–64.
8. Richter JE, Rubenstein JH. Presentation and epidemiology of gastroesophageal reflux disease. Gastroenterology 2018;154(2):267–76.
9. Johnson DA, Fennerty MB. Heartburn severity underestimates erosive esophagitis severity in elderly patients with gastroesophageal reflux disease. Gastroenterology 2004;126(3):660–4.
10. Lasch H, Castell DO, Castell JA. Evidence for diminished visceral pain with aging: studies using graded intraesophageal balloon distension. Am J Physiol 1997;272(1 Pt 1):G1–3.
11. Fass R, Pulliam G, Johnson C, et al. Symptom severity and oesophageal chemosensitivity to acid in older and young patients with gastro-oesophageal reflux. Age Ageing 2000;29(2):125–30.
12. Pilotto A, Franceschi M, Leandro G, et al. Clinical features of reflux esophagitis in older people: a study of 840 consecutive patients. J Am Geriatr Soc 2006; 54(10):1537–42.

13. Becher A, El-Serag H. Systematic review: the association between symptomatic response to proton pump inhibitors and health-related quality of life in patients with gastro-oesophageal reflux disease. Aliment Pharmacol Ther 2011;34(0). 618–27.

14. Marik PE, Kaplan D. Aspiration pneumonia and dysphagia in the elderly. Chest 2003;124(1):328–36.

15. Cock C, Omari T. Systematic review of pharyngeal and esophageal manometry in healthy or dysphagic older persons (>60 years). Geriatrics (Basel) 2018; 3(4):67.

16. Mei L, Dua A, Kern M, et al. Older age reduces upper esophageal sphincter and esophageal body responses to simulated slow and ultraslow reflux events and post-reflux residue. Gastroenterology 2018;155(3):760–70.e1.

17. Francis DO, Rymer JA, Slaughter JC, et al. High economic burden of caring for patients with suspected extraesophageal reflux. Am J Gastroenterol 2013; 108(6):905–11.

18. Mendelsohn AH. The effects of reflux on the elderly: the problems with medications and interventions. Otolaryngol Clin North Am 2018;51(4):779–87.

19. Khajanchee YS, Urbach DR, Butler N, et al. Laparoscopic antireflux surgery in the elderly. Surg Endosc 2002;16(1):25–30.

20. Achem SR, DeVault KR. Gastroesophageal reflux disease and the elderly. Gastroenterol Clin North Am 2014;43(1):147–60.

21. Hollis JB, Castell DO. Esophageal function in elderly man. A new look at "presbyesophagus". Ann Intern Med 1974;80(3):371–4.

22. Richter JE, Wu WC, Johns DN, et al. Esophageal manometry in 95 healthy adult volunteers. Variability of pressures with age and frequency of "abnormal" contractions. Dig Dis Sci 1987;32(6):583–92.

23. Grande L, Lacima G, Ros E, et al. Deterioration of esophageal motility with age: a manometric study of 79 healthy subjects. Am J Gastroenterol 1999;94(7): 1795–801.

24. Meshkinpour H, Haghighat P, Dutton C. Clinical spectrum of esophageal aperistalsis in the elderly. Am J Gastroenterol 1994;89(9):1480–3.

25. Ferriolli E, Oliveira RB, Matsuda NM, et al. Aging, esophageal motility, and gastroesophageal reflux. J Am Geriatr Soc 1998;46(12):1534–7.

26. Gutschow CA, Leers JM, Schroder W, et al. Effect of aging on esophageal motility in patients with and without GERD. Ger Med Sci 2011;9:Doc22.

27. Lee J, Anggiansah A, Anggiansah R, et al. Effects of age on the gastroesophageal junction, esophageal motility, and reflux disease. Clin Gastroenterol Hepatol 2007;5(12):1092–8.

28. Eckardt VF, LeCompte PM. Esophageal ganglia and smooth muscle in the elderly. Am J Dig Dis 1978;23(5):443–8.

29. Adams CW, Brain RH, Trounce JR. Ganglion cells in achalasia of the cardia. Virchows Arch A Pathol Anat Histol 1976;372(1):75–9.

30. Jacobson BC, Somers SC, Fuchs CS, et al. Body-mass index and symptoms of gastroesophageal reflux in women. N Engl J Med 2006;354(22):2340–8.

31. Schindlbeck NE, Klauser AG, Voderholzer WA, et al. Empiric therapy for gastroesophageal reflux disease. Arch Intern Med 1995;155(16):1808–12.

32. Gyawali CP, Kahrilas PJ, Savarino E, et al. Modern diagnosis of GERD: the Lyon consensus. Gut 2018;67(7):1351–62.

33. Jalal A, Payne HR, Jeyasingham K. The influence of age on gastro-oesophageal reflux: a re-appraisal of the DeMeester scoring system. Eur J Cardiothorac Surg 2000;18(4):411–7.

34. Zerbib F, Roman S, Bruley Des Varannes S, et al. Normal values of pharyngeal and esophageal 24-hour pH impedance in individuals on and off therapy and interobserver reproducibility. Clin Gastroenterol Hepatol 2013;11(4):366–72.

35. Baker ME. Role of the barium esophagram in antireflux surgery. Gastroenterol Hepatol (N Y) 2014;10(10):677–9.

36. Vaezi MF. New tests for the evaluation of laryngopharyngeal reflux. Gastroenterol Hepatol (N Y) 2013;9(2):115–7.

37. Stanciu C, Bennett JR. Effects of posture on gastro-oesophageal reflux. Digestion 1977;15(2):104–9.

38. Hamilton JW, Boisen RJ, Yamamoto DT, et al. Sleeping on a wedge diminishes exposure of the esophagus to refluxed acid. Dig Dis Sci 1988;33(5):518–22.

39. Pollmann H, Zillessen E, Pohl J, et al. [Effect of elevated head position in bed in therapy of gastroesophageal reflux]. Z Gastroenterol 1996;34(Suppl 2):93–9.

40. Tamanna S, Campbell D, Warren R, et al. Effect of CPAP therapy on symptoms of nocturnal gastroesophageal reflux among patients with obstructive sleep apnea. J Clin Sleep Med 2016;12(9):1257–61.

41. Duroux P, Bauerfeind P, Emde C, et al. Early dinner reduces nocturnal gastric acidity. Gut 1989;30(8):1063–7.

42. Leiman DA, Riff BP, Morgan S, et al. Alginate therapy is effective treatment for GERD symptoms: a systematic review and meta-analysis. Dis Esophagus 2017;30(5):1–9.

43. Tomljenovic L. Aluminum and Alzheimer's disease: after a century of controversy, is there a plausible link? J Alzheimers Dis 2011;23(4):567–98.

44. Colin-Jones DG. The role and limitations of H2-receptor antagonists in the treatment of gastro-oesophageal reflux disease. Aliment Pharmacol Ther 1995; 9(Suppl 1):9–14.

45. Fackler WK, Ours TM, Vaezi MF, et al. Long-term effect of H2RA therapy on nocturnal gastric acid breakthrough. Gastroenterology 2002;122(3):625–32.

46. Rodriguez S, Mattek N, Lieberman D, et al. Barrett's esophagus on repeat endoscopy: should we look more than once? Am J Gastroenterol 2008;103(8): 1892–7.

47. Huber R, Hartmann M, Bliesath H, et al. Pharmacokinetics of pantoprazole in man. Int J Clin Pharmacol Ther 1996;34(5):185–94.

48. Klinkenberg-Knol EC, Nelis F, Dent J, et al. Long-term omeprazole treatment in resistant gastroesophageal reflux disease: efficacy, safety, and influence on gastric mucosa. Gastroenterology 2000;118(4):661–9.

49. Dharmarajan TS, Kanagala MR, Murakonda P, et al. Do acid-lowering agents affect vitamin B12 status in older adults? J Am Med Dir Assoc 2008;9(3):162–7.

50. Valuck RJ, Ruscin JM. A case-control study on adverse effects: H2 blocker or proton pump inhibitor use and risk of vitamin B12 deficiency in older adults. J Clin Epidemiol 2004;57(4):422–8.

51. Rozgony NR, Fang C, Kuczmarski MF, et al. Vitamin B(12) deficiency is linked with long-term use of proton pump inhibitors in institutionalized older adults: could a cyanocobalamin nasal spray be beneficial? J Nutr Elder 2010;29(1): 87–99.

52. Sheen E, Triadafilopoulos G. Adverse effects of long-term proton pump inhibitor therapy. Dig Dis Sci 2011;56(4):931–50.

53. Sarkar M, Hennessy S, Yang YX. Proton-pump inhibitor use and the risk for community-acquired pneumonia. Ann Intern Med 2008;149(6):391–8.

54. Howell MD, Novack V, Grgurich P, et al. Iatrogenic gastric acid suppression and the risk of nosocomial Clostridium difficile infection. Arch Intern Med 2010; 170(9):784–90.
55. Haenisch B, von Holt K, Wiese B, et al. Risk of dementia in elderly patients with the use of proton pump inhibitors. Eur Arch Psychiatry Clin Neurosci 2015; 265(5):419–28.
56. Gomm W, Haenisch B. Proton pump inhibitors and dementia incidence-reply. JAMA Neurol 2016;73(8):1028–9.
57. Goldstein FC, Steenland K, Zhao L, et al. Proton pump inhibitors and risk of mild cognitive impairment and dementia. J Am Geriatr Soc 2017;65(9):1969–74.
58. Moledina DG, Perazella MA. PPIs and kidney disease: from AIN to CKD. J Nephrol 2016;29(5):611–6.
59. Edwards SJ, Lind T, Lundell L. Systematic review: proton pump inhibitors (PPIs) for the healing of reflux oesophagitis - a comparison of esomeprazole with other PPIs. Aliment Pharmacol Ther 2006;24(5):743–50.
60. Escourrou J, Deprez P, Saggioro A, et al. Maintenance therapy with pantoprazole 20 mg prevents relapse of reflux oesophagitis. Aliment Pharmacol Ther 1999;13(11):1481–91.
61. Carlsson R, Galmiche JP, Dent J, et al. Prognostic factors influencing relapse of oesophagitis during maintenance therapy with antisecretory drugs: a meta-analysis of long-term omeprazole trials. Aliment Pharmacol Ther 1997;11(3): 473–82.
62. Pasina L, Nobili A, Tettamanti M, et al. Prevalence and appropriateness of drug prescriptions for peptic ulcer and gastro-esophageal reflux disease in a cohort of hospitalized elderly. Eur J Intern Med 2011;22(2):205–10.
63. Lieberman DA, Keeffe EB. Treatment of severe reflux esophagitis with cimetidine and metoclopramide. Ann Intern Med 1986;104(1):21–6.
64. Verlinden M. Review article: a role for gastrointestinal prokinetic agents in the treatment of reflux oesophagitis? Aliment Pharmacol Ther 1989;3(2):113–31.
65. Brogden RN, Carmine AA, Heel RC, et al. Domperidone. A review of its pharmacological activity, pharmacokinetics and therapeutic efficacy in the symptomatic treatment of chronic dyspepsia and as an antiemetic. Drugs 1982;24(5): 360–400.
66. Galmiche JP, Hatlebakk J, Attwood S, et al. Laparoscopic antireflux surgery vs esomeprazole treatment for chronic GERD: the LOTUS randomized clinical trial. JAMA 2011;305(19):1969–77.
67. Grant AM, Boachie C, Cotton SC, et al. Clinical and economic evaluation of laparoscopic surgery compared with medical management for gastro-oesophageal reflux disease: 5-year follow-up of multicentre randomised trial (the REFLUX trial). Health Technol Assess 2013;17(22):1–167.
68. Grant KS, DeMeester SR, Kreger V, et al. Effect of Barrett's esophagus surveillance on esophageal preservation, tumor stage, and survival with esophageal adenocarcinoma. J Thorac Cardiovasc Surg 2013;146(1):31–7.
69. Aprea G, Ferronetti A, Canfora A, et al. GERD in elderly patients: surgical treatment with Nissen-Rossetti laparoscopic technique, outcome. BMC Surg 2012; 12(Suppl 1):S4.
70. Lundell L, Miettinen P, Myrvold HE, et al. Comparison of outcomes twelve years after antireflux surgery or omeprazole maintenance therapy for reflux esophagitis. Clin Gastroenterol Hepatol 2009;7(12):1292–8 [quiz: 60].
71. Anvari M, Allen C, Marshall J, et al. A randomized controlled trial of laparoscopic Nissen fundoplication versus proton pump inhibitors for the treatment of patients

with chronic gastroesophageal reflux disease (GERD): 3-year outcomes. Surg Endosc 2011;25(8):2547–54.

72. Maret-Ouda J, Wahlin K, El-Serag HB, et al. Association between laparoscopic antireflux surgery and recurrence of gastroesophageal reflux. JAMA 2017; 318(10):939–46.

73. Morgenthal CB, Shane MD, Stival A, et al. The durability of laparoscopic Nissen fundoplication: 11-year outcomes. J Gastrointest Surg 2007;11(6):693–700.

74. Dallemagne B, Arenas Sanchez M, Francart D, et al. Long-term results after laparoscopic reoperation for failed antireflux procedures. Br J Surg 2011; 98(11):1581–7.

75. Allen R, Rappaport W, Hixson L, et al. Referral patterns and the results of anti-reflux operations in patients more than sixty years of age. Surg Gynecol Obstet 1991;173(5):359–62.

76. Kamolz T, Bammer T, Granderath FA, et al. Quality of life and surgical outcome after laparoscopic antireflux surgery in the elderly gastroesophageal reflux disease patient. Scand J Gastroenterol 2001;36(2):116–20.

77. Tedesco P, Lobo E, Fisichella PM, et al. Laparoscopic fundoplication in elderly patients with gastroesophageal reflux disease. Arch Surg 2006;141(3):289–92 [discussion: 92].

78. Morganstern B, Anandasabapathy S. GERD and Barrett's esophagus: diagnostic and management strategies in the geriatric population. Geriatrics 2009; 64(7):9–12.

79. Zhu H, Pace F, Sangaletti O, et al. Features of symptomatic gastroesophageal reflux in elderly patients. Scand J Gastroenterol 1993;28(3):235–8.

80. Maekawa T, Kinoshita Y, Okada A, et al. Relationship between severity and symptoms of reflux oesophagitis in elderly patients in Japan. J Gastroenterol Hepatol 1998;13(9):927–30.

81. Jobe BA, Richter JE, Hoppo T, et al. Preoperative diagnostic workup before anti-reflux surgery: an evidence and experience-based consensus of the Esophageal Diagnostic Advisory Panel. J Am Coll Surg 2013;217(4):586–97.

82. Pech O, Gossner L, Manner H, et al. Prospective evaluation of the macroscopic types and location of early Barrett's neoplasia in 380 lesions. Endoscopy 2007; 39(7):588–93.

83. Ruigomez A, Garcia Rodriguez LA, Wallander MA, et al. Esophageal stricture: incidence, treatment patterns, and recurrence rate. Am J Gastroenterol 2006; 101(12):2685–92.

84. Kuipers EJ, Spaander MC. Natural history of Barrett's esophagus. Dig Dis Sci 2018;63(8):1997–2004.

85. Crane SJ, Talley NJ. Chronic gastrointestinal symptoms in the elderly. Clin Geriatr Med 2007;23(4):721–34, v.

86. Zimmerman J, Shohat V, Tsvang E, et al. Esophagitis is a major cause of upper gastrointestinal hemorrhage in the elderly. Scand J Gastroenterol 1997;32(9): 906–9.

87. Fitzgerald RC, di Pietro M, Ragunath K, et al. British Society of Gastroenterology guidelines on the diagnosis and management of Barrett's oesophagus. Gut 2014;63:7–42.

88. Shaheen NJ, Falk GW, Iyer PG, et al. ACG clinical guideline: diagnosis and management of Barrett's esophagus. Am J Gastroenterol 2016;111:30–50.

89. Asge Standards Of Practice C, Qumseya B, Sultan S, et al. ASGE guideline on screening and surveillance of Barrett's esophagus. Gastrointest Endosc 2019; 90(3):335–359 e2.

90. Ko MS, Fung KZ, Shi Y, et al. Barrett's esophagus commonly diagnosed in elderly men with limited life expectancy. J Am Geriatr Soc 2016;64(10):e109–11.

91. Bansal A, Fitzgerald RC. Biomarkers in Barrett's esophagus. Gastroenterol Clin North Am 2015;44:373–90.

92. Vennalaganti P, Kanakadandi V, Goldblum JR, et al. Discordance among pathologists in the United States and Europe in diagnosis of low-grade dysplasia for patients with Barrett's esophagus. Gastroenterology 2017;152(3):564–570 e4.

93. Cijs TM, Verhoef C, Steyerberg EW, et al. Outcome of esophagectomy for cancer in elderly patients. Ann Thorac Surg 2010;90(3):900–7.

94. Baranov NS, van Workum F, van der Maas J, et al. The influence of age on complications and overall survival after ivor Lewis totally minimally invasive esophagectomy. J Gastrointest Surg 2019;23(7):1293–300.

95. Cummings LC, Kou TD, Schluchter MD, et al. Outcomes after endoscopic versus surgical therapy for early esophageal cancers in an older population. Gastrointest Endosc 2016;84(2):232–40.e1.

96. Markar SR, Karthikesalingam A, Thrumurthy S, et al. Volume-outcome relationship in surgery for esophageal malignancy: systematic review and meta-analysis 2000-2011. J Gastrointest Surg 2012;16:1055–63.

97. Cole BF, Logan RF, Halabi S, et al. Aspirin for the chemoprevention of colorectal adenomas: meta-analysis of the randomized trials. J Natl Cancer Inst 2009; 101(4):256–66.

98. Rothwell PM, Fowkes FG, Belch JF, et al. Effect of daily aspirin on long-term risk of death due to cancer: analysis of individual patient data from randomised trials. Lancet 2011;377(9759):31–41.

99. Jankowski JAZ, de Caestecker J, Love SB, et al. Esomeprazole and aspirin in Barrett's oesophagus (AspECT): a randomised factorial trial. Lancet 2018; 392(10145):400–8.

100. Patrono C, Baigent C. Role of aspirin in primary prevention of cardiovascular disease. Nat Rev Cardiol 2019;16(11):675–86.

101. Whitlock EP, Burda BU, Williams SB, et al. Bleeding risks with aspirin use for primary prevention in adults: a systematic review for the U.S. Preventive Services Task Force. Ann Intern Med 2016;164(12):826–35.

102. Patrono C, Baigent C. Role of aspirin in primary prevention of cardiovascular disease. Nat Rev Cardiol 2019;16:675–86.

103. Bibbins-Domingo K. US Preventive Services Task Force. Aspirin Use for the Primary Prevention of Cardiovascular Disease and Colorectal Cancer: US Preventive Services Task Force Recommendation Statement. Ann Intern Med 2016 Jun 21,164(12).830–45. https://doi.org/10.7326/M16-0577. Epub 2016 Apr 12. PMID: 27064677.

Nonsteroidal Antiinflammatory Drugs, Anticoagulation, and Upper Gastrointestinal Bleeding

Mindy Winghin Lee, MD, Philip O. Katz, MD*

KEYWORDS

- Nonsteroidal antiinflammatory drugs (NSAIDs) • Anticoagulation • Elderly
- Upper GI bleeding • Peptic ulcer disease

KEY POINTS

- Advanced age, history of peptic ulcer disease, *Helicobacter pylori*, coadministration of nonsteroidal antiinflammatory drugs (NSAIDs), corticosteroids, anticoagulation, and antiplatelets are risk factors for gastrointestinal bleeding in the elderly.
- Awareness of these risks and appropriate use of NSAIDs, particularly in those needing antiplatelet or anticoagulant therapy, is critical to optimal management.
- Careful selection of elderly patients requiring antiplatelet, anticoagulation, or chronic NSAID therapy for cotherapy with proton pump inhibitors can significantly reduce morbidity and mortality from gastrointestinal bleeding.

INTRODUCTION

The elderly present constant challenges in medical management, particularly of pain and inflammation. Balancing the risk and benefits of medication requires extra vigilance on the part of care providers because symptoms are often subtle and side effects more frequent, with major adverse events always a concern. This tendency is particularly evident with the use of nonsteroidal antiinflammatory drugs (NSAIDs), anticoagulants, and antiplatelet agents because one of the major complications, gastrointestinal (GI) bleeding, can result in major morbidity in this population. This article discusses issues related to GI bleeding, NSAID complications, and issues related to anticoagulation in the elderly population.

Division of Gastroenterology and Hepatology, Weill Cornell Medical College, 1315 York Avenue, First Floor, New York, NY 10021, USA
* Corresponding author.
E-mail address: philipokatz@gmail.com

Clin Geriatr Med 37 (2021) 31–42
https://doi.org/10.1016/j.cger.2020.08.004   geriatric.theclinics.com

GASTROINTESTINAL BLEEDING

GI bleeding has been estimated to have a prevalence of around 3% in a large population based study in the elderly aged greater than or equal to 65 years.[1] Age has been suggested as a risk factor for GI bleeding, together with non–acetylsalicylic acid antiplatelet agents, index of comorbidity (Cumulative Illness Rating Scale) greater than 3, and liver cirrhosis. Peptic ulcer disease, hemorrhagic gastropathy, esophageal varices are the most common causes of upper GI bleeding, whereas diverticular bleeding and angiodysplasia are the most common causes of lower GI bleeding.[1–5] Peptic ulcer bleeding continues to be of major consequence in the elderly, with mortality reported to be 5% to 10% worldwide, predominantly related to nonbleeding causes.[6] One meta-analysis showed that increased peptic ulcer bleeding mortality is related to the number of comorbidities, with 3 or more comorbidities having a greater risk of death compared with 1 or 2. Hepatic, renal, and malignant comorbidities are associated with increased risk of death in peptic ulcer bleeding.[7]

NONSTEROIDAL ANTIINFLAMMATORY DRUGS

Studies have estimated the prevalence of NSAIDs and aspirin use to be 24.7% in the elderly.[8] Approximately half of the patients who regularly take NSAIDs have gastric erosions, and 15% to 30% have ulcers that are detected endoscopically. Clinical upper GI events (perforations, obstructions, bleeding, and uncomplicated ulcers) may occur in 3% to 4.5% of patients taking NSAIDs annually, and serious complicated events (perforation, obstruction, or major bleeding) develop in approximately 1.5%.[9]

NSAIDs can cause injury anywhere in the GI tract, although the upper GI tract seems most vulnerable. Injuries can be divided into gastroduodenal, small bowel, and colonic.

GASTRODUODENAL INJURY

NSAID-induced upper GI injury is a result of relative deficiency of mucosal prostaglandins leading to secondary acid-related ulceration in a compromised epithelial barrier.[10] Mucosal disruption, decreased bicarbonate secretion, and local vasoconstriction are consequences of cyclooxygenase (COX) inhibition.[10] This condition can lead to ulcer formation, hemorrhage, and perforation.

NSAIDs are divided into nonselective and selective COX inhibitors. Nonselective NSAIDs inhibit both COX-1 and COX-2, whereas selective COX inhibitors inhibit only COX-2. COX isoenzymes catalyze the rate-limiting step in the formation of prostaglandins, thromboxane, and levuloglandins. COX-1–derived prostaglandins play an important role in cytoprotection of the gastroduodenal mucosa, whereas COX-2 mediates tumor angiogenesis, inflammatory response, and thrombosis. Therefore, damage of gastroduodenal mucosa and resulting GI bleeding is associated with inhibition of COX-1, whereas COX-2 has been studied as a potential target for chemoprevention.[11]

It is of some surprise that the risk of GI bleeding has been reported to be higher in acute NSAID use compared with chronic use.[12] Up to 37% of patients develop severe gastric mucosal damage with short-term NSAID use, and 13% develop duodenal damage. Short-term use of NSAIDs may not be benign in the elderly.[13]

SMALL BOWEL INJURY

Small bowel injury, similar to gastroduodenal injury, involves both systemic and local mechanisms of injury. In addition to the decrease in prostaglandin cytoprotection, breach in local epithelial barrier, and changes in microcirculation, bile acids, pancreatic secretions, and bacteria can further exacerbate injury.[10]

Advances in small bowel imaging, capsule endoscopy, and enteroscopy have allowed the acute documentation of the spectrum of small bowel mucosal damage from NSAIDs. The so-called NSAID-induced enteropathy has various presentations, ranging from erythema, erosions, and ulcers to diaphragmlike strictures and small bowel bleeding.[14]

In healthy volunteers given a short course of nonselective NSAIDs (14 days), capsule endoscopy identified visible mucosal changes in 68% of volunteers. These changes included mucosal breaks (40%), erythema (35%), petechiae (33%), denuded mucosa (20%), and blood in lumen (8%).[15] In chronic NSAID use (>6 months), up to 8.4% of users developed small bowel ulcerations.[16] One study examined 120 asymptomatic patients on nonselective COX inhibitors and 40 patients on COX-2 inhibitors who underwent capsule endoscopy. Twenty-nine patients had mucosal breaks in the conventional NSAID group, whereas 22% had mucosal breaks in the COX-2 selective inhibitor group.[17] Strictures, obstruction, and perforation are far less common.

COLONIC INJURY

Although uncommon compared with gastroduodenal and small bowel injury, NSAID-induced colopathy has been reported in case reports. NSAID-induced colopathy can mimic symptoms of colorectal cancers, presenting with iron deficiency anemia, rectal bleeding, occult bleeding, and abdominal pain. When colonoscopy is performed, it can reveal fibrous strictures and ulcerations.

Risk Factors

Risk of NSAID-related injury and complications are influenced by demographic factors, duration of NSAID use, coadministration of medications, and comorbidities.

Age
Age has been shown to be a significant risk factor for adverse GI events related to NSAID use. Several age-related gastric changes, including reduced mucosal protective mechanisms and decreased gastric blood flow, compromise the mucosal barrier and further predispose the gastroduodenal mucosa to the adverse effects of NSAIDs.[18] A meta-analysis showed that elderly patients (defined as aged greater than or equal to 60 years) have an odds ratio (OR) of 5.52 versus 1.65 in younger patients for developing adverse events while on NSAIDs.[19]

Length of nonsteroidal antiinflammatory drug use
Short-term NSAID use is also associated with higher risk of NSAID-related adverse events. Surprisingly the odds of NSAID mucosa injury may decrease over time. The summary OR for less than 1 month of NSAID exposure was 8.00 (95% confidence interval [CI], 6.37–10.06); for more than 1 month but less than 3 months of exposure, the summary OR was 3.31 (95% CI, 2.27–4.82); and for more than 3 months of exposure, the summary OR was 1.92 (95% CI, 1.19–3.13).[19]

Prior history of gastrointestinal event
Prior upper GI bleeding is identified to be the strongest and most consistent risk factor for GI bleeding on antiplatelet therapy.[20] This finding forms the basis of several guidelines suggesting the use of gastroprotective prophylaxis in patients on chronic or dual antiplatelet therapy to prevent GI bleeding in those at risk, especially in those who require coadministration of long-term NSAID therapy.

Coadministration of medications

Prior studies have reported an increased risk of adverse GI events related to NSAID use in the setting of coadministration of corticosteroids, antiplatelets, and anticoagulants. Corticosteroids have not been shown to increase risk for peptic ulcer disease when used alone. When combined with NSAID, the estimated relative risk (RR) for development of peptic ulcer disease increases to 4.4 compared with using steroids alone.[21]

The risk of development of peptic ulcer disease is significantly lower with low-dose aspirin (81 mg) compared with full-dose aspirin (325 mg). The RR of low-dose aspirin has been shown to be 2.07 compared with full dose for major GI bleeding.[22] When low-dose aspirin is used with an NSAID, there is an additive increase risk of bleeding in patients in developing gastroduodenal ulcer.[23]

The risk of bleeding with anticoagulants is presumably caused by bleeding from clinically silent lesions caused by *Helicobacter pylori* or NSAID-induced ulcers. The risk of the combined effect of NSAIDs and anticoagulants has not been extensively studied. However, use of anticoagulants has been reported to confer double the risk of GI bleeding compared with low-dose aspirin.[24]

Helicobacter pylori

The risks of peptic ulcer disease with NSAID use and *H pylori* infection have been estimated to be 3-fold to 4-fold. Although these are independent risk factors, they seem to have synergistic and additive effects for development of peptic ulcer disease.[25]

Management of nonsteroidal antiinflammatory drug–related complications

Management of NSAID-induced injury depends on patient symptoms, acuity, and hemodynamic stability. Symptoms may range from dyspepsia and obstructive symptoms to life-threatening GI bleeding and perforation.

Dyspepsia

As previously mentioned, up to half of chronic NSAID users can be found to have endoscopic evidence of mucosal damage. Patients presenting with dyspepsia who do not require chronic NSAID therapy generally improve with cessation of NSAIDs. Patients who require chronic NSAID use should be considered for prophylaxis with gastroprotectants and *H pylori* testing (discussed later).

Bleeding

Initial assessment The most essential initial assessment is the evaluation of the patient's mental status and hemodynamics. Hypotension and/or tachycardia should prompt timely fluid resuscitation. Altered mental status and/or inability to protect the airway should lead to prompt assessment for airway protection or intubation. Several commonly used risk assessment tools (ie, Glasgow-Blatchford score and Rockall score) can assist in risk stratification regarding safety to discharge the patient. The Glasgow-Blatchford score ranges from 0 to 23, with higher score indicating higher risk. Various clinical variables, including blood urea nitrogen, hemoglobin, systolic blood pressure, heart rate, melena, syncope, hepatic disease, and cardiac failure, are included in the score. A low Glasgow-Blatchford score (defined as 0–1, 0–2 for patients younger than 70 years of age) has been shown to be associated with minimal risk of intervention and death.[26,27] Although care must be taken with the elderly, those with a low score can be considered for early discharge with close outpatient follow-up.

Initiation of proton pump inhibitors is a common practice across hospitals when patients present with symptoms of upper GI bleeding. The role of preendoscopic proton pump inhibitors (PPIs) has been studied and defined. A meta-analysis showed that preendoscopic PPI did not improve mortality, need for surgery, or further bleeding. However, it was found to decrease the frequency of high-risk endoscopic findings and the need for endoscopic therapy.[28]

Endoscopy assessment

Timing of endoscopy for nonvariceal bleeding For patients presenting with acute GI bleeding, most guidelines recommend endoscopy within 24 hours after adequate resuscitation has been achieved.[29] Data for urgent endoscopy (<6–12 hours) have been mixed. Some studies suggest that early endoscopy (<6–12 hours) confers worse outcomes,[30] whereas other studies suggest improvement of outcomes in high-risk patients.[31,32] This difference is likely related to degree of resuscitation and definition of high-risk patients. The general consensus is to perform endoscopy within 24 hours after adequate resuscitation and considers early endoscopy within 12 hours in patients with suspected variceal bleeding. A gastroenterology consult to evaluate the need for endoscopy is mandatory in patients presenting with GI bleeding. Endoscopic assessment for high-risk lesions and need for endoscopic intervention is based on Forrest classification and the risks of rebleeding associated with these lesions without therapy. Forrest classification categorizes ulcers into active bleeding (IA), oozing (IB), visible vessel (IIA), adherent clot (IIB), pigmented spot (IIC), and clean base (III). Ulcers with endoscopic features of active bleeding (IA), oozing (IB), and visible vessel (IIA) benefit from endoscopic therapy because of the high risk of recurrent bleeding without therapy (60%–100% for active bleeding ulcer and up to 35%–50% for nonbleeding visible vessel). Treatment of these high-risk lesions should involve dual endoscopic therapy with both injection (eg, epinephrine) and thermal therapy (eg, bipolar cautery or heater probe) rather than epinephrine alone whenever possible.

Postendoscopy proton pump inhibitors When NSAID ulcers with high-risk stigmata are identified during endoscopy, continuous intravenous infusion of PPIs for 72 hours has been shown to significantly reduce risks of further bleeding, the need for surgery, and mortality.[33,34] Subsequent studies have shown that intermittent oral and intermittent intravenous PPI therapy are noninferior to continuous intravenous PPI therapy, suggesting such therapy may be used as alternatives.[35]

On discharge, patients found to have ulcers with high-risk stigmata should receive twice-daily PPI therapy for 2 weeks, followed by a PPI once daily. In patients found to have low-risk ulcers and erosions, once-daily PPI for 6 to 8 weeks is sufficient for healing.[27] If NSAIDs are needed long term, PPI cotherapy to reduce bleeding risk is recommended, even if COX-selective NSAIDs are used.

Obscure bleeding In elderly patients on chronic NSAIDs with persistent bleeding symptoms where upper endoscopy and colonoscopy are unrevealing, small bowel bleeding should be suspected. NSAID-induced small bowel ulceration can usually be identified on capsule endoscopy. Small bowel enteroscopy and/or single-balloon enteroscopy may be needed for diagnosis or therapy. Multiple studies have shown that misoprostol is an effective treatment of small bowel ulcers and erosions in patients using low-dose aspirin and NSAIDs.[36,37]

Stricturing disease and obstruction Rarely, chronic NSAID use can cause a diaphragmlike stricture and/or small bowel obstruction. Double-balloon enteroscopy is an effective diagnostic and therapeutic tool in tissue sampling and balloon dilation in patients with persistent stricture.[38] Rarely, surgical intervention is required in cases of complete obstruction and recurrent obstruction refractory to endoscopic therapy.

Perforation Although perforated peptic ulcer (PPU) is uncommon compared with bleeding as a complication from NSAID-induced ulcer disease, short-term mortality can reach up to 30%.[39] Although there has been a decrease in prevalence of *H pylori* in many Western countries, there has been a proportional increase of PPU caused by NSAID use, especially in the elderly population.[40,41] Older age, presence of comorbidity (heart disease, liver disease, renal disease, diabetes mellitus), and surgical delay (>24 hours) have been associated with increased mortality in patients presenting with PPU.[40]

PREVENTION OF NONSTEROIDAL ANTIINFLAMMATORY DRUG–RELATED INJURY AND RISK MODIFICATIONS
Role of Helicobacter pylori

Eradication of *H pylori* has been shown to reduce risk of recurrent bleeding caused by peptic ulcer disease with and without NSAID use.

Early eradication of *H pylori* seems to be more effective in reducing the risk of rebleeding. One study compared early eradication (within 120 days of peptic ulcer diagnosis) and late eradication, and showed that the late eradication group had a higher rate of complicated recurrent peptic ulcers.[42]

Because of the synergistic effect on peptic ulcer formation in patients infected with *H pylori* on chronic NSAID therapy, current recommendation is eradication of *H pylori* without long-term antisecretory maintenance if there are no other indications for prophylaxis.

Role of Proton Pump Inhibitors, H2-Receptor Antagonists, Prostaglandin Analogue Prophylaxis

Numerous studies have examined the efficacy of various gastroprotective agents in prevention of NSAID complications. One large meta-analysis compared PPIs, prostaglandin analogues, and H2-receptor antagonists (H2RAs) with controls in prevention of NSAID-induced peptic ulcer disease. PPIs showed greater degree of reduction in upper GI bleeding (OR, 0.21; 99% CI, 0.12–0.36) compared with H2RA (OR, 0.49; 99% CI, 0.30–0.80) and prostaglandin analogues (OR, 0.63; 99% CI, 0.35–1.12).[43]

The American College of Cardiology Foundation (ACCF), the American College of Gastroenterology (ACG), and the American Heart Association (AHA) 2010 Consensus recommended cotherapy with PPIs in patients on antiplatelet therapy if there is a history of GI bleeding, and that it is appropriate to consider in patients with multiple risk factors (advanced age not specifically defined, concomitant use of warfarin, steroids, NSAIDs, and *H pylori* infection).[20] The American College of Cardiology (ACC)/AHA recommends PPI prophylaxis in patients with history of GI bleeding on dual antiplatelet therapy (**Tables 1** and **2**). PPI is reasonable and can be considered in patients at increased risk of GI bleeding, including advanced age, concomitant anticoagulation, and concomitant steroids or NSAIDs.[44]

Role of Selective Cyclooxygenase-2 Inhibitor

Selective COX-2 inhibitors, such as celecoxib, are associated with a lower risk of upper GI bleeding than are nonselective COX inhibitors; therefore, they are recommended for patients who require long-term NSAID therapy.[45–47]

Table 1
Consideration of cotherapy in reduction of gastrointestinal bleeding risk in patients on antiplatelet therapy

Risk Factors[a]	Consider
Prior history of peptic ulcer disease Prior history of GI bleeding Concomitant anticoagulation or antiplatelet Two or more of the following risk factors: • Age $\geq$ 60 y, steroid use, dyspepsia, or gastroesophageal reflux disease symptoms	Proton pump inhibitor daily

[a] ACCF/ACG/AHA consensus document.

ANTICOAGULATION
Risk of Gastrointestinal Bleeding

Vitamin K antagonists versus no anticoagulation
Anticoagulants do not seem to cause direct mucosal injury. The mechanism of GI bleeding is likely related to interference of the normal hemostatic process and conversion of otherwise subclinical bleeding into clinical bleeding.

The risk of major bleeding in patients taking vitamin K antagonists has been reported to have an OR of 3.2 (95% CI, 1.3–7.8) compared with no therapy.[48] The annualized rate of major bleeding with warfarin was estimated to be 3.43%.[49]

Warfarin versus novel oral anticoagulants
There have been newer anticoagulants introduced over the past 12 years, expanding the options for anticoagulation in the elderly. These anticoagulants include direct factor Xa inhibitors (apixaban, rivaroxaban, darexaban, edoxaban) and direct thrombin inhibitors (dabigatran). Many randomized trials compared the efficacy and safety of warfarin compared with direct oral anticoagulants (DOACs). The risk of fatal and major bleeding seems to be lower with DOACs than warfarin.[49,50] However, some novel oral anticoagulants NOACs have been suggested to confer a small increased risk of intracranial hemorrhage.[49] The risks of bleeding among various NOACs also seem to vary, with rivaroxaban showing the highest risk of bleeding complications, similar to or potentially higher than warfarin, whereas apixaban has been associated with lowest risk of any bleeding (RR, 0.73) and major bleeding (RR, 0.60).[51–55] Therefore, apixaban is recommended in patients at increased risk of bleeding.

Table 2
Consideration of cotherapy in reduction of gastrointestinal bleeding risk in patients on dual antiplatelet therapy

Risk Factors[a]	Consider
Prior history of GI bleeding Advanced age (age not specified) Concomitant anticoagulation Concomitant steroids or NSAIDs	Proton pump inhibitor daily

[a] ACC/AHA 2016 guidelines.

PREENDOSCOPIC MANAGEMENT OF ANTICOAGULATION (URGENT VS ELECTIVE ENDOSCOPY)

When planning an endoscopic procedure in patients on antithrombotics, the urgency or elective nature of the procedure should be balanced with (1) bleeding risk of the procedure, (2) the patient's thromboembolic risk, and (3) indication and duration of antithrombotic. In patients with urgent need for endoscopy (ie, clinically significant bleeding), several guidelines have provided recommendations on reversal agents to optimize bleeding risks. Note that NOACs depend on renal excretion and, therefore, timing for perioperative medication adjustment depends on creatinine clearance.

Several guidelines have slight variations in the perioperative management of antithrombotics. In cases of urgent or emergent endoscopic procedures in patients on chronic warfarin therapy, American Society for Gastrointestinal Endoscopy (ASGE) and AHA/ACC recommend 4-factor prothrombin complex concentrate (4F-PCC), which contains the human coagulation factors II, VII, IX, and X together with the endogenous inhibitor proteins S and C, and vitamin K or fresh frozen plasma for life-threatening GI bleeding, whereas American College of Chest Physicians (ACCP) only advocates 4F-PCC and vitamin K. International Normalized Ratio (INR) less than 2.5 is considered an acceptable threshold for endoscopic therapy and endoscopy should not be delayed. Unfractionated heparin can be used in patients with subtherapeutic INR at high risk of thromboembolic events.[56]

In elective procedures, patients who had recent acute coronary syndrome or recent placement of intracoronary stent should have their procedures deferred until minimum duration of antithrombotic therapy has been reached. Low-dose aspirin can be safely continued throughout the periendoscopic period. In patients at low risk of thromboembolic events, thienopyridines can be continued through low-risk endoscopic procedures, but discontinued for 5 to 7 days or switched to aspirin monotherapy before high-risk endoscopic procedures.[56]

Resumption of antithrombotics should depend on ability to achieve hemostasis during endoscopic therapy. Note that risk of cardiovascular event may increase after 1 to 2 weeks on discontinuation of aspirin indicated for secondary prevention, and therefore should be resumed within 7 days when hemostasis is achieved.[27,57] When hemostasis is achieved without significant risk of delayed bleeding or need for repeat intervention, warfarin can generally be safely resumed the same day given that the therapeutic level is not achieved for several days. Clopidogrel and NOACs can generally be safely restarted within 48 hours.[58]

In addition, risks of bleeding from antithrombotic and antiplatelet treatment should be continuously assessed and balanced with risks of thromboembolic events, especially in the geriatric population.

SUMMARY

Adverse events related to NSAIDs and anticoagulant-associated GI bleeding is of concern in elderly patients on these medications. Awareness of these risks and appropriate use of NSAIDs, particularly in patients needing antiplatelet or anticoagulant therapy, is critical to optimal management. Judicious use of proton pump inhibitor prophylaxis should be considered in chronic users, particularly those a higher risk for ulcer or GI bleeding. Management of antiplatelet/anticoagulants in patients needing diagnostic or therapeutic endoscopic procedures is in the purview of the geriatrician in conjunction with appropriate specialists. Complications of these excellent medications can be avoided (or treated) in the elderly.

CLINICS CARE POINTS

- Cotherapy with a proton pump inhibitor should be recommended in patients at risk for NSAID complications.
- Apixiban has the lowest risk for GI bleeding amongst the novel oral anticoagulants.
- Consider selective Cox2 inhibitors in patients at high risk for bleeding if the patient is not already on aspirin.
- NSAIDs can cause clinically important ulceration anyway in the GI tract though gastric ulceration is most common.

DISCLOSURE

Dr Katz is a Consultant for Phathom Pharma.

REFERENCES

1. Lenti M. Mortality rate and risk factors for gastrointestinal bleeding in elderly patients. Eur J Intern Med 2019;61:54–6155.
2. Yachimski P. Gastrointestinal bleeding in the elderly. Nat Clin Pract Gastroenterol Hepatol 2008;5:80–93.
3. Chait M. Lower gastrointestinal bleeding in the elderly. World J Gastrointest Endosc 2010;2(5):147–54.
4. Akhtar A. Lower gastrointestinal bleeding in elderly patients. J Am Med Dir Assoc 2003;4(6):320–32.
5. Charatcharoenwitthaya P. Characteristics and outcomes of acute upper gastrointestinal bleeding after therapeutic endoscopy in the elderly. World J Gastroenterol 2011;17(32):3724–32.
6. Sung JJ. Causes of mortality in patients with peptic ulcer bleeding: a prospective cohort study of 10,428 cases. Am J Gastroenterol 2010;105(1):84–9.
7. Leontiadis GI. Effect of comorbidity on mortality in patients with peptic ulcer bleeding: systematic review and meta-analysis. Am J Gastroenterol 2013;108(3):331–45.
8. Pilotto A, Franceschi M, Leandro G, et al. NSAID and aspirin use by the elderly in general practice: effect on gastrointestinal symptoms and therapies. Drugs Aging 2003;20(9):701–10.
9. Laine L. Approaches to nonsteroidal anti-inflammatory drug use in the high-risk patient. Gastroenterology 2001;120(3):594–606.
10. Scheiman JM. NSAID-induced gastrointestinal injury: a focused update for clinicians. J Clin Gastroenterol 2016;50(1):5–10.
11. Wang D. The role of prostaglandins and other eicosanoids in the gastrointestinal tract. Gastroenterology 2005;128:1445–61.
12. Pilotto A, Franceschi M, Leandro G, et al. The risk of upper gastrointestinal bleeding in elderly users of aspirin and other non-steroidal anti-inflammatory drugs: the role of gastroprotective drugs. Aging Clin Exp Res 2003;15(6):494–9.
13. Stalnikowicz R. NSAID-induced gastroduodenal damage: is prevention needed? A review and metaanalysis. J Clin Gastroenterol 1993;17(3):238–43.
14. Higuchi K. Present status and strategy of NSAIDs-induced small bowel injury. J Gastroenterol 2009;44(9):879–88.
15. Maiden L. A quantitative analysis of NSAID-induced small bowel pathology by capsule enteroscopy. Gastroenterology 2005;128(5):1172–8.

16. Allison MC, Howatson AG, Torrance CJ, et al. Gastrointestinal damage associated with the use of nonsteroidal antiinflammatory drugs. N Engl J Med 1992; 327:749–54.

17. Maiden L. Long-term effects of nonsteroidal anti-inflammatory drugs and cyclooxygenase-2 selective agents on the small bowel: a cross-sectional capsule enteroscopy study. Clin Gastroenterol Hepatol 2007;5(9):1040–5.

18. Dumic I. Gastrointestinal tract disorders in older age. Can J Gastroenterol Hepatol 2019;2019:6757524.

19. Gabriel SE. Risk for serious gastrointestinal complications related to use of nonsteroidal anti-inflammatory drugs. A meta-analysis. Ann Intern Med 1991; 115(10):787–96.

20. Abraham NS, Hlatky MA, Antman EM, et al. ACCF/ACG/AHA 2010 expert consensus document on the concomitant use of proton pump inhibitors and thienopyridines: a focused update of the ACCF/ACG/AHA 2008 expert consensus document on reducing the gastrointestinal risks of antiplatelet therapy and NSAID use. Am J Gastroenterol 2010;105(12):2533–49.

21. Piper JM. Corticosteroid use and peptic ulcer disease: role of nonsteroidal anti-inflammatory drugs. Ann Intern Med 1991;114(9):735–40.

22. McQuaid KR. Systematic review and meta-analysis of adverse events of low-dose aspirin and clopidogrel in randomized controlled trials. Am J Med 2006; 119(8):624–38.

23. Kawasaki K. Low-dose aspirin and non-steroidal anti-inflammatory drugs increase the risk of bleeding in patients with gastroduodenal ulcer. Dig Dis Sci 2015;60(4):1010–5.

24. Lanas A. Risk of upper and lower gastrointestinal bleeding in patients taking nonsteroidal anti-inflammatory drugs, antiplatelet agents, or anticoagulants. Clin Gastroenterol Hepatol 2015;13(5):906–12.e2.

25. Huang J. Role of Helicobacter pylori infection and non-steroidal anti-inflammatory drugs in peptic-ulcer disease: a meta-analysis. Lancet 2002;359(9300):14–22.

26. Laursen SB, Dalton HR, Murray IA, et al. Performance of new thresholds of the Glasgow Blatchford score in managing patients with upper gastrointestinal bleeding. Clin Gastroenterol Hepatol 2015;13(1):115–21.e2.

27. Laine L. Clinical practice. Upper gastrointestinal bleeding due to a peptic ulcer. N Engl J Med 2016;374:2367–76.

28. Sreedharan A, Martin J, Leontiadis GI, et al. Proton pump inhibitor treatment initiated prior to endoscopic diagnosis in upper gastrointestinal bleeding. Cochrane Database Syst Rev 2010;(7):CD005415.

29. Hwang JH, Fisher DA, Ben-Menachem T, et al. The role of endoscopy in the management of acute non-variceal upper GI bleeding. Gastrointest Endosc 2012;75: 1132.

30. Kumar NL, Cohen AJ, Nayor J, et al. Timing of upper endoscopy influences outcomes in patients with acute nonvariceal upper GI bleeding. Gastrointest Endosc 2017;85:945.

31. Cho SH, Lee YS, Kim YJ, et al. Outcomes and role of urgent endoscopy in high-risk patients with acute nonvariceal gastrointestinal bleeding. Clin Gastroenterol Hepatol 2018;16:370.

32. Lau JY, Sung JJ, Lam YH, et al. Endoscopic retreatment compared with surgery in patients with recurrent bleeding after initial endoscopic control of bleeding ulcers. N Engl J Med 1999;340:751–6.

33. Bour B, Pariente E, Hamelin B, et al. Orally administered omeprazole versus injection therapy in the prevention of rebleeding from peptic ulcer with visible vessel. A multicenter randomized study. Gastroenterol Clin Biol 1993;17:329–33.

34. Laine L, McQuaid KR. Endoscopic therapy for bleeding ulcers: an evidence based approach based on meta-analyses of randomized controlled trials. Clin Gastroenterol Hepatol 2009;7:33–47.

35. Sachar H, Vaidya K, Laine L. Intermittent vs continuous proton pump inhibitor therapy for high-risk bleeding ulcers: a systematic review and meta-analysis. JAMA Intern Med 2014;174:1755–62.

36. Taha AS, McCloskey C, McSkimming P, et al. Misoprostol for small bowel ulcers in patients with obscure bleeding taking aspirin and non-steroidal anti-inflammatory drugs (MASTERS): a randomised, double-blind, placebo-controlled, phase 3 trial. Lancet Gastroenterol Hepatol 2018;3(7):469–76.

37. Kyaw MH, Otani K, Ching JYL, et al. Misoprostol heals small bowel ulcers in aspirin users with small bowel bleeding. Gastroenterology 2018;155(4): 1090–7.e1.

38. Kroner PT, Brahmbhatt BS, Bartel MJ, et al. Yield of double-balloon enteroscopy in the diagnosis and treatment of small bowel strictures. Dig Liver Dis 2016;48(4): 446–8.

39. Møller MH, Adamsen S, Thomsen RW, et al. Multicentre trial of a perioperative protocol to reduce mortality in patients with peptic ulcer perforation. Br J Surg 2011;98(6):802–10.

40. Søreide K, Thorsen K, Harrison EM, et al. Perforated peptic ulcer. Lancet 2015; 386(10000):1288–98.

41. Ishikawa S, Inaba T, Mizuno M, et al. Characteristics of serious complicated gastroduodenal ulcers in Japan. Hepatogastroenterology 2012;59(113):147–54.

42. Chang SS, Hu HY. Helicobacter pylori eradication within 120 days is associated with decreased complicated recurrent peptic ulcers in peptic ulcer bleeding patients. Gut Liver 2015;9(3):346–52.

43. Scally B, Emberson JR, Spata E, et al. Effects of gastroprotectant drugs for the prevention and treatment of peptic ulcer disease and its complications: a meta-analysis of randomised trials. Lancet Gastroenterol Hepatol 2018;3(4): 231–41.

44. Levine GN, Bates ER, Bittl JA, et al. 2016 ACC/AHA guideline focused update on duration of dual antiplatelet therapy in patients with coronary artery disease: a report of the American College of Cardiology/American Heart Association task force on clinical practice guidelines: an update of the 2011 ACCF/AHA/SCAI guideline for percutaneous coronary intervention, 2011 ACCF/AHA guideline for coronary artery bypass graft surgery, 2012 ACC/AHA/ACP/AATS/PCNA/SCAI/ STS guideline for the diagnosis and management of patients with stable ischemic heart disease, 2013 ACCF/AHA guideline for the management of ST-elevation myocardial infarction, 2014 AHA/ACC guideline for the management of patients with non-ST-Elevation acute coronary syndromes, and 2014 ACC/AHA guideline on perioperative cardiovascular evaluation and management of patients undergoing noncardiac surgery. Circulation 2016;134(10):e123–55.

45. Nørgård B, Pedersen L, Johnsen SP, et al. COX-2-selective inhibitors and the risk of upper gastrointestinal bleeding in high-risk patients with previous gastrointestinal diseases: a population-based case-control study. Aliment Pharmacol Ther 2004;19(7):817–25.

46. Goldstein JL, Correa P, Zhao WW, et al. Reduced incidence of gastroduodenal ulcers with celecoxib, a novel cyclooxygenase-2 inhibitor, compared to naproxen in patients with arthritis. Am J Gastroenterol 2001;96(4):1019–27.

47. Goldstein JL, Aisenberg J, Lanza F, et al. A multicenter, randomized, double-blind, active-comparator, placebo-controlled, parallel-group comparison of the incidence of endoscopic gastric and duodenal ulcer rates with valdecoxib or naproxen in healthy subjects aged 65 to 75 years. Clin Ther 2006;28(3):340–51.

48. Coleman CL, Sobieraj DM, Winkler S, et al. Effect of pharmacological therapies for stroke prevention on major gastrointestinal bleeding in patients with atrial fibrillation. Int J Clin Pract 2012;66(1):53–63.

49. Giugliano RP, Ruff CT, Braunwald E, et al. Edoxaban versus warfarin in patients with atrial fibrillation. N Engl J Med 2013;369(22):2093–104.

50. Cangemi DJ, Krill T, Weideman R, et al. A comparison of the rate of gastrointestinal bleeding in patients taking non-vitamin K antagonist oral anticoagulants or warfarin. Am J Gastroenterol 2017;112(5):734–9.

51. Goodman SG, Wojdyla DM, Piccini JP, et al. Factors associated with major bleeding events: insights from the ROCKET AF trial (rivaroxaban once-daily oral direct factor Xa inhibition compared with vitamin K antagonism for prevention of stroke and embolism trial in atrial fibrillation). J Am Coll Cardiol 2014;63(9):891–900.

52. Halperin JL, Hankey GJ, Wojdyla DM, et al. Efficacy and safety of rivaroxaban compared with warfarin among elderly patients with nonvalvular atrial fibrillation in the rivaroxaban once daily, oral, direct factor Xa inhibition compared with Vitamin K Antagonism for Prevention of Stroke and Embolism Trial in Atrial Fibrillation (ROCKET AF). Circulation 2014;130(2):138–46.

53. Touma L, Filion KB, Atallah R, et al. A meta-analysis of randomized controlled trials of the risk of bleeding with apixaban versus vitamin K antagonists. Am J Cardiol 2015;115(4):533–41.

54. Hernandez I, Zhang Y, Saba S. Comparison of the effectiveness and safety of apixaban, dabigatran, rivaroxaban, and warfarin in newly diagnosed atrial fibrillation. Am J Cardiol 2017;120(10):1813–9.

55. Ruff CT, Giugliano RP, Braunwald E, et al. Comparison of the efficacy and safety of new oral anticoagulants with warfarin in patients with atrial fibrillation: a meta-analysis of randomised trials. Lancet 2014;383(9921):955–62.

56. ASGE Standards of Practice Committee, Acosta RD, Abraham NS, et al. The management of antithrombotic agents for patients undergoing GI endoscopy. Gastrointest Endosc 2016;83(1):3–16.

57. Gralnek IM, Dumonceau JM, Kuipers EJ, et al. Diagnosis and management of nonvariceal upper gastrointestinal hemorrhage: European Society of Gastrointestinal Endoscopy (ESGE) Guideline. Endoscopy 2015;47(10):a1–46.

58. Baron TH, Kamath PS, McBane RD. Management of antithrombotic therapy in patients undergoing invasive procedures. N Engl J Med 2013;368:2113–24.

Managing Gallstone Disease in the Elderly

Ankit Chhoda, MD[a], Saurabh S. Mukewar, MD[b], SriHari Mahadev, MD, MS[b],*

KEYWORDS

- Gallstone disease • Cholecystitis • Choledocholithiasis • Elderly
- Geriatric population

KEY POINTS

- Geriatric patients tend to have subtle presentations of biliary disorders and, if untreated, can decompensate acutely.
- Acute cholecystitis, a common complication of gallstones, is treated by conservative measures and cholecystectomy, laparoscopic or open, among patients with optimal surgical risk. High-risk patients undergo temporizing interventions, percutaneous or endoscopic, enabling definitive therapy. Acute cholecystitis with complications, including perforations, gangrene, and small bowel obstruction, warrants emergent cholecystectomy.
- Migration of gallstones into the biliary system can cause choledocholithiasis, which commonly results in complications, including biliary pancreatitis or cholangitis if not intervened. Therapy for common bile duct calculi is based on biliary clearance through endoscopic and, less commonly, surgical approaches.

INTRODUCTION

Gallstone disease is widely prevalent among the United States population and has been estimated to affect about 20 million people.[1] It is a leading cause of inpatient hospitalization in the United States and costs more than $6 billion annually.[2,3] Among the elderly population, the overall prevalence of gallstone disease ranges from 14% to 23% and can approach up to 80% for individuals more than 90 years old.[4] Advanced age has been considered an independent risk factor for incidence of gallstones. The prolongation of life expectancy is expected to alter patient demographics, causing more individuals with advanced age and, subsequently, an incremental increase in gallstone burden.

[a] Department of Internal Medicine, Bridgeport Hospital, Yale New Haven Hospital System, 267 Grant Street Bridgeport, CT, USA; [b] Advanced Endoscopy, Division of Gastroenterology & Hepatology, Weill Cornell Medicine, 1283 York Avenue, 9th Floor, New York, NY 10065, USA
* Corresponding author.
E-mail address: srm9005@med.cornell.edu

Clin Geriatr Med 37 (2021) 43–69
https://doi.org/10.1016/j.cger.2020.08.005
geriatric.theclinics.com

With progression of age, the biliary tract undergoes anatomic and physiologic changes[5–8] (**Fig. 1**). Geriatric patients tend to have subtle presentation of biliary disorders and can decompensate acutely if untreated.[9] They have higher rates of complications and slower recovery because of delayed healing, comorbidities, and weaker immune systems. The management of gallstones must incorporate therapeutic goals ranging from improvement of quality of life and maintenance of independence to absolute cure.[10] This article reviews the management of gallstone disease involving both the gallbladder and associated ductal system among the elderly.

ASYMPTOMATIC CHOLELITHIASIS

Gallstones are asymptomatic in most individuals and incidentally diagnosed through imaging. A recent study by Shabanzadeh and colleagues[11] included 664 patients with gallstones with a median age of 60 years, among whom 19.6% of participants developed gallstone-related events (8.0% complicated and 11.6% uncomplicated). The study showed a negative association between age and gallstone-related events. Similar trends have been observed in prior cohort studies.[12,13]

Management

Prophylactic surgery
No prospective trial has been performed to establish the efficacy of surgical or medical therapy among asymptomatic gallstone carriers. In a decision-analysis study, prophylactic surgery had a negative survival impact.[14] Its role is limited to individuals with primary risk factors of gallbladder cancer.[15]

Expectant management
Although consensus is lacking, observation and annual follow-up of asymptomatic gallstones have been suggested by some guidelines.[16]

Medical therapy
Gallstones with smaller sizes (<10 mm) and lower calcium concentrations (radiolucent stones) are amenable to therapy by ursodeoxycholic acid. They act by inhibiting

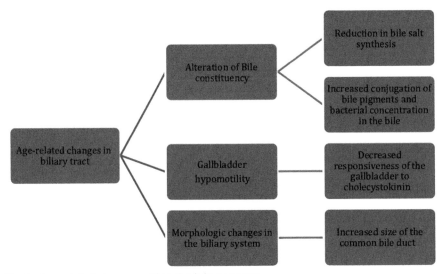

Fig. 1. Age-related changes within the biliary system.

intestinal cholesterol absorption and subsequent fragmentation and expulsion of stones and can be used for primary prophylaxis for gallstones.[17,18]

BILIARY COLIC

Gallbladder contraction against the cystic duct opening may cause right upper quadrant or epigastric pain of variable severity, associated with postprandial exacerbations and nocturnal variations.[19–21] Elderly patients may present with altered mental status, falls, or incontinence.[22]

Among symptomatic patients, gallstones are commonly diagnosed through ultrasonography (US) and appear as acoustic shadows (**Fig. 2**A, B). Biliary sludge observed on US may indicate microlithiasis and has resulted in complications warranting cholecystectomy.[23] Despite omission of small stones or sludge, US has a diagnostic sensitivity and specificity of 84% (95% confidence interval [CI], 0.76–0.92) and 99% (95% CI, 0.97–1.00) respectively.[24]

Treatment

Elective cholecystectomy
Natural history studies have shown occurrence of complications among untreated symptomatic gallstones.[25] Elderly patients with symptomatic gallstones must be considered for an elective cholecystectomy based on their surgical risk. A minimally invasive approach is preferred except in patients with gallbladder architectural distortion or associated gallbladder cancer risks.[26] Postponing cholecystectomy may cause accumulation of comorbidities with age and a higher surgical risk. Furthermore, late presentations and complications may warrant emergent cholecystectomy, which is associated with worse outcomes and has associated mortality of 6% to 15%.[27,28]

Medical resolution therapy
Reduction in biliary pain and risk of cholecystitis have been shown among patients with biliary colic with medical therapy, including bile acid therapy and extracorporeal shock wave lithotripsy.[29] A meta-analysis showed a 37% dissolution rate among individuals with gallstones.[30] However, medical therapy should be reserved for patients who refuse or are unfit for surgery.

ACUTE CHOLECYSTITIS

Acute cholecystitis refers to acute inflammation of the gallbladder, which in most cases results from gallstones, except among 5% to 10% of patients with acalculous

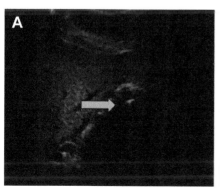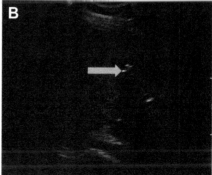

Fig. 2. (*A*) Sagittal and (*B*) axial views of a stone in 75-year-old woman with biliary colic. The arrow points to the stone.

cholecystitis. Acute calculous cholecystitis results from cystic duct obstruction and increased intraluminal pressure and congestion. In addition, lysolecithin, an enzyme arising from mucosal irritation by gallstones, causes gallbladder inflammation.[31,32] Superimposed infections may also contribute, as shown among patients with gallstones with positive cultures found in 22% to 46% of bile samples from the gallbladder and common bile duct (CBD).[33]

Clinical Presentation

Patients with acute cholecystitis generally present with right upper quadrant or epigastric pain. Proximity to the parietal peritoneum may cause local inflammation, guarding, and a positive Murphy sign. However, among the geriatric population, the symptoms are atypical and physical signs may be masked by neuropathy. The Murphy sign has a lower sensitivity of 48% among the elderly, compared with 65% among the general population.[34,35]

Diagnostic Approach

Laboratory findings

Typical leukocytosis and bandemia may be obscured among the elderly; thus, a higher index of clinical suspicion is imperative. Marked increases in bilirubin level and liver chemistry are seldom observed and often indicate complications such as cholangitis, choledocholithiasis, or Mirizzi syndrome (an extrinsic compression of CBD by the neck of the gallbladder).

Imaging modality

1. US is the most common imaging modality for the diagnosis of acute cholecystitis. A systematic review suggested the adjusted sensitivity and specificity for sonographic diagnosis of acute cholecystitis to be 88% and 80% respectively. The features on US that support acute cholecystitis include gallbladder wall thickening, pericholecystic fluid, and sonographic Murphy sign.[24]
2. Cross-sectional imaging is rarely used for diagnosis of acute cholecystitis, except for detection of its complications or ruling out alternate differentials (**Fig. 3**A–C).
3. Cholescintigraphy (99mTc-heaptoiminodiacetic acid [HIDA] scanning) is used for diagnosis of acute cholecystitis among individuals with negative US results. A large study compared HIDA scan with abdominal US among patients with acute cholecystitis and revealed significantly higher sensitivity (90.7% vs 64.0%, $P<.001$) and specificity (71.4% vs 58.4%, $P = .005$).[36]

Complications

Gangrenous cholecystitis

Gangrenous cholecystitis (GC) is the most common complication of acute cholecystitis. Prevalent in around 20% of patients with acute cholecystitis, GC results from transmural inflammation and gallbladder ischemia. It occurs particularly among individuals with a prolonged course and those with vasculopathy.[37] Radiologically, GC is diagnosed through computed tomography (CT) findings of the gallbladder and is associated with gallbladder distention greater than 4.0 cm, mural striations, and decreased mural enhancement. GC warrants urgent cholecystectomy and is associated with higher rates of conversion from laparoscopic to open cholecystectomy. A cohort study showed significantly higher mortality (1%–2% vs 0.8%) and complication rates (10.8% vs 8.0%) among individuals with GC (n = 7017) compared with the entire cohort (n = 141,970).[38]

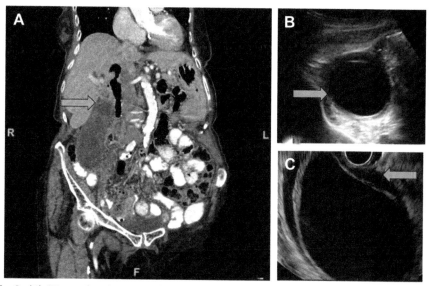

Fig. 3. (*A*) CT scan showing acute cholecystitis (*arrows*) in a 102-year-old woman. (*B*) US and (*C*) endoscopic US (EUS) visualization of acute cholecystitis including pericholecystic fluid.

Gallbladder perforation

Ongoing gallbladder inflammation from delayed diagnosis or failed therapy may result in gallbladder perforation. Gallbladder perforation is classified into 4 types based on the Niemeier classification and its modification: type 1, free perforation; type 2, perforation with abscess; type 3, chronic perforation with cholecystoenteric fistula; or type 4, perforation into biliary tree resulting in formation of cholecystobiliary fistulae.[39,40]

Emphysematous cholecystitis

Emphysematous cholecystitis (EC), a fulminant complication of acute cholecystitis, is characterized by accumulation of gas within the gallbladder wall or lumen or its biliary duct extension. It is caused by secondary infection by gas-forming organisms such as *Clostridium welchii*. EC commonly occurs in the setting of gallbladder ischemia, and among individuals with advanced age, diabetes, or nephropathy. On US, detection of air within the gallbladder wall has high specificity but may obscure visualization of the gallbladder. CT imaging is accurate in the diagnosis of gas within the gallbladder wall and surrounding structures and enables gradation based on the extent of spread. EC is managed by emergent cholecystectomy. Open cholecystectomy is preferred for patients with peritoneal involvement.

Cholecystoenteric fistula

Cholecystoenteric fistula occurs because of pressure necrosis from long-standing gallbladder stones and perforation of the gallbladder wall into the intestinal lumen. Cholecystoenteric fistula presents as bilious diarrhea or, rarely, may result in gallstone ileus.

Gallstone ileus

Gallstone ileus is defined as small bowel obstruction caused by impacted gallstones, which are generally 2 to 2.5 cm in size. Gallstone ileus is commonly found among frail elderly individuals (average age of incidence, 74 years) and is found in up to 25% of elderly individuals with small bowel obstruction.[41,42] It is classically associated with the Rigler triad: pneumobilia, small bowel obstruction, and ectopic radio-opaque gall-stones, which is incident in about 15% of the cases.[43] CT scan of the abdomen has variable sensitivity in diagnosing gallstones but has high diagnostic sensitivity for bowel obstruction.[44] Besides management for obstruction, gallstone ileus is treated surgically by enterolithotomy, with or without cholecystectomy.[42,45]

Treatment of Acute Cholecystitis

Supportive care

Patients with acute calculous cholecystitis require inpatient care with supportive measures such as intravenous hydration and analgesia through nonsteroidal antiinflammatory drugs (NSAIDs). Opioids increase sphincter of Oddi pressure and are used when NSAIDs have inadequate response or are contraindicated.[46] Antibiotics are indicated for acute cholecystitis with complications or among frail and immunocompromised individuals.[47] They prevent septic complications before surgery and can be discontinued 24 hours after gallbladder removal or clinical resolution.

Risk stratification

Patients with acute cholecystitis warrant definitive therapy. Although cholecystectomy is the gold standard, patients must undergo risk stratification to determine the choice of therapy. The following systems facilitate guidance for surgical candidacy of patients with acute cholecystitis:

- Tokyo Guidelines 2018: grade I to III cholecystitis.[48]
- American Association of Surgery of Trauma (AAST) System: grade I to V cholecystitis.[49]
- Parkland Grading Scale for Cholecystitis: based on the intraoperative appearance of the gallbladder.[50]
- American Society of Anesthesiologists (ASA): patients with low-risk (ASA I/II) or high-risk (ASA III–V) cholecystitis.

Cholecystectomy

Cholecystectomy is the preferred procedure for patients with acute cholecystitis with low surgical risk.[51]

Methods of surgery

- Laparoscopic cholecystectomy: this approach has become the standard modality for surgical resection among elderly patients with mild to moderate acute cholecystitis.[52] It has better perioperative survival and fewer complications, including wound infections and pneumonia.[53] However, patients with acute cholecystitis have higher technical requirements because of acute inflammation, causing adhesions and altered anatomy.

    Acute cholecystitis may also cause so-called difficult gallbladder, a term for cholecystectomy procedures with increased procedural risk from bleeding (eg, liver cirrhosis) or anatomic distortion.[54] Difficult dissection should prompt surgeons to choose a fundus-first approach, subtotal cholecystectomy, or conversion into open cholecystectomy.[55,56]
- Open cholecystectomy: although associated with higher local complications, an open approach enables more vascular and duct control. It must be attempted for patients with porcelain gallbladder and contraindications to pneumoperitoneum.
- Natural orifice transluminal endoscopic surgery (NOTES): this procedure has a limited role in acute cholecystitis because of altered surgical anatomy and higher dissection requirements. The procedure involves gallbladder access through

natural orifices, including transvaginal or transgastric approach. It has been attempted in limited medical centers and promises faster recovery and better cosmetic outcomes.[57,58]

Timing of surgery

Current evidence favors early cholecystectomy (0–3 days) rather than delayed cholecystectomy among surgically fit individuals.[59,60] A recent meta-analysis of studies of early cholecystectomy among the geriatric population reports perioperative morbidity of 24% and mortality of 3.5%.[61]

Safety

1. Morbidity and mortality: elderly individuals tend to have higher ASA grades and comorbidity burden (assessed through the Charlson Comorbidity Index). In a recent systematic review, a significantly higher morbidity rate was observed among the geriatric population compared with younger individuals. No significant difference in intraoperative complications was observed; however, lower conversion rates were observed among younger individuals (relative risk, 0.96; 0.94–0.98).[62]
2. Biliary and vascular injury: higher rates of biliary injury were noted among elderly patients undergoing gallbladder surgery. In a cross-sectional analysis based on the National Inpatient Survey, the rate of bile duct injury among individuals aged less than 50 years was 0.10%, 60 to 79 years was 0.13%, and greater than or equal to 80 years was 0.14% ($P<.003$).[63] Laparoscopic cholecystectomy is associated with higher rates of bile duct injury compared with open cholecystectomy.[64,65] During surgical procedures, a critical view of safety should be performed in order to prevent biliary and vascular injury during cholecystectomy.[66,67]

Emergency cholecystectomy

In addition to supportive measures, emergent cholecystectomy is indicated for acute cholecystitis with complications. It is also indicated in patients with acute cholecystitis with hemodynamic instability and sepsis.

Percutaneous cholecystostomy

Patients with acute cholecystitis with increased surgical risk who are septic or critically ill, and those lacking clinical response to antibiotics with greater than 72 hours of symptom onset, warrant gallbladder drainage through percutaneous cholecystostomy.[68,69] The procedure can be performed through transperitoneal or transhepatic routes and has a technical success rate of around 85%.[70] Although transhepatic approach is preferred because of its better safety profile, it is challenging among individuals with cirrhosis. It is contraindicated among individuals with coagulopathy and can be complicated by vascular injury, biliary leak, peritonitis, and catheter dislodgement.[71] High-quality evidence supporting its use as a definitive drainage procedure is lacking. Recent evidence shows higher complication rates, disease recurrence, reintervention, and median hospital stay among individuals undergoing percutaneous interventions.[72,73]

Endoscopic gallbladder drainage

Endoscopic techniques can be used as a bridge to surgery or destination therapy among high-risk patients, especially those with coagulopathy and suboptimal anatomy, including inaccessible gallbladder, ascites, and advanced cirrhosis.[74] Endoscopic gallbladder drainage is attempted through transpapillary or transmural approaches.

- Endoscopic transpapillary gallbladder drainage involves passage of a drainage catheter through the cystic duct under fluoroscopic guidance to access the gallbladder. The other end of the catheter is passed through the nose or drains into the duodenum. This technique is limited by tortuosity of the cystic duct and dependence on fluoroscopic visualization. Its pooled technical success rate has been estimated to be 80% to 91%.[75,76]
- Endoscopic US (EUS)–guided transmural gallbladder drainage (GBD) enables access to the gallbladder through the transgastric or transduodenal passage of a needle and placement of either a drain or stent. Self-expanding stents have now been replaced by lumen-apposing metallic stents (LAMSs) (**Fig. 4A–F**). They provide reliable anchorage because of double-walled flanges perpendicular to the lumen and have lesser complications. The technical success of EUS-GBD via LAMS has been observed to be as high as 95.2%.[77] Compared with percutaneous interventions, EUS-GBD showed fewer adverse events (odds ratio [OR], 0.43; 95% CI, 0.18–1.00), shorter hospitalizations (2.53 days; 95% CI, −4.28 to −0.78), and fewer reinterventions (OR, 0.16; 95% CI, 0.04–0.042) and readmissions (OR, 0.16; 95% CI, 0.05–0.53).[78] Significantly better clinical success and safety have been observed in EUS-guided drainage vis-à-vis transpapillary drainage.[79]

Post–gallbladder drainage care

Clinical resolution after a percutaneous or endoscopic procedure warrants risk stratification. Low-risk patients can be considered for elective cholecystectomy.[80,81] Individuals with high surgical risk have the following options:

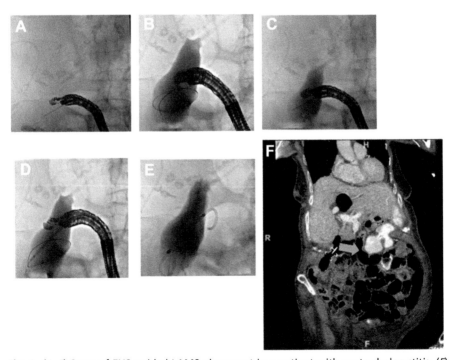

Fig. 4. (*A–E*) Steps of EUS-guided LAMS placement in a patient with acute cholecystitis. (*F*) CT image of a patient after LAMS placement. *Arrow* denotes GB Drainage through LAMS.

- Clinical decompensation at any time warrants emergent cholecystectomy.
- Expectant management and interval cholecystectomy: one of the approaches for patients with high surgical risk is to follow them and attempt cholecystectomy only among those with recurrent acute cholecystitis.[82]
- Percutaneous stone extraction: after maturation of cholecystostomy tract (2–3 weeks after percutaneous drainage), dilation through graded dilators under fluoroscopic guidance and stone extraction is performed.[83,84]
- Extracorporeal lithotripsy: this procedure involves passage of shockwaves and enables breaking the stones in the gallbladder and their passage through biliary system.
- Endoscopic gallstone extraction: endoscopic removal of gallstones has been successfully shown through the use of LAMSs.[85]

CHRONIC CHOLECYSTITIS

Long-standing gallstones or prior episodes of acute cholecystitis may cause indolent gallbladder inflammation, also called chronic cholecystitis. On histology, gallbladder wall thickening, serosal adhesions, smooth muscle hypertrophy, and pathognomonic Rokitansky-Aschoff sinuses are observed.[86] The chronic inflammation may cause gallbladder calcification and porcelain gallbladder, the mechanism of which is unclear.[87]

Clinical Presentation

These patients generally present with insidious biliary colic, which may progress over the chronic course. Older individuals may have an uncomfortable feeling or loss of appetite prompting clinical evaluation.

Diagnosis

US is a noninvasive diagnostic modality that may reveal a thickened gallbladder wall or shrunken fibrotic gallbladder with gallstones. HIDA scan can also be used for confirmation of the diagnosis.

Treatment

Conservative therapy
For biliary colic, NSAIDs are preferred as analgesics. Antibiotics should be started in patients who have evidence of sepsis.

Definitive therapy
Cholecystectomy is considered when the acute symptoms have subsided. Chronic cholecystitis can be treated by cholecystectomy, through a laparoscopic or open approach. Laparoscopic cholecystectomy has lower complication rates and faster recovery. An open approach should be used on suspicion of gallbladder cancer.[88] Altered surgical anatomy caused by prior surgeries or adhesions also supports open methods.[89]

Expectant management
Patients with high surgical risk may also be managed conservatively through dietary restriction and medical resolution therapy.

CHOLEDOCHOLITHIASIS

Choledocholithiasis refers to the presence of gallstones in the CBD. Although associated with up to 5% to 20% of patients with gallstones, the exact incidence and prevalence of choledocholithiasis is unknown.[90] Among the elderly, most calculi originate from the gallbladder and migrate into the CBD.[91] Alternatively, primary choledocholithiasis may result from long-standing biliary stasis associated with conditions including CBD dilatation and periampullary diverticulum (PAD).[92]

Asymptomatic Choledocholithiasis

Asymptomatic choledocholithiasis is diagnosed in up to half of patients with choledocholithiasis through abnormal laboratory values, radiologic findings, or intraoperative cholangiography (IOC) during cholecystectomy.[93]

Risk of progression

Because of the paucity of studies investigating the natural history of asymptomatic choledocholithiasis, the risk of progression to symptomatic and complicated CBD stones remains elusive. A study of patients undergoing laparoscopic cholecystectomy with IOC and delayed postoperative cholangiography revealed persistence of CBD calculi in only about 50% of individuals.[94–96]

In contrast, a study on Swedish Registry for Gallstone Surgery and Endoscopic Retrograde Cholangiopancreatography (GallRiks) reported unfavorable outcomes in 25.3% of the individuals with choledocholithiasis who did not undergo any intervention.[97] A significantly lower risk was observed among patients in whom any measures for biliary ductal clearance were taken (12.7%; OR, 0.44 [0.35–0.55]).

Symptomatic Choledocholithiasis

Patients with choledocholithiasis may be asymptomatic, have epigastric or right upper quadrant pain, or present with complications including cholangitis or biliary pancreatitis.

Complications of Choledocholithiasis

Acute cholangitis

Acute cholangitis results from CBD inflammation caused by biliary stasis and superimposed infection, most probably from gram-negative bacteria.[98,99] Presentation of cholangitis among the geriatric population is atypical and lacks correlation with severity.[100] The diagnostic criteria for cholangitis include evidence of systemic inflammation, cholestasis, and imaging (**Box 1**).[101]

The imaging modalities for evaluation of cholangitis include US and, if negative, CT scan for detection of biliary dilatation or evidence of underlying obstructive cause. In case of diagnostic dilemma, MRI/magnetic resonance cholangiopancreatography (MRCP) and EUS can also be used[102] (**Figs. 5**A, B and **6**).

Old age is an important risk factor for mortality among patients with acute cholangitis.[103] Among the elderly, acute cholangitis is associated with delayed medical care from masked presentation and significantly higher rates of hypotension, peritonism, renal failure.[104]

The assessment for severity is based on concomitant organ dysfunction, as described in **Box 2**.[101]

Acute biliary pancreatitis

Among the elderly, age-related biliary dilatation and incremental incidence of gallstones result in predominance of a biliary cause of acute pancreatitis. Age is an independent criterion for severity scoring systems of acute pancreatitis, including the Glasgow scoring system, Ranson scoring system, and Acute Physiology and Chronic Health Evaluation (APACHE II).[105–107] Among geriatric patients, higher comorbidity burden is associated with mortality from acute pancreatitis.[108] Acute biliary

---

Box 1
Diagnostic criteria for cholangitis

A. Systemic inflammation
   A1. Fever (>38°C) and/or shaking chills
   A2. Laboratory data. Evidence of inflammatory response: leukocytosis (<4000 or >10,000), increased C-reactive protein levels (≥1 mg/dL), and other changes indicating inflammation

B. Cholestasis
   B1. Jaundice (≥2 mg/dL)
   B2. Laboratory data: abnormal liver function tests (≥1.5 upper limit of normal)

C. Imaging:
   C1. Biliary dilatation
   C2. Evidence of the cause on imaging (eg, stricture, stone, stent)

Suspected diagnosis: 1 item in A plus 1 item in either B or C. Definite diagnosis: 1 item in A, 1 item in B, and 1 item in C.

---

pancreatitis (ABP) presents similarly to other causes of acute pancreatitis and is diagnosed by biochemical alteration of pancreatitis; namely, increased serum amylase/lipase level in the setting of gallstones.

Management of Choledocholithiasis

American Society for Gastrointestinal Endoscopy risk stratification
Risk stratification for choledocholithiasis has been proposed by the Practice Committee of the American Society for Gastrointestinal Endoscopy (ASGE).[109,110] The predictor for choledocholithiasis is based on biochemical and imaging parameters (summarized in **Box 3**).

Laboratory findings
Patients with choledocholithiasis tend to have a cholestatic pattern of liver tests. CBD dilatation and alteration of liver chemistry are moderate predictors in ASGE guidelines in preprocedural diagnosis of choledocholithiasis.[109,110] A meta-analysis of 22 studies revealed diagnostic sensitivity of 69% and a specificity of 88% for increased serum bilirubin level in the diagnosis of CBD stone.[111]

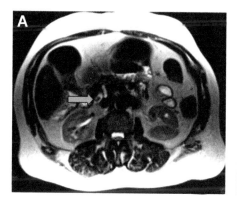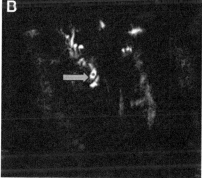

Fig. 5. CBD stone on (*A*) T2-MRI and (*B*) three-dimensional reconstruction images.

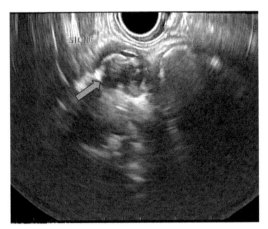

Fig. 6. CBD stone (*arrow*) on EUS.

Imaging

1. US: choledocholithiasis warrants initial work-up through transabdominal US. A meta-analysis investigated the diagnostic accuracy of liver enzymes and US for diagnosis of choledocholithiasis and showed pooled sensitivity of 73% (95% CI, 44%–95%) and specificity of 91% (95% CI, 84%–95%). Current ASGE guidelines include visualization of a stone or biliary duct dilatation on cross-sectional or sonographic imaging and total bilirubin level increase greater than4 mg/dL (strong predictors).[109,110] Although practice guidelines suggest 6 mm as a cutoff for choledocholithiasis, the CBD diameter varies with the patient's age.[112] A study by Bachar and colleagues[113] showed significantly greater CBD sizes among patients aged more than 50 years. This study revealed gradual ductal dilation of 0.04 mm/y and proposed an upper normal limit of 8.5 mm among the elderly. Nondilated CBD does not equate with no CBD stones, and each CBD dimension has an associated choledocholithiasis probability necessitating its application to overall clinical context.[114]

Box 2
Classification of severity of cholangitis

Grade III (severe) acute cholangitis: acute cholangitis in any of the following organs:
1. Cardiovascular: hypotension requiring dopamine greater than or equal to 5 μg/kg/min, or any dose of norepinephrine
2. Neurologic: altered consciousness
3. Respiratory: Pao_2/fraction of inspired oxygen less than 300
4. Renal: oliguria, serum creatinine level greater than 2.0 mg/dL
5. Hepatic: prothrombin time–International Normalized Ratio greater than 1.5
6. Hematological: platelet count less than 1 million/mm^3

Grade II (moderate) acute cholangitis associated with any 2 of the following:
1. Abnormal white blood cell count (>12,000/mm^3, <4000/mm^3)
2. High fever (≥39°C)
3. Age (≥75 years)
4. Hyperbilirubinemia (total bilirubin ≥5 mg/dL)
5. Hypoalbuminemia (<Upper limit of Normal Value × 0.7)

Grade I (mild): acute cholangitis not meeting the criteria for grade II/III acute cholangitis.

Box 3
American Society for Gastrointestinal Endoscopy risk criterion

Strong:
- CBD stones on transabdominal US
- Clinical ascending cholangitis
- Bilirubin level greater than 4 mg/dL and dilated CBD on US (>6 mm with gall bladder in situ and >8 mm after cholecystectomy)

Moderate
- Abnormal liver tests other than bilirubin
- Age>55 years
- Dilated CBD on US

Low
- Lack of intermediate and high risk factors

Adapted from ASGE Standards of Practice Committee, Buxbaum JL, Abbas Fehmi SM, et al. ASGE guideline on the role of endoscopy in the evaluation and management of choledocholithiasis. Gastrointest Endosc. 2019;89(6):1099; with permission.

---

2. Intraoperative cholangiography and intraoperative US: during cholecystectomy (open or laparoscopic), the bile duct system can be delineated through IOC. The procedure involves injection of water-soluble dye and subsequent radiologic visualization through fluoroscopy. Although its performance during surgeries is debated, anatomic characterization of the biliary tree by IOC can prevent biliary injury.[115] A systematic review showed higher summary sensitivity of 0.99 (95% CI, 0.83–1.00) versus 0.83(95% CI, 0.72–0.90) and specificity of 0.99 (95% CI, 0.95–1.00) versus 0.99 (95% CI, 0.94–1.00) for IOC compared with endoscopic retrograde cholangiopancreatography (ERCP).[116] In addition, intraoperative US (IUS) can be performed through insertion of the US probe into the peritoneal cavity. It has diagnostic sensitivity and specificity of 95% and 100%, reduces the need for IOC, and prevents bile duct injury.
3. EUS and MRCP: patients with intermediate risk should undergo EUS or MRCP. Although EUS can diagnose smaller stones (0.1 mm) compared with MRCP (1.5 mm), it is more invasive and associated with sedation and procedural risks (bleeding, perforations). Both modalities have high diagnostic sensitivity (EUS 0.95, 95% CI 0.91–0.97 versus MRCP 0.93, 95% CI 0.87–0.96) and specificity (EUS 0.97, 95% CI 0.94–0.99 versus MRCP 0.96, 95% CI 0.90–0.98) for choledocholithiasis.[117] The selection of these modalities is based on technical expertise, costs, availability, and sedation risks.
4. ERCP: among patients with suspected choledocholithiasis, ERCP can be used as a diagnostic and therapeutic modality. It is reserved for individuals with high likelihood of choledocholithiasis[118] (**Fig. 7A–F**).

Treatment

Uncomplicated choledocholithiasis is managed through CBD stone extraction via endoscopic or, in certain circumstances, surgical routes. Endoscopic and surgical CBD stone extraction have similar safety profiles, although the surgical approach is more invasive.[119] The technique of choice for CBD calculi extraction is based on institutional practice and availability of expertise.

Surgery Intraoperative CBD exploration through laparoscopic or open methods is commonly performed with cholecystectomy. The choice of surgical exploration is

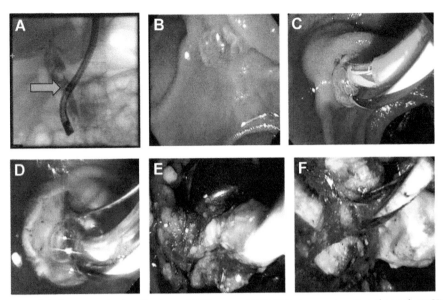

Fig. 7. (*A*) Fluoroscopic visualization of CBD stone. (*B–F*) CBD stone extraction through ERCP.

based on expertise and preference. Open CBD exploration has higher surgical morbidity, operative blood loss, and length of hospitalization.[120]

Endoscopic modality Patients with high risk for choledocholithiasis should be considered for ERCP for extraction of the calculi. Patients at moderate risk should undergo IOC/IUS, MRI, or EUS, followed by cholecystectomy (**Fig. 8**).

- ERCP technique involves deep cannulation of the bile duct via the major papilla, or, if cannulation is challenging, use of needle papillotome, called precut papillotomy.
- CBD stone clearance is attained through sphincterotomy (ie, incision through the deep muscle layer of the sphincter to maximize access to CBD stone) and/or balloon dilation and subsequent extraction through extraction balloons and baskets.
- For stones too large to remove en bloc, lithotripsy via mechanical baskets or cholangioscopic application of laser or electrohydraulic energy enables breaking down stones for removal (**Fig. 9A–C**).

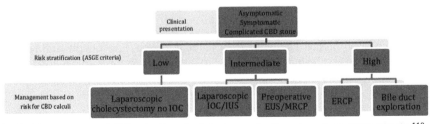

Fig. 8. Management of CBD calculi and related complications based on ASGE criteria.[110]

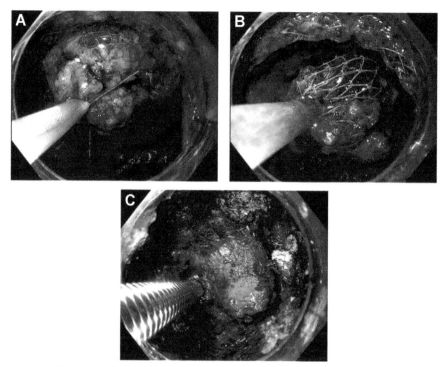

Fig. 9. (*A–C*) Endoscopic gallstone clearance via lithotripsy and stone extraction with Roth net through the LAMS.

Safety and outcomes of endoscopic retrograde cholangiopancreatography

Although performed routinely, ERCP has risks, which have been reported in up to 5% to 10% of cases. Their predisposing factors, outcomes, and preventive strategies are outlined in **Table 1**. Post-ERCP pancreatitis (PEP) is the most common complication of ERCP, although individuals aged greater than or equal to 65 years have a lower incidence than younger individuals.[121] The presence of choledocholithiasis is also protective against PEP, although the exact mechanism is not clear.[122] Age has been postulated as a protective factor for PEP. With advanced age, histologic alterations within the pancreatic parenchyma occur, including replacement of ductal epithelium with stratified squamous epithelium, fatty infiltration, and fibrosis.[123] Decreased perfusion, fibrosis, and atrophy may also cause age-related pancreatic exocrine insufficiency.[124] However, risks of bleeding and cardiopulmonary complications have been shown as predominant adverse effects among the elderly.[125] Risk of bleeding is attributable to higher rates of anticoagulant use, performance of precut sphincterotomy, therapeutic maneuvers, and PADs. Cardiopulmonary events can be hypothesized to result from higher ASA grading, comorbidity burden, and sensitivity to sedation.

Treatment of complications
Cholangitis

- Conservative management: conservative management for acute cholangitis includes volume expansion, correction of electrolyte abnormalities, and, especially among elderly patients, monitoring for organ dysfunction. Advanced age greater

Table 1
Post–endoscopic retrograde cholangiopancreatography complications, their predispositions, age-related cumulative incidence, and preventive strategies

Adverse Events	Predisposing Factor	Outcomes in Elderly[a]	Preventive Strategies
Post-ERCP pancreatitis	Patient-related factors: younger age, female, history of PEP, nondilated ducts, normal bilirubin, suspected SOD Procedure-related factors: difficult pancreatic cannulation, sphincterotomy, injections or sampling, precut sphincterotomy	Age ≥ 65 y: 13.1 (11.0–15.5) Age ≥ 80 y: 18.1 (14.0–23.0) Age ≥ 90 y: 12.2 (5.6–23.1)	Prophylactic pancreatic duct stenting Aggressive fluid hydration Chemoprophylaxis rectal indomethacin
Bleeding	Patient-related factors: coagulopathy or thrombocytopenia, anticoagulant therapy within 3 d after the sphincterotomy, active cholangitis, ampullary stone impaction, periampullary diverticula Procedure-related factors: low endoscopist experience, uncontrolled cutting (the so-called zipper cut), needle-knife sphincterotomy, degree of intraprocedural bleeding	Age ≥ 65 y: 7.7 (5.7–10.1) Age ≥ 80 y: 11.1 (7.7–15.4) Age ≥ 90 y: 28.6 (17.8–43.3)	• Blood products transfusion among patients with thrombocytopenia or coagulopathy, delay anticoagulation within 3 d of ERCP performance • Avoid sphincterotomy by balloon sphincteroplasty. Balloon tamponade using standard stone extraction or by balloon tamponade. Prophylactic epinephrine injection, intraprocedural usage of blended current, thermal coaptive coagulation using either a multipolar probe or heater probe device, endoscopic clip placement
Perforation • Free wall • Retroperitoneal • Perforation of the bile or pancreatic duct	Patient-related factors: esophageal stricture, Zenker diverticulum, postsurgical altered anatomy gastric outlet obstruction caused by pancreatic cancer, PAD, SOD, biliary or pancreatic duct strictures Procedure-related factors: mechanical pressure from a rigid duodenoscope, guidewire-related ductal perforation, knife precut access, use of a large extraction balloon in a small-caliber duct	Age ≥ 65 y: 3.8 (1.8–7.0) Age ≥ 80 y: 4.5 (2.2–8.0) Age ≥ 90 y: 1.3 (0–7.5)	—

(continued on next page)

		Outcomes in	Preventive
Adverse Events	**Predisposing Factor**	**Elderly**[a]	**Strategies**
Infection	Patient-related factors: jaundice, especially if caused by malignancy; primary sclerosing cholangitis Procedure-related factors: failed or incomplete biliary drainage, endoscopist inexperience, performance of a rendezvous (combined percutaneous/endoscopic) procedure	Age ≥ 65 y: 16.1 (11.7–21.7) Age ≥ 80 y: 4.1 (2.0–7.5) Age ≥ 90 y: 6.8 (2.2–15.8)	• Before contrast injection, aspiration and lavage of infected bile from an obstructed biliary system • Prompt endoscopic (and, if not possible, percutaneous) decompression • Minimize contrast volume
Cardiopulmonary events	Elderly patients with multiple comorbidities risk aspiration from concomitant gastric outlet obstruction in patients with advanced pancreaticobiliary malignancies	Age ≥ 65 y: 3.7 (1.5–7.6) Age ≥ 80 y: 39.6 (29.7–51.6) Age ≥ 90 y: 8.3 (3.0–17.9)	• Appropriate risk-assessment to minimize cardiopulmonary and sedation-related adverse events • Endotracheal intubation with general anesthesia should be used when indicated

Abbreviations: PEP, post-ERCP pancreatitis; SOD, sphincter of Oddi dysfunction.

[a] Cumulative incidence shown as events more than 1000 ERCPs.

than or equal to 70 years, the presence of medical comorbidities, immunocompromised state, extensive peritoneal involvement, delay in or inadequate source control, and presence of sepsis predispose patients to higher risk of adverse outcomes and warrant broad antimicrobial coverage (**Table 2**).[47] Prior isolation of resistant organisms, health care infections, or recent travel to regions with high prevalence of multidrug-resistant organisms require broader coverage.[126]

- Biliary drainage: timing of interventions is based on severity at diagnosis.[127] Although patients with mild cholangitis need conservative measures, biliary drainage is indicated on failure or inadequate response within 24 hours. Patients with moderate to severe cholangitis need immediate biliary drainage plus conservative measures. Patients with severe cholangitis must be monitored for and require support for organ dysfunction. The choice of drainage procedures includes the following:

1. Endoscopic drainage has much lower complication rates compared with surgical biliary compression. A study of 207 patients with cholangitis (102 aged ≥80 years vs 105 controls) showed its safety among the elderly, in whom comparable technical success rates, procedural times, and complications rates were observed.[128]

2. Percutaneous biliary drainage and extraction of CBD calculi is attempted on failure or unavailability of endoscopic interventions.

Table 2
Antibiotic regimen for gallbladder and bile duct infection

Infection	Regimen
Community-acquired acute cholecystitis of mild to moderate severity	Cefazolin, cefuroxime, or ceftriaxone
Community-acquired acute cholecystitis with severe physiologic disturbance, advanced age, or immunocompromised state	meropenem, imipenem-cilastatin, doripenem, or piperacillin-tazobactam alone; or ciprofloxacin, levofloxacin, or ceftazidime or cefepime, each in combination with metronidazole
Acute cholangitis following bilioenteric anastomosis of any severity	Imipenem-cilastatin, meropenem, doripenem, piperacillin-tazobactam, ciprofloxacin, levofloxacin, or cefepime, each in combination with metronidazole
Health care–associated biliary infection of any severity	Imipenem-cilastatin, meropenem, doripenem, piperacillin-tazobactam, ciprofloxacin, levofloxacin, or cefepime, each in combination with metronidazole, vancomycin added to each regimen

3. Surgical CBD exploration and subsequent stone extraction is attempted among individuals with failed endoscopic or percutaneous interventions.

Acute biliary pancreatitis Along with conservative management, stone extraction is indicated via endoscopic intervention (ie, ERCP) among suitable ABP candidates.[129,130] Although earlier convention supported endoscopic removal, recent evidence challenges the performance of routine ERCP, and its benefit is substantiated only among patients with ABP with concomitant cholangitis. Early cholecystectomy in the index admission was supported among patients with mild ABP.[131,132] Delay in cholecystectomy has been associated with complications including colic, pancreatitis, and hospitalizations among these individuals. However, among patients with moderate to severe ABP, cholecystectomy should be delayed.[133,134]

ROLE FOR SPHINCTEROTOMY AMONG NONSURGICAL CANDIDATES

Age and comorbidities may render geriatric individuals with ABP unsuitable for cholecystectomy and subsequently cause recurrent biliary events. Endoscopic sphincterotomy (ES) has been used for prophylaxis among these patients and mitigates the risk of recurrent ABP, biliary events, readmissions, and mortality.[135,136] A recent study showed the protective role of ES for ABP recurrence (adjusted hazard ratio [HR], 0.29; 95% CI, 0.08–0.92; $P = .037$) and any gallstone-related event (HR, 0.46; 95% CI, 0.21–0.98; $P = .043$).[137] Although randomized trials supporting ES among nonsurgical candidates are lacking, a randomized study (Endoscopic Sphincterotomy for Delaying Cholecystectomy in Mild Acute Biliary Pancreatitis [EMILY]) designed to evaluate ES in delaying cholecystectomy is underway.[138]

SUMMARY

With advanced age demographics, gallstone disease and associated complications are projected to have a much higher prevalence. Current advancements in diagnostic and therapeutic modalities have enabled inclusion of geriatric individuals for biliary interventions. However, each procedure needs appraisal for efficacy, therapeutic targets, safety, and cost-effectiveness. With risk/benefit ratio in mind, formulation of an individualized treatment plan with a multidisciplinary approach is imperative. Accumulating data from cohort studies and randomized trials will address knowledge gaps in various biliary disorders and their response to treatment modalities.

CLINICS CARE POINTS

- Among the geriatric population with acute cholecystitis, symptoms are atypical and physical signs may be masked by neuropathy. For e.g. Murphy sign has a lower sensitivity of 48% among the elderly. Typical leukocytosis and bandemia may be also obscured. Diagnostic sensitivity and specificity of acute cholecystitis was found to be 88% and 80% respectively.[24]Patients with acute cholecystitis warrant risk stratification followed by definitive drainage. Cholecystectomy is preferred treatment and high risk patients need temporizing measures.[48-50] Elderly individuals with higher ASA grades and comorbidity burden, have high peri-operative morbidity and biliary and vascular injury.[62,63]Acute cholecystitis with complications, sepsis and hemodynamic instability warrant emergent cholecystectomy.

- Among the elderly with CBD calculi, 'current evidence supports a significantly lower risk among patients in whom any measures for biliary ductal clearance were taken (12.7%; OR, 0.44 [0.35–0.55]).[97] Risk stratification for choledocholithiasis has been proposed by the Practice Committee of the American Society for Gastrointestinal Endoscopy (ASGE).[109,110]

- Uncomplicated choledocholithiasis is managed through CBD stone extraction via endoscopic or, in certain circumstances, surgical routes. Endoscopic and surgical CBD stone extraction have similar safety, although the surgical approach is more invasive.[119] For stones too large to remove en-bloc, lithotripsy via mechanical baskets or cholangioscopic application of laser or electrohydraulic energy enables breaking down stones for removal Acute Cholangitis is diagnosed through evidence of systemic inflammation, cholestasis, and imaging.[101]Among the elderly, acute cholangitis is associated with delayed medical care from masked presentation and significantly higher rates of hypotension, peritonism, renal failure.[104] They are managed through antibiotics, fluids and prompt biliary clearance.

- Among patients with acute biliary pancreatitis, pancreatitis is managed conservatively and undergo risk stratification before biliary clearance. Among mild ABP, ERCP benefits among only patients with concomitant cholangitis. Early cholecystectomy in the index admission was supported among patients with mild ABP and delays have been associated with colic, pancreatitis, and hospitalizations.[131,132]However, among patients with moderate to severe ABP, cholecystectomy should be delayed.[133,134]

ACKNOWLEDGMENTS

The authors would like to thank Mr Todd-Allen Lane, Chief, Library & Multimedia Services, Bridgeport Hospital for his help in literature search and multimedia services.

DISCLOSURE

The authors have nothing to disclose.

REFERENCES

1. Shaheen NJ, Hansen RA, Morgan DR, et al. The burden of gastrointestinal and liver diseases, 2006. Am J Gastroenterol 2006;101(9):2128–38.
2. Everhart JE, Ruhl CE. Burden of digestive diseases in the United States part I: overall and upper gastrointestinal diseases. Gastroenterology 2009;136(2): 376–86.
3. Everhart JE, Khare M, Hill M, et al. Prevalence and ethnic differences in gall-bladder disease in the United States. Gastroenterology 1999;117(3):632–9.
4. Ratner J, Lisbona A, Rosenbloom M, et al. The prevalence of gallstone disease in very old institutionalized persons. JAMA 1991;265(7):902–3.
5. Ross SO, Forsmark CE. Pancreatic and biliary disorders in the elderly. Gastro-enterol Clin North Am 2001;30(2):531–45, x.
6. Einarsson K, Nilsell K, Leijd B, et al. Influence of age on secretion of cholesterol and synthesis of bile acids by the liver. N Engl J Med 1985;313(5):277–82.
7. Khalil T, Walker JP, Wiener I, et al. Effect of aging on gallbladder contraction and release of cholecystokinin-33 in humans. Surgery 1985;98(3):423–9.
8. Kaim A, Steinke K, Frank M, et al. Diameter of the common bile duct in the elderly patient: measurement by ultrasound. Eur Radiol 1998;8(8):1413–5.
9. Magidson PD, Martinez JP. Abdominal pain in the geriatric patient. Emerg Med Clin North Am 2016;34(3):559–74.
10. Campion EW. The value of geriatric interventions. N Engl J Med 1995;332(20): 1376–8.
11. Shabanzadeh DM, Sorensen LT, Jorgensen T. A prediction rule for risk stratifica-tion of incidentally discovered gallstones: results from a large cohort study. Gastroenterology 2016;150(1):156–67.e1.
12. McSherry CK, Ferstenberg H, Calhoun WF, et al. The natural history of diag-nosed gallstone disease in symptomatic and asymptomatic patients. Ann Surg 1985;202(1):59–63.
13. Halldestam I, Enell EL, Kullman E, et al. Development of symptoms and compli-cations in individuals with asymptomatic gallstones. Br J Surg 2004;91(6): 734–8.
14. Ransohoff DF, Gracie WA, Wolfenson LB, et al. Prophylactic cholecystectomy or expectant management for silent gallstones. A decision analysis to assess sur-vival. Ann Intern Med 1983;99(2):199–204.
15. Kapoor VK. Cholecystectomy in patients with asymptomatic gallstones to pre-vent gall bladder cancer–the case against. Indian J Gastroenterol 2006;25(3): 152–4.
16. Tazuma S, Unno M, Igarashi Y, et al. Evidence-based clinical practice guidelines for cholelithiasis 2016. J Gastroenterol 2017;52(3):276–300.
17. Portincasa P, Moschetta A, Palasciano G. Cholesterol gallstone disease. Lancet 2006;368(9531):230–9.
18. Villanova N, Bazzoli F, Taroni F, et al. Gallstone recurrence after successful oral bile acid treatment. A 12-year follow-up study and evaluation of long-term post-dissolution treatment. Gastroenterology 1989;97(3):726–31.
19. Diehl AK, Sugarek NJ, Todd KH. Clinical evaluation for gallstone disease: use-fulness of symptoms and signs in diagnosis. Am J Med 1990;89(1):29–33.
20. Festi D, Sottili S, Colecchia A, et al. Clinical manifestations of gallstone disease: evidence from the multicenter Italian study on cholelithiasis (MICOL). Hepatol-ogy 1999;30(4):839–46.

21. Minoli G, Imperiale G, Spinzi GC, et al. Circadian periodicity and other clinical features of biliary pain. J Clin Gastroenterol 1991;13(5):546–8.
22. Cobden I, Lendrum R, Venables CW, et al. Gallstones presenting as mental and physical debility in the elderly. Lancet 1984;1(8385):1062–4.
23. Shaffer EA. Gallbladder sludge: what is its clinical significance? Curr Gastroenterol Rep 2001;3(2):166–73.
24. Shea JA, Berlin JA, Escarce JJ, et al. Revised estimates of diagnostic test sensitivity and specificity in suspected biliary tract disease. Arch Intern Med 1994; 154(22):2573–81.
25. Gurusamy KS, Samraj K, Fusai G, et al. Early versus delayed laparoscopic cholecystectomy for biliary colic. Cochrane Database Syst Rev 2008;(4):CD007196.
26. Antoniou SA, Antoniou GA, Koch OO, et al. Meta-analysis of laparoscopic vs open cholecystectomy in elderly patients. World J Gastroenterol 2014;20(46): 17626–34.
27. Kahng KU, Roslyn JJ. Surgical issues for the elderly patient with hepatobiliary disease. Surg Clin North Am 1994;74(2):345–73.
28. Glenn F, Hays DM. The age factor in the mortality rate of patients undergoing surgery of the biliary tract. Surg Gynecol Obstet 1955;100(1):11–8.
29. Tomida S, Abei M, Yamaguchi T, et al. Long-term ursodeoxycholic acid therapy is associated with reduced risk of biliary pain and acute cholecystitis in patients with gallbladder stones: a cohort analysis. Hepatology 1999;30(1):6–13.
30. Rubin RA, Kowalski TE, Khandelwal M, et al. Ursodiol for hepatobiliary disorders. Ann Intern Med 1994;121(3):207–18.
31. Kaminski DL. Arachidonic acid metabolites in hepatobiliary physiology and disease. Gastroenterology 1989;97(3):781–92.
32. Jivegard L, Thornell E, Svanvik J. Pathophysiology of acute obstructive cholecystitis: implications for non-operative management. Br J Surg 1987;74(12): 1084–6.
33. Csendes A, Burdiles P, Maluenda F, et al. Simultaneous bacteriologic assessment of bile from gallbladder and common bile duct in control subjects and patients with gallstones and common duct stones. Arch Surg 1996;131(4):389–94.
34. Adedeji OA, McAdam WA. Murphy's sign, acute cholecystitis and elderly people. J R Coll Surg Edinb 1996;41(2):88–9.
35. Trowbridge RL, Rutkowski NK, Shojania KG. Does this patient have acute cholecystitis? JAMA 2003;289(1):80–6.
36. Kaoutzanis C, Davies E, Leichtle SW, et al. Is hepato-imino diacetic acid scan a better imaging modality than abdominal ultrasound for diagnosing acute cholecystitis? Am J Surg 2015;210(3):473–82.
37. Reiss R, Nudelman I, Gutman C, et al. Changing trends in surgery for acute cholecystitis. World J Surg 1990;14(5):567–70 [discussion: 570–1].
38. Ganapathi AM, Speicher PJ, Englum BR, et al. Gangrenous cholecystitis: a contemporary review. J Surg Res 2015;197(1):18–24.
39. Niemeier OW. Acute free perforation of the gall-bladder. Ann Surg 1934;99(6): 922–4.
40. Anderson BB, Nazem A. Perforations of the gallbladder and cholecystobiliary fistulae: a review of management and a new classification. J Natl Med Assoc 1987;79(4):393–9.
41. Ploneda-Valencia CF, Gallo-Morales M, Rinchon C, et al. Gallstone ileus: an overview of the literature. Rev Gastroenterol Mex 2017;82(3):248–54.

42. Mallipeddi MK, Pappas TN, Shapiro ML, et al. Gallstone ileus: revisiting surgical outcomes using National Surgical Quality Improvement Program data. J Surg Res 2013;184(1):84–8.

43. Lassandro F, Gagliardi N, Scuderi M, et al. Gallstone ileus analysis of radiological findings in 27 patients. Eur J Radiol 2004;50(1):23–9.

44. Liang X, Li W, Zhao B, et al. Comparative analysis of MDCT and MRI in diagnosing chronic gallstone perforation and ileus. Eur J Radiol 2015;84(10): 1835–42.

45. Reisner RM, Cohen JR. Gallstone ileus: a review of 1001 reported cases. Am Surg 1994;60(6):441–6.

46. Thompson DR. Narcotic analgesic effects on the sphincter of Oddi: a review of the data and therapeutic implications in treating pancreatitis. Am J Gastroenterol 2001;96(4):1266–72.

47. Solomkin JS, Mazuski JE, Bradley JS, et al. Diagnosis and management of complicated intra-abdominal infection in adults and children: guidelines by the Surgical Infection Society and the Infectious Diseases Society of America. Clin Infect Dis 2010;50(2):133–64.

48. Yokoe M, Hata J, Takada T, et al. Tokyo Guidelines 2018: diagnostic criteria and severity grading of acute cholecystitis (with videos). J Hepatobiliary Pancreat Sci 2018;25(1):41–54.

49. Hernandez M, Murphy B, Aho JM, et al. Validation of the AAST EGS acute cholecystitis grade and comparison with the Tokyo guidelines. Surgery 2018;163(4): 739–46.

50. Madni TD, Nakonezny PA, Barrios E, et al. Prospective validation of the Parkland grading Scale for cholecystitis. Am J Surg 2019;217(1):90–7.

51. Ansaloni L, Pisano M, Coccolini F, et al. 2016 WSES guidelines on acute calculous cholecystitis. World J Emerg Surg 2016;11:25.

52. Bingener J, Richards ML, Schwesinger WH, et al. Laparoscopic cholecystectomy for elderly patients: gold standard for golden years? Arch Surg 2003; 138(5):531–5 [discussion: 535–6].

53. Coccolini F, Catena F, Pisano M, et al. Open versus laparoscopic cholecystectomy in acute cholecystitis. Systematic review and meta-analysis. Int J Surg 2015;18:196–204.

54. Salky BA, Edye MB. The difficult cholecystectomy: problems related to concomitant diseases. Semin Laparosc Surg 1998;5(2):107–14.

55. Mahmud S, Masaud M, Canna K, et al. Fundus-first laparoscopic cholecystectomy. Surg Endosc 2002;16(4):581–4.

56. Henneman D, da Costa DW, Vrouenraets BC, et al. Laparoscopic partial cholecystectomy for the difficult gallbladder: a systematic review. Surg Endosc 2013; 27(2):351–8.

57. Auyang ED, Santos BF, Enter DH, et al. Natural orifice translumenal endoscopic surgery (NOTES(®)): a technical review. Surg Endosc 2011;25(10):3135–48.

58. Rattner DW, Hawes R, Schwaitzberg S, et al. The Second SAGES/ASGE White Paper on natural orifice transluminal endoscopic surgery: 5 years of progress. Surg Endosc 2011;25(8):2441–8.

59. Gutt CN, Encke J, Koninger J, et al. Acute cholecystitis: early versus delayed cholecystectomy, a multicenter randomized trial (ACDC study, NCT00447304). Ann Surg 2013;258(3):385–93.

60. Gurusamy KS, Davidson C, Gluud C, et al. Early versus delayed laparoscopic cholecystectomy for people with acute cholecystitis. Cochrane Database Syst Rev 2013;(6):CD005440.

61. Loozen CS, van Ramshorst B, van Santvoort HC, et al. Early cholecystectomy for acute cholecystitis in the elderly population: a systematic review and meta-analysis. Dig Surg 2017;34(5):371–9.

62. Lord AC, Hicks G, Pearce B, et al. Safety and outcomes of laparoscopic cholecystectomy in the extremely elderly: a systematic review and meta-analysis. Acta Chir Belg 2019;119:349–56.

63. Kuy S, Sosa JA, Roman SA, et al. Age matters: a study of clinical and economic outcomes following cholecystectomy in elderly Americans. Am J Surg 2011; 201(6):789–96.

64. Waage A, Nilsson M. Iatrogenic bile duct injury: a population-based study of 152 776 cholecystectomies in the Swedish Inpatient Registry. Arch Surg 2006; 141(12):1207–13.

65. Flum DR, Cheadle A, Prela C, et al. Bile duct injury during cholecystectomy and survival in medicare beneficiaries. JAMA 2003;290(16):2168–73.

66. Strasberg SM, Hertl M, Soper NJ. An analysis of the problem of biliary injury during laparoscopic cholecystectomy. J Am Coll Surg 1995;180(1):101–25.

67. Sanjay P, Kulli C, Polignano FM, et al. Optimal surgical technique, use of intraoperative cholangiography (IOC), and management of acute gallbladder disease: the results of a nation-wide survey in the UK and Ireland. Ann R Coll Surg Engl 2010;92(4):302–6.

68. Spira RM, Nissan A, Zamir O, et al. Percutaneous transhepatic cholecystostomy and delayed laparoscopic cholecystectomy in critically ill patients with acute calculus cholecystitis. Am J Surg 2002;183(1):62–6.

69. Horn T, Christensen SD, Kirkegard J, et al. Percutaneous cholecystostomy is an effective treatment option for acute calculous cholecystitis: a 10-year experience. HPB (Oxford) 2015;17(4):326–31.

70. Bakkaloglu H, Yanar H, Guloglu R, et al. Ultrasound guided percutaneous cholecystostomy in high-risk patients for surgical intervention. World J Gastroenterol 2006;12(44):7179–82.

71. Venara A, Carretier V, Lebigot J, et al. Technique and indications of percutaneous cholecystostomy in the management of cholecystitis in 2014. J Visc Surg 2014;151(6):435–9.

72. Loozen CS, van Santvoort HC, van Duijvendijk P, et al. Laparoscopic cholecystectomy versus percutaneous catheter drainage for acute cholecystitis in high risk patients (CHOCOLATE): multicentre randomised clinical trial. BMJ 2018; 363:k3965.

73. Dimou FM, Adhikari D, Mehta HB, et al. Outcomes in older patients with grade III cholecystitis and cholecystostomy tube placement: a propensity score analysis. J Am Coll Surg 2017;224(4):502–11.e1.

74. James TW, Krafft M, Croglio M, et al. EUS-guided gallbladder drainage in patients with cirrhosis: results of a multicenter retrospective study. Endosc Int Open 2019;7(9):E1099–104.

75. Widmer J, Alvarez P, Sharaiha RZ, et al. Endoscopic gallbladder drainage for acute cholecystitis. Clin Endosc 2015;48(5):411–20.

76. Itoi T, Coelho-Prabhu N, Baron TH. Endoscopic gallbladder drainage for management of acute cholecystitis. Gastrointest Endosc 2010;71(6):1038–45.

77. Jain D, Bhandari BS, Agrawal N, et al. Endoscopic ultrasound-guided gallbladder drainage using a lumen-apposing metal stent for acute cholecystitis: a systematic review. Clin Endosc 2018;51(5):450–62.

78. Luk SW, Irani S, Krishnamoorthi R, et al. Endoscopic ultrasound-guided gallbladder drainage versus percutaneous cholecystostomy for high risk surgical

patients with acute cholecystitis: a systematic review and meta-analysis. Endoscopy 2019;51(8):722–32.

79. Higa JT, Sahar N, Kozarek RA, et al. EUS-guided gallbladder drainage with a lumen-apposing metal stent versus endoscopic transpapillary gallbladder drainage for the treatment of acute cholecystitis (with videos). Gastrointest Endosc 2019;90(3):483–92.

80. Molavi I, Schellenberg A, Christian F. Clinical and operative outcomes of patients with acute cholecystitis who are treated initially with image-guided cholecystostomy. Can J Surg 2018;61(3):195–9.

81. Akyurek N, Salman B, Yuksel O, et al. Management of acute calculous cholecystitis in high-risk patients: percutaneous cholecystotomy followed by early laparoscopic cholecystectomy. Surg Laparosc Endosc Percutan Tech 2005;15(6):315–20.

82. Stanek A, Dohan A, Barkun J, et al. Percutaneous cholecystostomy: a simple bridge to surgery or an alternative option for the management of acute cholecystitis? Am J Surg 2018;216(3):595–603.

83. Goodacre B, vanSonnenberg E, D'Agostino H, et al. Interventional radiology in gallstone disease. Gastroenterol Clin North Am 1991;20(1):209–27.

84. Burhenne HJ, Stoller JL. Minicholecystostomy and radiologic stone extraction in high-risk cholelithiasis patients. Preliminary experience. Am J Surg 1985;149(5):632–5.

85. Teoh AY, Perez-Miranda M, Kunda R, et al. Outcomes of an international multicenter registry on EUS-guided gallbladder drainage in patients at high risk for cholecystectomy. Endosc Int Open 2019;7(8):E964–73.

86. Jones MW, Ferguson T. Chronic cholecystitis. In: StatPearls. Treasure Island (FL): 2019.

87. Stephen AE, Berger DL. Carcinoma in the porcelain gallbladder: a relationship revisited. Surgery 2001;129(6):699–703.

88. Sheth S, Bedford A, Chopra S. Primary gallbladder cancer: recognition of risk factors and the role of prophylactic cholecystectomy. Am J Gastroenterol 2000;95(6):1402–10.

89. Welch NT, Fitzgibbons RJ Jr, Hinder RA. Beware of the porcelain gallbladder during laparoscopic cholecystectomy. Surg Laparosc Endosc 1991;1(3):202–5.

90. Siegel JH, Kasmin FE. Biliary tract diseases in the elderly: management and outcomes. Gut 1997;41(4):433–5.

91. Krasman ML, Gracie WA, Strasius SR. Biliary tract disease in the aged. Clin Geriatr Med 1991;7(2):347–70.

92. Lee JJ, Brahm G, Bruni SG, et al. Biliary dilatation in the presence of a periampullary duodenal diverticulum. Br J Radiol 2015;88(1053):20150149.

93. Sarli L, Costi R, Gobbi S, et al. Asymptomatic bile duct stones: selection criteria for intravenous cholangiography and/or endoscopic retrograde cholangiography prior to laparoscopic cholecystectomy. Eur J Gastroenterol Hepatol 2000;12(11):1175–80.

94. Frossard JL, Hadengue A, Amouyal G, et al. Choledocholithiasis: a prospective study of spontaneous common bile duct stone migration. Gastrointest Endosc 2000;51(2):175–9.

95. Collins C, Maguire D, Ireland A, et al. A prospective study of common bile duct calculi in patients undergoing laparoscopic cholecystectomy: natural history of choledocholithiasis revisited. Ann Surg 2004;239(1):28–33.

96. Caddy GR, Kirby J, Kirk SJ, et al. Natural history of asymptomatic bile duct stones at time of cholecystectomy. Ulster Med J 2005;74(2):108–12.

97. Moller M, Gustafsson U, Rasmussen F, et al. Natural course vs interventions to clear common bile duct stones: data from the Swedish Registry for Gallstone Surgery and Endoscopic Retrograde Cholangiopancreatography (GallRiks). JAMA Surg 2014;149(10):1008–13.
98. Cooper GS, Shlaes DM, Salata RA. Intraabdominal infection: differences in presentation and outcome between younger patients and the elderly. Clin Infect Dis 1994;19(1):146–8.
99. Kimura Y, Takada T, Kawarada Y, et al. Definitions, pathophysiology, and epidemiology of acute cholangitis and cholecystitis: Tokyo Guidelines. J Hepatobiliary Pancreat Surg 2007;14(1):15–26.
100. Sugiyama M, Atomi Y. Treatment of acute cholangitis due to choledocholithiasis in elderly and younger patients. Arch Surg 1997;132(10):1129–33.
101. Kiriyama S, Takada T, Strasberg SM, et al. New diagnostic criteria and severity assessment of acute cholangitis in revised Tokyo Guidelines. J Hepatobiliary Pancreat Sci 2012;19(5):548–56.
102. Eun HW, Kim JH, Hong SS, et al. Assessment of acute cholangitis by MR imaging. Eur J Radiol 2012;81(10):2476–80.
103. Pitt HA, Cameron JL, Postier RG, et al. Factors affecting mortality in biliary tract surgery. Am J Surg 1981;141(1):66–72.
104. Agarwal N, Sharma BC, Sarin SK. Endoscopic management of acute cholangitis in elderly patients. World J Gastroenterol 2006;12(40):6551–5.
105. Ranson JH, Rifkind KM, Roses DF, et al. Prognostic signs and the role of operative management in acute pancreatitis. Surg Gynecol Obstet 1974;139(1):69–81.
106. Blamey SL, Imrie CW, O'Neill J, et al. Prognostic factors in acute pancreatitis. Gut 1984;25(12):1340–6.
107. Wilson C, Heath DI, Imrie CW. Prediction of outcome in acute pancreatitis: a comparative study of Apache II, clinical assessment and multiple factor scoring systems. Br J Surg 1990;77(11):1260–4.
108. Frey C, Zhou H, Harvey D, et al. Co-morbidity is a strong predictor of early death and multi-organ system failure among patients with acute pancreatitis. J Gastrointest Surg 2007;11(6):733–42.
109. ASGE Standards of Practice Committee, Maple JT, Ben-Menachem T, et al. The role of endoscopy in the evaluation of suspected choledocholithiasis. Gastrointest Endosc 2010;71(1):1–9.
110. ASGE Standards of Practice Committee, Buxbaum JL, Abbas Fehmi SM, et al. ASGE guideline on the role of endoscopy in the evaluation and management of choledocholithiasis. Gastrointest Endosc 2019;89(6):1075 105.e5.
111. Abboud PA, Malet PF, Berlin JA, et al. Predictors of common bile duct stones prior to cholecystectomy: a meta-analysis. Gastrointest Endosc 1996;44(4):450–5.
112. Urquhart P, Speer T, Gibson R. Challenging clinical paradigms of common bile duct diameter. Gastrointest Endosc 2011;74(2):378–9.
113. Bachar GN, Cohen M, Belenky A, et al. Effect of aging on the adult extrahepatic bile duct: a sonographic study. J Ultrasound Med 2003;22(9):879–82 [quiz: 883–5].
114. Hunt DR. Common bile duct stones in non-dilated bile ducts? An ultrasound study. Australas Radiol 1996;40(3):221–2.
115. Massarweh NN, Devlin A, Elrod JA, et al. Surgeon knowledge, behavior, and opinions regarding intraoperative cholangiography. J Am Coll Surg 2008;207(6):821–30.

116. Gurusamy KS, Giljaca V, Takwoingi Y, et al. Endoscopic retrograde cholangio-pancreatography versus intraoperative cholangiography for diagnosis of common bile duct stones. Cochrane Database Syst Rev 2015;(2):CD010339.

117. Giljaca V, Gurusamy KS, Takwoingi Y, et al. Endoscopic ultrasound versus magnetic resonance cholangiopancreatography for common bile duct stones. Cochrane Database Syst Rev 2015;(2):CD011549.

118. Freeman ML, Nelson DB, Sherman S, et al. Complications of endoscopic biliary sphincterotomy. N Engl J Med 1996;335(13):909–18.

119. Dasari BV, Tan CJ, Gurusamy KS, et al. Surgical versus endoscopic treatment of bile duct stones. Cochrane Database Syst Rev 2013;(9):CD003327.

120. Grubnik VV, Tkachenko AI, Ilyashenko VV, et al. Laparoscopic common bile duct exploration versus open surgery: comparative prospective randomized trial. Surg Endosc 2012;26(8):2165–71.

121. Lillemoe KD. Pancreatic disease in the elderly patient. Surg Clin North Am 1994; 74(2):317–44.

122. Mehta SN, Pavone E, Barkun JS, et al. Predictors of post-ERCP complications in patients with suspected choledocholithiasis. Endoscopy 1998;30(5):457–63.

123. Schmitz-Moormann P, Himmelmann GW, Brandes JW, et al. Comparative radiological and morphological study of human pancreas. Pancreatitis like changes in postmortem ductograms and their morphological pattern. Possible implication for ERCP. Gut 1985;26(4):406–14.

124. Lohr JM, Panic N, Vujasinovic M, et al. The ageing pancreas: a systematic review of the evidence and analysis of the consequences. J Intern Med 2018; 283(5):446–60.

125. Day LW, Lin L, Somsouk M. Adverse events in older patients undergoing ERCP: a systematic review and meta-analysis. Endosc Int Open 2014;2(1):E28–36.

126. Woerther PL, Burdet C, Chachaty E, et al. Trends in human fecal carriage of extended-spectrum beta-lactamases in the community: toward the globalization of CTX-M. Clin Microbiol Rev 2013;26(4):744–58.

127. Mayumi T, Okamoto K, Takada T, et al. Tokyo Guidelines 2018: management bundles for acute cholangitis and cholecystitis. J Hepatobiliary Pancreat Sci 2018;25(1):96–100.

128. Tohda G, Ohtani M, Dochin M. Efficacy and safety of emergency endoscopic retrograde cholangiopancreatography for acute cholangitis in the elderly. World J Gastroenterol 2016;22(37):8382–8.

129. Schepers NJ, Bakker OJ, Besselink MG, et al. Early biliary decompression versus conservative treatment in acute biliary pancreatitis (APEC trial): study protocol for a randomized controlled trial. Trials 2016;17:5.

130. Coutinho LMA, Bernardo WM, Rocha RS, et al. Early endoscopic retrograde cholangiopancreatography versus conservative treatment in patients with acute biliary pancreatitis: systematic review and meta-analysis of randomized controlled trials. Pancreas 2018;47(4):444–53.

131. da Costa DW, Bouwense SA, Schepers NJ, et al. Same-admission versus interval cholecystectomy for mild gallstone pancreatitis (PONCHO): a multicentre randomised controlled trial. Lancet 2015;386(10000):1261–8.

132. Moody N, Adiamah A, Yanni F, et al. Meta-analysis of randomized clinical trials of early versus delayed cholecystectomy for mild gallstone pancreatitis. Br J Surg 2019;106(11):1442–51.

133. Uhl W, Muller CA, Krahenbuhl L, et al. Acute gallstone pancreatitis: timing of laparoscopic cholecystectomy in mild and severe disease. Surg Endosc 1999;13(11):1070–6.

134. Nealon WH, Bawduniak J, Walser EM. Appropriate timing of cholecystectomy in patients who present with moderate to severe gallstone-associated acute pancreatitis with peripancreatic fluid collections. Ann Surg 2004;239(6):741–9 [discussion: 749–51].

135. Hwang SS, Li BH, Haigh PI. Gallstone pancreatitis without cholecystectomy. JAMA Surg 2013;148(9):867–72.

136. Qayed E, Shah R, Haddad YK. Endoscopic retrograde cholangiopancreatography decreases all-cause and pancreatitis readmissions in patients with acute gallstone pancreatitis who do not undergo cholecystectomy: a nationwide 5-year analysis. Pancreas 2018;47(4):425–35.

137. Garcia de la Filia Molina I, Garcia Garcia de Paredes A, Martinez Ortega A, et al. Biliary sphincterotomy reduces the risk of acute gallstone pancreatitis recurrence in non-candidates for cholecystectomy. Dig Liver Dis 2019;51(11): 1567–73.

138. Kucserik LP, Marta K, Vincze A, et al. Endoscopic sphincterotoMy for delayIng choLecystectomy in mild acute biliarY pancreatitis (EMILY study): protocol of a multicentre randomised clinical trial. BMJ Open 2019;9(7):e025551.

Fecal Incontinence in the Elderly

Trisha Pasricha, MD, Kyle Staller, MD, MPH*

KEYWORDS

- Fecal incontinence • Elderly • Diarrhea • Fecal seepage • Sacral nerve stimulation
- Algorithm • Rectal examination

KEY POINTS

- Fecal incontinence can be a challenging and stigmatizing disease with a high prevalence in the elderly population.
- Despite effective treatment options, most patients with fecal incontinence are never asked by providers about the condition and do not receive care.
- Clues in the history and physical examination can assist the provider in establishing a diagnosis for fecal incontinence.
- Treating underlying bowel disturbances are one of the most effective first-line treatments for fecal incontinence.

INTRODUCTION

Fecal incontinence (FI) can be a challenging, stigmatizing disease for elderly patients to manage alone. Fortunately, a variety of treatment options exist for patients once the diagnosis is established, with more promising therapies in development. Despite its potentially devastating psychosocial and economic impact, most patients do not receive care for FI. As the population in the United States ages, the prevalence of FI will increase in turn. Health care providers must therefore remain vigilance to assess for FI in their aging patients while directing sufferers to appropriate treatment resources. In this article, we review the epidemiology, risk factors, diagnosis, and management of FI in the elderly population.

EPIDEMIOLOGY AND IMPACT
Definition

FI is the unintentional passage of solid or liquid stool. It can coexist with diarrhea and constipation, as well as urinary incontinence. By the Rome IV criteria,[1] FI is no longer

[a] Division of Gastroenterology, Massachusetts General Hospital, Wang 5, Boston, MA 02114, USA; [b] Department of Gastroenterology, Massachusetts General Hospital, 165 Cambridge Street, CRP 9, Boston, MA 02114, USA
* Corresponding author.
E-mail address: kstaller@mgh.harvard.edu
Twitter: @DrKyleStaller (K.S.)

Clin Geriatr Med 37 (2021) 71–83
https://doi.org/10.1016/j.cger.2020.08.006
0749-0690/21/© 2020 Elsevier Inc. All rights reserved.

described as functional (as in the Rome III criteria),[2] and there is no distinction as to the presumed etiology in making the diagnosis. For research purposes, FI is now defined as at least 2 episodes in a 4-week period, whereas previous definitions were less stringent.[3]

Three subtypes have been described[4,5]:

Passive incontinence: The unintentional passage of stool or gas without awareness of its occurrence.

Urge incontinence: The discharge of fecal matter despite active attempts to retain contents. These patients may describe constantly being unable to reach the bathroom in time.

Fecal seepage: The unintentional passage of stool that can follow an otherwise normal defecation, often presenting with fecal staining of undergarments. These patients may demonstrate dyssynergia with impaired rectal sensation.

Risk Factors

Several factors drive FI. Anatomic factors involved in maintenance of continence include anorectal sensation, muscle strength, rectal compliance, and neurologic integrity.[6] Anal resting tone is composed 70% of the circular smooth muscle of the internal anal sphincter and 30% of the striated muscle of the external anal sphincter. At rest, the puborectalis component of the levator ani complex helps to form the rectoanal angle to provide an additional barrier to incontinence with resting anal sphincter tone serving as an important barrier to passive incontinence (**Fig. 1**). In healthy individuals, both the puborectalis and the external anal sphincter can be voluntarily contracted to avoid defecation. Aging results in several related neuromuscular changes, including decreased anal resting and squeeze pressures, decreased rectal compliance, decreased rectal sensation, and an increased threshold to sense volume[7,8]— all physiologic alterations that can predispose to FI.

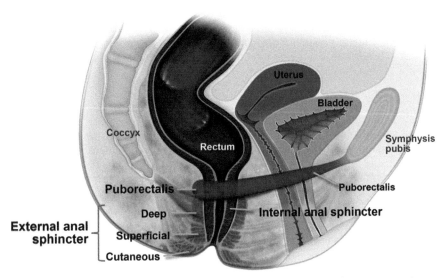

Fig. 1. Anorectal anatomy relevant to FI. (*From* Rao SS, Bharucha AE, Chiarioni G, et al. Anorectal disorders. Gastroenterology. 2016;150(6):1432; with permission.)

There has been much debate over the role of obstetric injury in the development of FI. Vaginal delivery has been shown to cause anal sphincter injury despite the initial absence of clinical symptoms,[9] It was therefore previously thought that obstetric injury may be major contributing risk factor in FI in older women.[10] However, more recent data indicate that bowel disturbances such as diarrhea and Irritable bowel syndrome with diarrhea are the main risk factors for FI in the elderly, rather than obstetric history.[11] Such injuries likely remain an important risk factor in immediate post-partum FI,[12] rather than late-onset FI, although obstetric injuries may nevertheless work synergistically with the aforementioned neuromuscular changes to increase risk of FI with aging. In the elderly, recognition of bowel disturbances driving FI can have tremendous therapeutic implications, because they are relatively easier to correct than neuromuscular injuries to the pelvic floor.

Several important medical comorbidities are associated with FI. Among neurologic disorders, diabetes mellitus as well as stroke are correlated with FI in older patients,[13] and FI in patients with multiple sclerosis is common.[14] Within gastrointestinal disorders, FI is more common in patients with inflammatory bowel disease than controls without inflammatory bowel disease (odds ratio, 7.73) in a meta-analysis of 17 studies and 4671 patients, with a likely multifactorial etiology heightened by local inflammation during a flare.[15] In patients with ulcerative colitis who have undergone a curative colectomy with ileal pouch anal anastomosis, FI symptoms are a common complication. Of these patients, 19% suffer occasional daytime incontinence and 49% suffer nocturnal incontinence at 12 months after the procedure.[16] Other gastrointestinal disorders, including celiac disease and irritable bowel syndrome, are also more commonly associated with FI.[17] Among those with preexisting bowel disturbances and predisposing medical conditions and demographics, more aggressive screening for FI is warranted.

Demographic risk factors for FI remain murky. A cross-sectional survey found an increased likelihood of FI in Hispanic and male patients, although these patients may not frequently present for FI care. Alternatively, another study found that white women (not including those identifying as Hispanic) were more likely to develop incident FI compared with black male and female patients.[18] Those seeking care seem to be predominantly women,[19,20] which may have previously driven the assumption that obstetric injuries were the main risk factor for FI. Nonetheless, the sex split for FI remains controversial, with some arguing for an even distribution among men and women,[19,21,22] and others arguing for a strong female predominance.[23]

Furthermore, lifestyle factors such as obesity and smoking[17,24] have been demonstrated as modifiable risk factors for FI. Similarly, higher levels of physical activity have been associated with a 25% risk reduction in new FI.[25] Anal intercourse, in both men and women, increases risk of FI (prevalence odds ratios of 2.8 and 1.5, respectively), although this is an area that has received comparatively little research.[26] Dietary factors have been shown to decrease the risk for the development of FI, namely, fiber intake. Our group demonstrated a modestly decreased risk of new FI, primarily from liquid stool, with increased long-term fiber intake in older women.[27] This finding may in turn reflect an improvement in stool consistency among those with bowel disturbances and FI, with the benefit seen at current guideline-recommended fiber intake levels (25 g/d).[28]

Last, and of particular relevance to the elderly population, additional risk factors include cognition and neurologic diseases such as dementia or a compromised ability to communicate, and poor mobility.[29] Not surprisingly, patients with limitations in their ability to perform activities of daily living have a higher odds of FI than those without (odds ratio, 2.54 for mobility, 4.03 for dressing, and 7.37 for toilet use).[30] Prompted toileting and fitness training among nursing home residents with these issues have had mixed results.[31,32]

Prevalence

Studies from the 1980s to the 1990s cite FI estimates at 2% of the population (and 10%–13% of elderly community residents).[23,33] However, the prevalence of this disease is likely more common than previously appreciated, with a recent large population-based study reporting that 1 in 7 Americans have experienced FI,[34] and a cross-sectional survey finding self-reported FI in 36.2% of respondents.[35]

Estimates of FI prevalence increase with age, hospitalization, and most with institutionalization. In people over age 50, the incidence of FI has been estimated at 7% per 10 years,[22] and age is independently associated with FI for both men and women other analyses.[36] Among hospitalized patients, the incidence of FI increases to 16% (12% of all patients have FI daily),[37] and this is estimated to be as high as 33% among the acutely ill.[38] Once institutionalized, nearly one-half of all residents have FI according to a recent systemic review on older people in care homes.[39]

Impact

Given these estimates, the overall burden of FI is significant. Medical complications of particular concern in the elderly are skin breakdown and pressure ulcers. FI can create excess moisture on the skin and enhances the permeability of irritants, including enteric enzymes, increasing the risk of pressure ulcer formation.[40] In elderly patients, pressure ulcer incidence is independently associated with FI within the first 48 hours of hospitalization.[41]

Economically, FI plays a major role in the $12 billion adult diaper market, projected to reach a value of $19 billion by 2023, with a growth far surpassing baby diapers.[42] An American mail-based study that analyzed the use of medical and nonmedical resources for FI as well as lost productivity found that the average annual total cost for FI is $4110 per person.[43] Finally, patients with FI have more frequent health care visits per year than those without (average difference of 4.21 visits per year), and more severe symptoms are associated with increased cost.[35]

Several studies have demonstrated an increased risk for institutionalization among patients with FI.[44–46] FI is associated with an increased likelihood of geriatrician referral to a skilled nursing facility, ranking among mobility restrictions, cognitive decline, and multiple chronic illnesses as major factors in the risk for nursing home referral.[47] Moreover, FI disproportionately increases the burden on caregivers, increasing the likelihood for the institutionalization of a relative.[48,49]

Beyond its economic impact, the psychosocial burden of FI cannot be overstated. Major areas of restriction caused by FI include social life, physical activities, hygiene, fear, and embarrassment.[50] Interviews of patients with FI highlight poor self-esteem and feeling that others perceive them as repulsive and impolite.[51] The perceived shame of FI can lead to increased social isolation and job loss.[52] Understandably, FI is linked to increased depression and anxiety as well as decreased quality of life.[53] An association between FI and the likelihood of mortality has even been described in community-dwelling elderly adults, even after adjustment for variables otherwise linked to mortality.[54]

WORKUP FOR FECAL INCONTINENCE
History

Asking the patient directly about FI is the most essential, yet frequently underused, aspect of the history. Despite its high prevalence, only 10% to 30% of patients with FI discuss treatment options with their physicians.[55,56] Part of this stems from a lack of systemic screening for FI in the primary care setting.[35] Only 13% of patients report being screened by the primary care doctors. Among those who consulted with their doctors about FI, 88% say the discussion was initiated by themselves.[57] The same study noted that some patients do not consult their doctors about FI because they are unaware that effective treatments exist.

The language providers use to broach a conversation about FI is also important. Physicians can try asking the question using other terms such as "accidental bowel leakage," which has been shown to be a preferred term by women when discussing FI.[58] Additionally, providers should take the health literacy of their patients into consideration with these questions, because many patients may not have ever heard of FI, or know this is a condition others experience, despite having symptoms themselves.[59] During the initial history, a physician should probe further if a patient endorses diarrhea, because this may be an intentional mislabeling of FI owing to embarrassment.

If FI is suspected, it should be better characterized to elucidate potential underlying, correctable causes. Providers should ask about the onset, frequency, volume, presence of blood, and pattern (gas vs liquid vs solid) of the patient's FI. Incontinence of urgent liquid stools may suggest the presence of a treatable bowel disturbance, such as irritable bowel syndrome, with symptom improvement possible with conservative measures before referral to specialized care. Passive incontinence of solid stool may suggest more severe neuromuscular dysfunction of the pelvic floor, requiring early referral for specialized management. It is also crucial to ask about vision loss, difficulty with communication, and gait impairment, because these factors may point to an overall neurologic or cognitive decline in the elderly.

Next, a thorough medical history should be taken with special attention to diseases that affect the gastrointestinal tract, cognition, and the central or peripheral nervous systems. Dementia, stroke, multiple sclerosis, diabetes mellitus, Parkinson's disease, inflammatory bowel disease, microscopic colitis, and chronic constipation are among the many age-related conditions that can increase risk of FI. These conditions deserve special mention because bowel disturbances are among the most important risk factors for developing FI. Approximately one-fourth of patients with inflammatory bowel disease experience FI,[15] and 10% to 15% of new cases of inflammatory bowel disease are diagnosed after the age of 60, despite commonly being seen as a young person's disease.[60,61] Evidence of anemia, rectal bleeding, and bloody diarrhea as well as an increased fecal calprotectin or fecal lactoferrin should prompt further evaluation with colonoscopy or flexible sigmoidoscopy.

Microscopic colitis is an important cause of chronic diarrhea in the elderly population with an average age at diagnosis of 66 years and a female predilection.[62] Patients with microscopic colitis report new-onset watery diarrhea and the disease is associated with certain drugs (nonsteroidal anti-inflammatory drugs, selective serotonin reuptake inhibitors) and autoimmune disorders. Endoscopically, the mucosa typically seems to be normal; however, the diagnosis of microscopic colitis is based on characteristic pathology.[63] Therefore, it is important to communicate to the gastroenterologist performing the colonoscopy that random colonic biopsies are requested with this condition on the differential.

Fecal impaction owing to constipation can be complicated by FI, as seen with an overflow diarrhea. This diagnosis is supported by a history of constipation mixed with diarrhea, abdominal discomfort, and evidence of impaction of rectal examination. Although a kidney, ureter, and bowel examination demonstrating severe fecal loading can help to determine the etiology of symptoms, the clinical presentation may be the best predictor of this diagnosis.[64] Our patients frequently describe several days of constipation followed by a "dam breaking" sensation with hard stools progressing to looser stools over a short time period.

In addition to a thorough surgical and obstetric history, the provider should focus on the patient's diet and medications. New medications (with special attention to recent antibiotics), herbal supplements, or changes in dosing can provide clues to causes of bowel disturbances. Especially in the elderly, side effects as well as drug–drug interactions of all medications should be considered. With an FI prevalence of 22% in patients with diabetes,[65] providers should give careful attention to dietary and medication changes in this population. Artificial sweeteners such as sorbitol can aggravate diarrhea, as can medications such as metformin, with their effects on FI compounded by neuropathy-associated rectal hyposensitivity. Physicians should assess dietary fiber intake and evaluate for possible food triggers causing bowel disturbances such as lactose, fructose, or gluten.

Physical Examination

The physical examination should encompass several aspects, including a complete neurologic examination to encompass cognition, vision, and mobility. The rectal examination will be reviewed here. It is worth noting that confidence in making a diagnosis with rectal examination is strongly associated with the number of rectal examinations performed annually, and that patient refusal rates negatively correlate with the comfort level of the physician.[66]

With the patient on their left side with knees and hips flexed, inspect the perianal region for lesions, including skin tags, ulcers or skin breakdown, hemorrhoids, rashes, fissures, and warts or frank masses. Residual stool is frequently seen surrounding the anal opening in patients with FI. A gaping or patulous anal orifice can suggest a neuromuscular etiology of FI and often indicates internal anal sphincter dysfunction.[67]

Eliciting an anal wink can serve as a helpful (although insensitive) measure of S2 to S4 nerve root or pudendal nerve function.[5,68] The examiner gently strokes toward the anus with a finger or cotton swab in all 4 quadrants to assess for a brisk, involuntary anal contraction. Its absence may indicate a potential neuropathic problem.[69]

Rectal prolapse can contribute to FI and can be assessed by asking the patient to bear down—preferably in the standing position to take advantage of gravity. Prolapsed rectal mucosa through the anus appears as a rosette of red tissue with care to note whether only radiating folds (suggestive of milder prolapse) or concentrically circular folds appear (suggestive of larger prolapse involving the entire bowel wall).[70] Having the patient bear down will similarly expose prolapsing internal hemorrhoids that may prevent an adequate seal of the anal canal and lead to seepage.

Inserting a gloved fingertip into the anal canal allows for an assessment of sphincter tone at rest and when asking the patient to squeeze voluntarily. The former maneuver primarily assesses the function of the internal anal sphincter and the latter the function of the external anal sphincter (under voluntary control). Next, the provider should request that the patient try to expel the inserted finger as the provider observes the degree of perineal descent (3 cm or greater is considered abnormal). Lack of coordination between the rectal push and the anal relaxation is suggestive of dyssynergic defecation, which can predispose to incomplete rectal evacuation and subsequent leakage through a weakened anal sphincter.

Further Testing

As described, if bowel disturbances are present, stool studies and colonoscopy or flexible sigmoidoscopy should be considered to evaluate for an underlying etiology. A kidney, ureter, and bowel examination assessing for stool burden can also be valuable when considering overflow incontinence or megarectum. Other more specific tests include anorectal manometry, balloon expulsion testing, and defecography.

These test can help to identify and characterize structural or sensory abnormalities. However, additional testing in FI does not always change management,[71] and therefore should not delay initial treatment or subspecialty referral.

MANAGEMENT

There are several effective treatment options for the management of FI and referral to a gastroenterologist or colorectal surgeon (depending on local expertise) is essential to further determine the optimal treatment options for the patient. Conservative treatment, however, should begin immediately at the primary care level. As a rule, correcting bowel disturbances associated with loose stools and liquid stool incontinence is much easier, less invasive—and in many cases more effective—than invasive options targeting the anal sphincter. Dietary modifications such as increased fiber intake or fiber supplementation as well as decreasing foods that can prompt loose stools like

Table 1
Common bowel disturbances, workup, and first-line treatments

Bowel Disturbance	Diagnostic Workup	First-Line Treatment
IBS-D	History (suggestive features include absence of red flag symptoms, association with defecation), negative infectious and inflammatory work-up	Fiber supplementation, loperamide, antispasmodics (caution in elderly)
Bile acid diarrhea	History (suggestive features include history of cholecystectomy or suspicion of IBS-D)	Cholestyramine, colesevelam, colestipol (caution about spacing out from other medications)
Microscopic colitis	Pathology from endoscopic biopsies	Frequently directed by GI: budesonide (9 mg daily), smoking and NSAID cessation (may contribute to disease)
Chronic infectious diarrhea	History (suggestive features include recent travel or immunocompromise), fecal giardia/stool ova and parasites/stool culture, fecal leukocyte	Targeted antimicrobial therapy
Inflammatory bowel disease	Fecal calprotectin, endoscopy, iron studies	Treatment directed by GI
Lactose intolerance	Dietary history, note that prevalence increases with age	Lactose-free diet, lactase enzyme supplementation
Celiac disease	Dietary history, IgA/tissue transglutaminase	Gluten-free diet
Small bowel bacterial overgrowth	Breath testing, although significant accuracy issues	Antibiotics (preference for nonabsorbable agents, ie, rifaximin)
Constipation with overflow incontinence	History, kidney, ureter, and bowel examination	Laxatives, pelvic floor biofeedback

Abbreviations: IBS-D, irritable bowel syndrome with diarrhea; NSAID, nonsteroidal anti-inflammatory drug.

coffee or fructose can markedly improve FI.[72] Loperamide for diarrhea-associated FI[73] or laxatives for constipation or fecal impaction-associated FI are common first-line treatments,[64] with assessment and treatment of the underlying etiology initiated in the primary care office. For example, FI being driven by bile acid malabsorption can often be treated with cholestyramine effectively whereas FI resulting from an inability to reach the toilet in a patient with Parkinson's disease can be reduced by ordering a bedside commode. **Table 1** lists etiologies of common bowel disturbances, the diagnostic workup, and first-line treatments.

The current anorectum-specific treatments with the best evidence to date are sacral nerve stimulation, a type of neuromodulation involving outpatient surgical implantation of electrodes adjacent to the sacral nerves,[74] and biofeedback, which is performed with the assistance of a therapist to retrain a patient's neuromuscular coordination and improve rectal sensation.[75,76] These treatment modalities have been reviewed in depth,[77] and typically require subspecialty guidance. In all cases, treatment success is generally defined as a 50% or greater decrease in weekly FI episodes.[78]

It must be noted that, in women with normal stool consistency, loperamide was recently shown to be no more effective than placebo or an educational pamphlet on FI.[79] The same randomized controlled trial did not show a significant difference between biofeedback and an educational pamphlet in this population. This lack of improvement with some of the long-used, traditional interventions in FI with normal stool consistency suggests a patient population with more severe damage to the continence mechanism, warranting earlier subspecialty evaluation.

Nonetheless, conservative management by the primary care physician plays an integral role in FI, yielding a 60% improvement in symptoms and continence in 20% of patients.[80] It is therefore insufficient to merely make a diagnosis of FI. Rather, it is paramount that a plan is implemented to address it with our suggested algorithmic approach (**Fig. 2**), expediently involving specialists if needed.

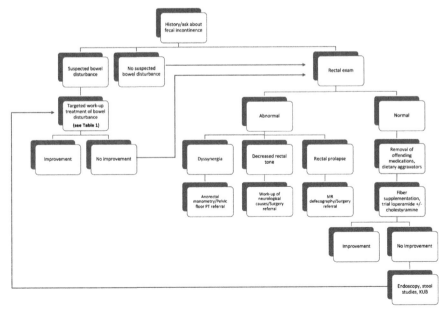

Fig. 2. Suggested treatment algorithm for the evaluation of FI in the elderly. KUB, kidney, ureter, and bowel examination; MR, magnetic resonance.

SUMMARY

FI is a widespread issue among the elderly with a significant toll on patients and society. With a purposeful history and physical examination, physicians can make the diagnosis and start effective FI treatments, which can be life changing. Although we still have much to learn about the pathophysiology of FI, several exciting new therapies are on the horizon.

Our institution is currently collaborating in a randomized clinical trial for translumbosacral neuromodulation therapy for FI. Translumbosacral neuromodulation therapy is a novel technique that delivers magnetic energy to the lumbosacral nerves, which, unlike sacral nerve stimulation, is noninvasive. As with other options for FI, it remains to be seen if a sham control clinical trial will demonstrate long-term efficacy.

A number of promising preclinical and observational studies have investigated local injections to the anal sphincter of muscle-derived or mesenchymal stem cells.[81] A recent phase II, randomized clinical trial using autologous myoblasts demonstrated sustained improvement in FI severity at 12 months.[82]

Despite these strides, stigma reduction remains an enormous barrier in FI. On an individual provider level, however, the first step in the right direction is as simple as asking the patient.

DISCLOSURE

K. Staller has received research support from AstraZeneca, Gelesis, and Takeda; he has served as a consultant to Arena, Bayer, Shire, and Synergy; he has served as a speaker for Shire. T. Pasricha has nothing to disclose.

REFERENCES

1. Rao SS, Bharucha AE, Chiaroni G, et al. Functional anorectal disorders. Gastroenterology 2016;150(6):143–1442.
2. Bharucha AE, Wald A, Enck P, et al. Functional anorectal disorders. Gastroenterology 2006;130(5):1510–8.
3. Whitehead WE, Simren M, Busby-Whitehead J, et al. Fecal incontinence diagnosed by the Rome IV criteria in the United States, Canada, and the United Kingdom. Clin Gastroenterol Hepatol 2020;18(2):385–91.
4. Rao SS, Ozturk R, Stessman M. Investigation of the pathophysiology of fecal seepage. Am J Gastroenterol 2004;99:2204–9.
5. Rao SS. Diagnosis and management of fecal incontinence. American College of Gastroenterology Practice Parameters Committee. Am J Gastroenterol 2004; 99(8).1585–604.
6. Bharucha AE, Dunivan G, Goode PS, et al. Epidemiology, pathophysiology, and classification of fecal incontinence: state of the science summary for the national institute of diabetes and digestive and kidney diseases (NIDDK) workshop. Am J Gastroenterol 2015;110:127–36.
7. Fox JC, Fletcher JG, Zinmeister AR, et al. Effect of aging on anorectal and pelvic floor functions in females. Dis Colon Rectum 2006;49:1726–35.
8. Ryhammer AM, Laurberg S, Bek KM. Age and anorectal sensibility in normal women. Scand J Gastroenterol 1998;32:278–84.
9. Dudding TCC, Vaizey CJ, Kamm MA. Obstetric anal sphincter injury: incidence, risk factors, and management. Ann Surg 2008;247:224–37.
10. Melville JL, Fan MY, Newton K, et al. Fecal incontinence in US women: a population-based study. Am J Obstet Gynecol 2005;193:2071–6.

11. Bharucha A, Zinmeister A, Schleck CD, et al. Bowel disturbances are the most important risk factors for late onset fecal incontinence: a population-based case-control study in women. Gastroenterology 2010;139:1559–66.

12. Sultan AH, Kamm MA, Hudson CN, et al. Anal-sphincter disruption during vaginal delivery. N Engl J Med 1993;329:1905–11.

13. Quander CR, Morris MC, Melson J, et al. Prevalence of and factors associated with fecal incontinence in a large community study of older individuals. Am J Gastroenterol 2005;100(4):905–9.

14. Preziosi G, Gordon-Dixon A, Emmanuel A. Neurogenic bowel dysfunction in patients with multiple sclerosis: prevalence, impact, and management strategies. Degener Neurol Neuromuscul Dis 2018;8:79–90.

15. Gu P, Kuenzig ME, Kaplan GG, et al. Fecal incontinence in inflammatory bowel disease: a systemic review and meta-analysis. Inflamm Bowel Dis 2018;24(6):1280–90.

16. Meagher AP, Farouk R, Dozois RR, et al. J ileal pouch-anal anastomosis for chronic ulcerative colitis: complications and long-term outcome in 1310 patients. Br J Surg 1998;85(6):800–3.

17. Townsend MK, Matthews CA, Whitehead WE, et al. Risk factors for fecal incontinence in older women. Am J Gastroenterol 2013;108(1):113–9.

18. Markland AD, Goode PS, Burgio KL, et al. Incidence and risk factors for fecal incontinence in black and white older adults: a population-based study. J Am Geriatr Soc 2010;58(7):1341–6.

19. Madoff RD, Parker SC, Varma MG, et al. Faecal incontinence in adults. Lancet 2004;364:621–32.

20. Perry S, Shaw C, McGrother C, et al. Prevalence of faecal incontinence in adults aged 40 years or more living in the community. Gut 2002;50:480–4.

21. Talley NJ, O'Keefe EA, Zinmeister AR, et al. Prevalence of gastrointestinal symptoms in the elderly: a population-based study. Gastroenterology 1992;102:895–901.

22. Rey E, Choung RS, Schleck CD, et al. Onset and risk factors for fecal incontinence in a US community. Am J Gastroenterol 2010;105:412–9.

23. Nelson R, Norton N, Cautley E, et al. Community-based prevalence of anal incontinence. JAMA 1995;274:559–61.

24. Varma MG, Brown JS, Creasman JM, et al. Fecal incontinence in females older than aged 40 years: who is at risk? Dis Colon Rectum 2006;49(6):841–51.

25. Staller K, Song M, Grodstein F, et al. Physical activity, BMI, and risk of fecal incontinence in the Nurses' health Study. Clin Transl Gastroenterol 2018;9(10):200.

26. Markland AD, Dunivan GC, Vaughan CP. Anal intercourse and fecal incontinence: evidence from the 2009-2010 national health and nutrition examination survey. Am J Gastroenterol 2016;111(2):269–74.

27. Staller K, Song M, Grodstein F, et al. Increased long-term dietary fiber intake is associated with a decrease in fecal incontinence in older women. Gastroenterology 2018;155(3):661–7.

28. Dietary Guidelines for Americans. 2010. U.S. department of agriculture and U.S. department of health and human services. 7th edition. Washington, DC: U.S. Government Printing Office; 2010.

29. Chassagne P, Landrin I, Neveu C, et al. Fecal incontinence in the institutionalized elderly: incidence , risk factors, and prognosis. Am J Med 1999;106(2):185–90.

30. Saga S, Vinsnes AG, Morkved S, et al. Prevalence and correlates of fecal incontinence among nursing home residents: a population-based cross-sectional study. BMC Geriatr 2013;13:87.

31. Ouslander JG, Simmons S, Schnelle J, et al. Effects of prompted voiding on fecal continence among nursing home residents. J Am Geriatr Soc 1996;44:424–8.
32. Schnelle JF, Leung FW, Rao SSC, et al. A controlled trial of an intervention to improve urinary and fecal incontinence and constipation. J Am Geriatr Soc 2010;58:1504–11.
33. Thomas TM, Egan M, Walgrove A, et al. The prevalence of faecal and double incontinence. Community Med 1984;6:216–20.
34. Menees SB, Almario CV, Spiegel BM, et al. Prevalence of and factors associated with fecal incontinence: results from a population-based survey. Gastroenterology 2018;154:1672–81.
35. Dunivan GC, Heyman S, Palsson OS, et al. Fecal incontinence in primary care: prevalence, diagnosis, and health care utilization. Am J Obstet Gynecol 2010; 202:493.e1–6.
36. Whitehead WE, Borrud L, Goode PS, et al. Fecal incontinence in US adults: epidemiology and risk factors. Gastroenterology 2009;137:512–7, 517.e1-2.
37. Hughes BT, Chepyala P, Hendon S, et al. Fecal incontinence in an inpatient population: a not uncommon finding. Dig Dis Sci 2009;54:2215–9.
38. Bliss DZ, Johnson S, Savik K, et al. Fecal incontinence in hospitalized patients who are acutely ill. Nurse Res 2000;49(2):101–8.
39. Musa MK, Saga S, Blekken LE, et al. The prevalence, incidence, and correlates of fecal incontinence among older people living in care homes: a systemic review. J Am Med Dir Assoc 2019;20(8):956–62.
40. Coleman S, Nixon J, Keen J, et al. A new pressure ulcer conceptual framework. J Adv Nurs 2014;70(10):2222–34.
41. Baumgarten M, Margolis DJ, Localio AR, et al. Pressure ulcers among elderly patients early in the hospital stay. J Gerontol A Biol Sci Med Sci 2006;61(7):749–54.
42. Research and Markets. "Global adult diaper market to 2023." PR newswire: press release distribution, targeting, monitoring, and marketing. 2018. Available at: https://www.prnewswire.com/news-releases/global-adult-diaper-market-to-2023-300686415.html. Accessed October 26, 2019.
43. Xu X, Menees SB, Zochowski MK. Economic cost of fecal incontinence. Dis Colon Rectum 2012;55(5):586–98.
44. AlAmeel T, Andrew MK, MacKnight C. The association of fecal incontinence with institutionalization and mortality in older adults. Am J Gastroenterol 2010;105(8): 1830–4.
45. Nelson R, Furner S, Jusdason V. Fecal incontinence in Wisconsin nursing homes: prevalence and associations. Dis Colon Rectum 1998;41:1126–229.
46. O'Donnell BF, Drachman DA, Barnes HJ, et al. Incontinence and troublesome behaviors predict institutionalization in dementia. J Geriatr Psychiatry Neurol 1992; 5:45–52.
47. Grover M, Busby-Whitehead J, Palmer MH, et al. Survey of geriatricians on the effect of fecal incontinence on nursing home referral. J Am Geriatr Soc 2010; 58(6):1058–62.
48. Noelker LS. Incontinence in elderly cared for by family. Gerontologist 1987;27: 194–200.
49. Ouslander JG, Zarit SH, Orr NK, et al. Incontinence among elderly community-dwelling dementia patients. Characteristics, management, and impact on caregivers. J Am Geriatr Soc 1990;38:440–5.
50. Cotterill N, Norton C, Avery KN, et al. A patient-centered approach to developing a comprehensive symptom and quality of life assessment of anal incontinence. Dis Colon Rectum 2007;51:82–7.

51. Olsson F, Bertero C. Living with faecal incontinence: trying to control the daily life that is out of control. J Clin Nurs 2015;24(1–2):141–50.
52. Norton NJ. The perspective of the patient. Gastroenterology 2004;126:S175–9.
53. Miner PB. Economic and personal impact of fecal and urinary incontinence. Gastroenterology 2004;126(1 suppl 1):S8–13.
54. Jamieson HA, Schluter PJ, Pyun J, et al. Fecal incontinence is associated with mortality among older adults with complex needs: an observational cohort study. Am J Gastroenterol 2017;112:1431–7.
55. Bharucha AE, Zinsmeister AR, Locke GR, et al. Prevalence and burden of fecal incontinence: a population-based study in women. Gastroenterology 2005; 129:42–9.
56. Johanson JF, Lafferty J. Epidemiology of fecal incontinence: the silent affliction. Am J Gastroenterol 1996;91:33–6.
57. Kunduru L, Kim SM, Heymen S, et al. Factors that affect consultation and screening for fecal incontinence. Clin Gastroenterol Hepatol 2015;13(4):709–16.
58. Brown HW, Wexner SD, Lukacz ES. Factors associated with care seeking among women with accidental bowel leakage. Female Pelvic Med Reconstr Surg 2013; 19(2):66–71.
59. Brown HW, Rogers RG, Wise ME. Barriers to seeking care for accidental bowel leakage: a qualitative study. Int Urogynecol J 2017;28(4):543–51.
60. Loftus eV, Silvertstein MD, Sandbord WF, et al. Ulcerative colitis in Olmstead County, Minnesota, 1940-1993: incidence, prevalence, and survival. Gut 2000; 46:336–43.
61. Loftus eV, Silvertstein MD, Sandbord WF, et al. Crohn's disease in Olmstead County, Minnesota, 1940-1993: incidence, prevalence, and survival. Gastroenterology 1998;114:1161–8.
62. Gentile NM, Khanna S, Loftus EV, et al. The epidemiology of microscopic colitis in Olmsted Count from 2002-2010: a population-based study. Clin Gastroenterol Hepatol 2014;12(5):838–42.
63. Storr MA. Microscopic colitis: epidemiology, pathophysiology, diagnosis, and management-an update 2013. ISRN Gastroenterol 2013;2013:352718.
64. Arasaradhnam RP, Brown S, Forbes A. Guidelines for the investigation of chronic diarrhea in adults: British Society of Gastroenterology, 3rd edition. Gut 2018; 67(8):1380–99.
65. Schiller LR, Santa Ana CA, Schmulen AC, et al. Pathogenesis of fecal incontinence in diabetes mellitus: evidence for internal-anal-sphincter dysfunction. N Engl J Med 1982;307:1666–71.
66. Wong RK, Drossman DA, Bharucha AE, et al. The digital rectal examination: a multicenter survey of physicians' and students' perceptions and practice patterns. Am J Gastroenterol 2012;107(8):1157–63.
67. Dobben AC, Terra MP, Deutekom M, et al. Anal inspection and digital rectal examination compared to anorectal physiology tests and endoanal ultrasonography in evaluating fecal incontinence. Int J Colorectal Dis 2007;22:783–90.
68. Schmidt RA, Senn E, Tanagho EA. Functional evaluation of sacral nerve root integrity. Report of a technique. Urology 1990;35(5):388–92.
69. Talley NJ. How to do and interpret a rectal examination in gastroenterology. Am J Gastroenterol 2008;103(4):820–2.
70. Bickley LS, Szilagyi PG. "Abnormalities of the Anus, Surrounding Skin, and Rectum." Bate's Guide to Physical Examination: And History Taking. Philadelphia: Lippincott Williams & Wilkins; 2007. p. 561–9.

71. Wexner SD, Jorge JM. Colorectal physiological tests: use or abuse of technology? Eur J Surg 1994;160:167–74.
72. Wald A. Clinical practice. Fecal incontinence in adults. N Engl J Med 2007; 356(16):1648–55.
73. Sun WM, Read NW, Barber DC, et al. Effects of loperamide on anal sphincter function in patients complaining of chronic diarrhea with fecal incontinence and urgency. Dig Dis Sci 1982;27(9):807–14.
74. Thaha MA, Abukar AA, Thin NN, et al. Sacral nerve stimulation for faecal incontinence and constipation in adults. Cochrane Database Syst Rev 2015;(8):CD004464.
75. Rao SS. The technical aspects of biofeedback therapy for defecation. Gastroenterologist 1998;6(2):96–103.
76. Norton C, Chelvanayagam S, Wilson-Barnett J, et al. Randomized controlled trial of biofeedback for fecal incontinence. Gastroenterology 2003;125:1320–9.
77. Whitehead WE, Rao SSC, Lowry A, et al. Treatment of fecal incontinence: state of the science summary for the national institute of diabetes and digestive and kidney diseases workshop. Am J Gastroenterol 2015;110:138–46.
78. Barker A, Hurley J. Novel treatment options for fecal incontinence. Clin Colon Rectal Surg 2014;27(3):116–20.
79. Jelovsek JE, Markland AD, Whitehead WE, et al. Controlling faecal incontinence in women by performing anal exercises with biofeedback or loperamide: a randomized clinical trial. Lancet Gastroenterol Hepatol 2019;4(9):698–710.
80. Whitehead WE. Treating fecal incontinence: an unmet need in primary care medicine. N C Med J 2016;77(3):221–5.
81. Trebol J, Carabias-Orgaz A, Garcia-arranz M, et al. Stem cell therapy for faecal incontinence: current state and future perspectives. World J Stem Cells 2018; 10(7):82–105.
82. Boyer O, Bridoux V, Giverne C, et al. Autologous myoblasts for the treatment of fecal incontinence: results of a phase 2 randomized placebo-controlled study (MIAS). Ann Surg 2018;267:443–50.

Evaluation and Treatment of Constipation in the Geriatric Population

Susan Lucak, MD[a,1], Tisha N. Lunsford, MD[b],
Lucinda A. Harris, MS, MD[b,*]

KEYWORDS

- Constipation • Elderly • Bowel training • Laxatives • Linaclotide • Lubiprostone
- Plecanatide • Tegaserod

KEY POINTS

- Chronic constipation, a common gastrointestinal disorder, has increased prevalence in elderly individuals because of polypharmacy, immobility, and physiologic changes in the intestinal tract and pelvic floor function caused by aging.
- A thorough history and physical examination including pelvic floor evaluation is necessary for assessment of severity and causation of constipation to guide the diagnostic work-up.
- Initial treatment approaches should include diet and lifestyle changes as well as review of medications, but recognition and treatment of pelvic floor dysfunction may be an important aspect of early treatment.
- Pharmacologic treatments include over-the-counter medications as well as newer prescription medications targeting various physiologic receptors, but few data are available regarding their safety in the elderly.

INTRODUCTION

Constipation is estimated to affect 33 million individuals in the United States alone and it is nearly twice as common in women compared with men.[1] The prevalence of constipation in women more than 65 years of age is 26% and 16% in men.[2] This prevalence may be influenced by a variety of factors, such as whether the patient is in a community setting versus institutional setting, the patient's diet, comorbidities, socioeconomic status, polypharmacy, and pelvic floor sensorimotor defecation disorders. The prevalence continues to increase with increasing age, to 34% in

[a] Weill Cornell Medicine, Columbia University Medical Center; [b] Division of Gastroenterology & Hepatology, Alix School of Medicine, Mayo Clinic, 13400 East Shea Boulevard, Scottsdale, AZ 85259, USA
[1] Present address: 930 Park Avenue, First Floor, New York, NY 10075.
* Corresponding author. LucindaHarris@LucindaHarris16
E-mail address: Harris.Lucinda@mayo.edu

Clin Geriatr Med 37 (2021) 85–102
https://doi.org/10.1016/j.cger.2020.08.007
0749-0690/21/© 2020 Elsevier Inc. All rights reserved.

women and 26% in men more than 85 years of age.[2] In long-term care facilities, the prevalence of constipation may increase to almost 80%.[1,3] It is important to recognize that management of constipation in older individuals has inherent challenges that must be recognized in order to properly diagnose and treat this condition more effectively. This article discusses the definition of constipation, outlines the epidemiology of this disorder, as well as providing an understanding of the physiology of constipation in older individuals. Diagnostic approach as well as the non-pharmacologic and pharmacologic aspects of treatment, including evolving treatments, are discussed.

DEFINITION OF CONSTIPATION

The Rome criteria for constipation have recently been modified and define constipation as having 2 or more of the following features: less than 3 bowel movements per week, or for at least 25% of bowel movements having hard or lumpy stools, straining at stool, use of digital maneuvers, sensation of incomplete evaluation, or sensation of anorectal obstruction.[4] Loose stools should rarely be present without the use of laxatives and the criteria listed earlier should be fulfilled for the last 3 months with symptom onset starting at least 6 months before diagnosis. Although this newest definition states that there should be insufficient criteria for a diagnosis of irritable bowel syndrome, it does acknowledge that patients with constipation may have pain or bloating but that these should not be the predominant symptoms. The new criteria do recognize that these disorders should be thought of as a continuum rather than a distinct entity.

Constipation can be further divided into primary and secondary causes. Primary causes include slow transit constipation, pelvic floor dysfunction, and normal transit constipation. Patients with slow transit constipation have delayed transit of stool through the colon and this may be caused by primary defects in innervation of the gut (neuropathic) and/or the colonic smooth muscle (myopathic). Patients with pelvic floor dysfunction have difficulty expelling bowel movements because of inability to relax pelvic floor muscle, or improper coordination of abdominal and pelvic floor muscles while defecating, or the inability to produce the necessary propulsive forces in the rectum. Patients with normal transit constipation may also include patients with irritable bowel syndrome with constipation (IBS-C), for whom pain or discomfort is predominant and is relieved with defecation.[2] Irritable bowel syndrome may be less common in the elderly but it is still part of the spectrum of constipation in this age group. Also, it is important to realize that pelvic floor disorders may overlap in both normal and slow transit defecation.

Secondary causes of constipation can include neurologic disorders, medications, endocrine and metabolic disorders, myopathic disorders, cancer, paraneoplastic conditions, and medications (**Table 1**). Diet, psychological factors, and lifestyle may be additional contributory factors.

SPECIAL CONSIDERATIONS IN THE ELDERLY

A variety of pathophysiologic changes occur in the colon, sphincter muscles, and rectum in elderly individuals. **Table 2** summarizes these pathophysiologic changes and their clinical significance. These changes involve receptors in the colon as well as anatomic changes in the rectum resulting in changes in sensation, motor function, and reservoir function.[5]

Table 1
Common causes of constipation in the elderly

Lifestyle	Diet (low fiber, low intake, very high fiber, high protein), sedentary lifestyle, travel, dehydration, ignoring the urge to defecate, anorexia
Medications	Anabolic steroids, analgesics (NSAIDs and opioids), antacids containing aluminum or calcium, anticholinergics, anticonvulsants, antidepressants (TCAs, NSRIs), antihistamines, antihypertensives (eg, calcium channel blockers, clonidine), anti-Parkinson medications, bile-binding agents (eg, cholestyramine), calcium or iron supplements, diuretics
Metabolic	Hypokalemia, hypercalcemia, hyperglycemia, chronic renal insufficiency
Endocrine disorders	Diabetes mellitus, hypothyroidism, pregnancy, porphyria, panhypopituitarism
Neuropathic disorders	Autonomic neuropathy, chronic intestinal pseudo-obstruction, Hirschsprung disease, multiple sclerosis, Parkinson disease, spinal cord injury
Myopathic	Amyloidosis, chronic intestinal pseudo-obstruction, dermatomyositis, scleroderma, myotonic dystrophy
Idiopathic	Ischemia, stroke
Intestinal disorders	Adenoma, cancer (colon or metastatic), diverticulitis/diverticulosis, adhesions, obstruction, hernia, foreign bodies, fecal impaction, inflammatory bowel disease, stenosis
Anorectal abnormalities	Rectocele, anal fissures/fistula, anal stenosis, proctitis, inflamed or thrombosed hemorrhoids

Abbreviations: NSAIDs, nonsteroidal antiinflammatory drugs; TCAs, tricyclic antidepressants; NSRI, Serotonin and Norepinephrine Reuptake Inhibitor.

DIAGNOSTIC CONSIDERATIONS
History and Physical Examination

Although many individuals more than 65 years of age are intact mentally and physically, history taking can be challenging when problems with vision, hearing, and memory occur. Clinicians must be vigilant and thorough. For instance, ascertaining what the patient means by constipation is particularly important: questions about stool form; frequency; straining; use of manual maneuvers; and occurrence of fecal impaction, seepage, and incontinence all are important. Elderly patients may have seepage or incontinence that reflects possible watery stool around solid stool but also reflects the physiologic changes noted earlier. It is also essential to take a social history and inquire about diet, living conditions, social supports, stressors, psychiatric comorbidities, and the patient's ability to do activities of daily living. Clinicians must screen also for alarm symptoms such as loss of appetite, weight loss, and sudden change in bowel function or bleeding.

Table 2
Physiologic changes in the elderly colon/rectum

Anatomic Structure	Defect	Pathophysiologic Change	Clinical Result
Colon			
Number of HAPCs	Decreased	Colonic propulsion decreased	Constipation
Transit time	Slowed	Colon transit slowed	
Anus			
Anal sphincter length	Decreased	Sphincter is weakened	Seepage/urgency/incontinence
Internal anal sphincter	Thinned/atrophic	Sphincter is weakened	Seepage/incontinence
External anal sphincter	Thinned/atrophic	Sphincter is weakened	Urgency/incontinence
Rectum			
Sensation	Decreased	Colorectal sensorimotor function is impaired	Seepage/incontinence
Compliance	Decreased	Reservoir function is impaired	Urgency/incontinence
Capacity	Decreased	Reservoir function is impaired	Urgency/incontinence
Pudendal Nerve			
—	Decreased function	Colorectal sensorimotor function is impaired	Seepage/incontinence

Abbreviation: HAPCs, high-amplitude propagating contractions.

When doing the physical examination, the clinician should observe the patient for general condition and mobility. A careful abdominal examination should involve looking for distention, feeling for palpable masses or stool, and inquiring and examining for hernias. The importance of the digital rectal examination cannot be overemphasized. The examination should be performed in the left lateral decubitus position. The perianal region should be inspected for skin lesions, hemorrhoids, and fissures. On digital examination, clinicians should be attentive to resting anal tone and ask the patient to squeeze and bear down to assess for pelvic floor dyssynergia or evidence of excessive perineal descent. Sensation can be assessed by using a Q-tip to stroke the perineal skin around the anus in a 4-quadrant fashion looking for the so-called anal wink. Neuropathy should be suspected if this does not occur.

Diagnostics

Basic blood work, such as complete blood count, comprehensive metabolic profile (includes calcium), and thyroid function tests, can be performed to rule out anemia and a metabolic disorder. Structural testing, such as a flexible sigmoidoscopy or colonoscopy, should be performed to rule out malignancy, inflammatory bowel disease, or solitary rectal ulcer syndrome. Mucosal findings of melanosis coli might provide evidence of chronic laxative use. Recent guidelines suggest that colon cancer screening should be started at age 45 years; at advanced ages, routine colon cancer screening may not be warranted and should be tailored to the individual.[6] Other structural examinations include radiologic procedures such as computed tomography (CT) scan of the abdomen and pelvis and pelvic ultrasonography (abdominal and transvaginal), which may help exclude malignancies. Ovarian tumors may present as bloating and change in bowel habits.[7] The abdominal flat plate radiograph may be helpful to assess stool burden, obstruction, and impaction.

Physiologic tests are particularly helpful in diagnosing disorders of pelvic floor dysfunction or slow transit constipation. The primary test used to evaluate the pelvic floor is anal rectal manometry. This test can provide information on strength, tone, and sensation in the anus and rectum.[8] In addition, the balloon expulsion test, which is a 4-cm balloon filled with 50 mL of warm water or a silicon-filled stool-like device (fecom), is used to test function.[9] Most individuals can expel the balloon within 1 minute, and inability to do so is highly correlated with dyssynergic defecation.

Barium defecography or dynamic pelvic MRI defecography study not only provides information on pelvic floor function but can reveal structural abnormalities such as rectoceles, enteroceles, or pelvic organ prolapse that are also contributing to constipation.

Transit through the colon can be assessed with a Sitzmark capsule study, which contains 24 radio-opaque markers. The patient swallows the capsule on day 1 and an abdominal radiograph is taken on day 6. In patients with normal transit, fewer than 5 markers should be present.[10] The presence of 6 or more markers spread throughout the colon is suggestive of slow transit constipation.[10] An additional modality to assess transit is the wireless motility capsule. This swallowed device can assess both regional and whole-gut transit, and a recent study has confirmed its safety in the elderly.[11] Nuclear scintigraphy can be used to measure gastric, colonic, or whole-gut transit, but only a few centers in the United States perform the study.

LIFESTYLE AND DIETARY MODIFICATION

First-line therapies for the treatment of constipation consist of discussing diet, exercise, and bowel management techniques. Physicians may find it challenging to cover all of these issues in a single visit, so use of a nurse practitioner or a physician's assistant to perform dedicated counseling may be helpful in educating patients about this condition. **Box 1** covers important features of the nurse/physician assistant education material. Patients can also bring a significant other/caretaker to assist with remembering important teaching points. Helping patients understand the anatomy of the colon and pelvic floor may be the first step in empowering the patients to understand their conditions. In addition, the physician extender can review medications and also help identify issues that are interfering with patient compliance, such as visual impairments, hearing deficits, dietary habits, and declining cognitive function. Patients are encouraged to set up a schedule for defecation and take advantage of the stronger physiologic contractions that occur early in the morning. These contractions can be further stimulated by physical activity, eating a meal that includes fiber, and a hot beverage with caffeine (if feasible), which can intensify the gastrocolic reflex. Patients are encouraged to keep a stool diary that documents bowel movements, stool form based on the Bristol stool form scale,[12] and need to strain or use manual maneuvers and medications taken to improve defecation. Such visits can also be used to properly teach breathing techniques and use of manual maneuvers to facilitate defecation, such as splinting.

Dietary fiber in the average Western diet is often inadequate and usually about half the recommended dose.[13] Current recommendations suggest that women get 20 to 28 g of fiber and men get 30 to 38 g of fiber in their diets.[14] Patients should be encouraged to increase dietary fiber in the forms of nuts, fruits, and vegetables. Soluble fiber can create less gas and bloating than insoluble fiber. The goal is to increase fiber slowly by no more than 5 g/wk and to increase it as tolerated. Patients with slow transit

> **Box 1**
> **Tips for teaching bowel management techniques**
>
> - Assess the patient's functional status: cognitive abilities, visual and hearing impairments.
> - Review patient medications, both prescription and nonprescription (do not forget to ask about supplements), to identify medications that may exacerbate constipation.
> - Discuss diet and encourage increasing fiber to appropriate levels (20–28 g/d for women, 30–38 g/d for men) and also increasing fluids (5–8 235-mL [8 oz] glasses of water/hydrating fluids per day) as allowed.
> - Encourage patient to keep a diary of diet and bowel movements and form over 1 week, which may indicate dietary and fluid intake (a diary incorporating Bristol stool form may be helpful).
> - Encourage patient to eat breakfast with a hot beverage to help with the gastrocolic reflex.
> - Encourage daily physical activity if the patient is able.
> - Encourage patients to listen to their bodies and go to the bathroom when the urge occurs.
> - Use of anatomic drawings may aide in patients' understanding of their condition, especially pelvic floor maneuvers to assist with defecation.
> - When sitting on the toilet, patients should sit tall and use a small stool under their feet. Ideal toileting time is 3 to 5 minutes, but definitely not more than 10 minutes.
> - To assist with pelvic floor function and increasing intra-abdominal pressure, patients should use diaphragmatic breathing, which involves taking a deep breath and exhaling slowly over 10 seconds while pushing the stomach forward and relaxing the anus. Allow 20 seconds between breaths.
> - Patients should be instructed not to strain because this creates pelvic floor congestion. Relaxation of strain reverses the congestion.

constipation may not be able to reach the desired goals, and some patients with excessive bloating may respond better with alternative diets, such as the low-FODMAP (fermentable oligosaccharides, disaccharides, monosaccharides and polyols) diet. There is also evidence that prunes and kiwi fruit specifically can be efficacious in increasing gut motility.[15,16]

PHARMACOLOGIC TREATMENTS FOR CHRONIC CONSTIPATION

If dietary and lifestyle modifications do not successfully, or only partially, relieve symptoms, pharmacologic therapies should be considered as the next therapeutic option. In addition to appropriate classification into normal or slow transit constipation with or without pelvic floor dysfunction, treatment in the elderly should be individualized with special consideration of the patient's medical history (cardiac, neurologic, and renal comorbidities), mobility and functional status, level of independence of living, cost of therapy, medications, and potential adverse effects and interactions.[17] The treatment of chronic constipation in the elderly may also be challenging because older adults who have a cumulative incidence of chronic constipation for many years, or even decades, compared with younger patients, may have more treatment-refractory symptoms.[18] Elderly adults may also be more at risk of constipation because they may be on constipating medications such as calcium channel blockers, antidepressants, analgesics, antiparkinsonian drugs, antacids, and diuretics.[19] Moreover, with pharmacotherapy for constipation, elderly patients are at a higher risk of fecal incontinence in response to catharsis, an under-reported symptom, compared with younger patients.[20,21] It is important to consider all these factors before proceeding to pharmacotherapy. Commonly used over-the-counter treatments for chronic constipation are listed in **Table 3**.

Soluble fiber supplements are bulk-forming agents that have been shown to improve constipation and should be used as the first-line treatment. Bowel function is facilitated by increasing water absorbency of the stool.[22] Synthetic bulking agents include psyllium, methylcellulose, calcium polycarbophil, and wheat dextrin (US trade name Benefiber). Despite widespread use of bulking agents, the evidence regarding their efficacy has been inconsistent.[23,24] The dose of these agents may be increased gradually on a weekly basis to maximize efficacy and minimize adverse side effects, such as bloating, flatulence, abdominal cramping, and (rarely) diarrhea. They may be used alone or in combination with laxatives or other cathartic medications. Patients with slow transit constipation or anatomic or functional issues with evacuation are likely not to benefit from fiber supplementation and may experience exacerbation of symptoms.[19]

In patients not responding to bulk laxatives alone, the addition of osmotic laxatives should be considered as a next step. High-molecular-weight polyethylene glycol (PEG) is a large polymer with substantial osmotic activity that holds on to intraluminal

Table 3
Over-the-counter treatments for constipation

Medication	Mechanism of Action	Recommended Dosing	Efficacy (NNT)	Possible Side Effects
Calcium polycarbophil Or Methylcellulose Or Wheat dextrin	Bulking agent	Variable: titrate to effect	NA	Bloating, abdominal cramps, flatulence, or rarely diarrhea
Psyllium	Bulking agent	Variable: titrate to effect	1–3	Bloating, abdominal cramps, diarrhea
PEG	Osmotic agent	17 g	2–4	Nausea, bloating, diarrhea, flatulence, abdominal cramps
Magnesium-based laxatives	Osmotic agent	Variable	NA	Nausea, vomiting, electrolyte disturbances in CKD
Bisacodyl (5 mg)	Stimulant	Two 5-mg tablets	4	Nausea, abdominal cramps, diarrhea
Senna (8.6 mg) Anthraquinone	Stimulant	2 tablets daily to 2 tablets twice a day	NA	Nausea, abdominal cramps, bloating, diarrhea, flatulence, melanosis coli
Cascara sagrada	Stimulant	2 tablets daily	NA	Nausea, abdominal cramps, bloating, diarrhea

Abbreviations: CKD, chronic kidney disease; NA, not available; NNT, number needed to treat; PEG, polyethylene glycol.

water by creating an osmotic gradient. By retaining or drawing water into the gut lumen, PEG use leads to increased bowel motility.[25] Several controlled trials, lasting up to 6 months, have revealed that this treatment is effective,[26] and studies up to 24 months have confirmed its safety.[27] The major side effects of PEG are bloating and flatulence.

Saline laxatives, including magnesium citrate, are also available over the counter and work by an osmotic effect with retention of fluid to increase stool frequency and consistency.[28] Magnesium-based laxatives should be used with caution in patients with kidney disease because they may develop hypermagnesemia, which may lead to prolongation of the QT interval, bradycardia, and hypotension.[29]

Stimulant laxatives such as bisacodyl and senna exert their primary effects through alteration of electrolyte transport in intestinal mucosa and enhancement of colonic motility.[30]

They can be used safely as rescue laxatives if patients have no bowel movements for 2 to 3 days[31]; however, long-term safety of stimulant laxatives has not been confirmed. Side effects include abdominal cramping, distention, nausea, and diarrhea. Although long-term use of stimulant laxatives that contain anthraquinone, such as senna, can cause melanosis coli, they do not seem to impair the enteric nervous system based on studies in animal models.[32,33] This knowledge should be used to dispel the notion that chronic use of these agents causes nerve damage and worsening constipation.

Although stool softeners, suppositories, enemas, and probiotics are commonly used, the evidence to support their use is lackluster. Bisacodyl or glycerin suppositories may be helpful in the elderly with a defecation disorder to aid in evacuation. The suppository should be given 30 minutes after breakfast in order to take advantage of the gastrocolic reflex.[34]

When over-the-counter treatments are ineffective in remedying chronic constipation, there are several prescription therapies available. Current prescription and US Food and Drug Administration (FDA)–approved pharmacologic treatments for chronic constipation are listed in **Table 4**. Studies investigating the efficacy and safety of pharmacologic agents used for treatment of chronic constipation in the elderly are limited. Trials of adult patients often include only a limited number of study subjects aged more than 65 years.

Lactulose is a prescription osmotic laxative that has been in use since the 1950s. It is a nonabsorbable carbohydrate that exerts its effect by altering intestinal osmolality. It is safe at a dose of 20 g (30 mL) once daily. Lactulose can cause significant abdominal bloating, discomfort, and flatulence, which may decrease patient acceptance and, because it contains lactose and galactose, caution must be used in patients with diabetes.[35]

Linaclotide and plecanatide are intestinal secretagogues approved by the FDA for treatment of chronic constipation. They are minimally absorbed peptide agonists of guanylate cyclase C receptor that bind on the apical side of intestinal epithelial cells, resulting in generation of cyclic guanosine monophosphate (cGMP). The increase of cGMP levels within the intestinal cells triggers a signal transduction cascade that activates the cystic fibrosis transmembrane conductance regulator. This activation causes secretion of chloride and bicarbonate into the intestinal lumen, increasing luminal fluid secretion and accelerating intestinal transit.[36,37] Linaclotide works in a pH-independent manner and is active in both the small and large intestines at a broad pH of 5 to 8, whereas plecanatide works in a pH-dependent way at more acidic pH of 5.5 to 7, and causes fluid secretion mostly in the upper small intestine. Linaclotide is available in 3 doses: 72, 145, and 290 μg daily. In elderly patients, a lower starting dose

Table 4
Prescription agents for constipation

Treatment	Mechanism of Action	Recommended Dose	Efficacy (NNT)	Potential Side Effects
Lactulose	Osmotic	20 g daily	NA	Bloating, cramping, diarrhea, flatulence, nausea, vomiting High doses may cause electrolyte disturbances
Linaclotide	GC receptor agonist	72 or 145 µg (CIC) or 290 µg (IBS-C) daily	10	Diarrhea, cramping, flatulence, headache
Plecanatide	GC receptor agonist	3 mg daily	11–12	Diarrhea
Lubiprostone	Chloride channel activator	8 µg BID (IBS-C, women only) 24 µg BID (CIC)	3–6	Nausea,[a] diarrhea, SOB
Prucalopride	Serotonin (5-HT4) receptor agonist	2 mg daily, 1 mg for severe renal disease or ESRD	5–9	Diarrhea, headache, <1% suicidal ideation/depression
Tepanor	Inhibitor of sodium/hydrogen exchanger 3	50 mg BID (IBS-C only)	NA	Diarrhea, bloating, flatulence

Abbreviations: 5-HT4, 5-hydroxytryptamine 4; BID, twice daily; CIC, chronic idiopathic constipation; ESRD, end-stage renal disease; GC, guanylate cyclase; IBS-C, irritable bowel syndrome with constipation; SOB, Shortness of breath; NNT, number needed to treat.

[a] Nausea: higher incidence at 24-µg dose (31%); at 8-µg dose, nausea occurred in 8%. Recommended to take medication with food.

may be prudent. Plecanatide is available in the single dose of 3 mg daily. The main adverse reaction to both linaclotide and plecanatide is diarrhea, occurring at a rate of 16% to 19% and 5% respectively.[37–39] Reassuring data from a recent pooled analysis of 451 patients more than 65 years of age with both chronic idiopathic constipation and IBS-C confirmed that plecanatide is well tolerated in the elderly demographic and no serious events of diarrhea occurred.[40]

Lubiprostone, another intestinal secretagogue approved by the FDA for chronic constipation at a dose of 24 µg twice a day and IBS-C–predominant constipation at 8 µg twice a day, is a bicyclic fatty acid derivative of prostaglandin E1 that increases fluid secretion into the lumen of the intestine by activating apical chloride channel 2. By increasing intestinal fluid secretion, transit time in both small and large intestines is accelerated.[41] The dose for chronic constipation is 24 µg twice a day. The main side effect is nausea, which can be mitigated when the medication is taken with meals. Lubiprostone has been also approved by the FDA for treatment of opioid-induced constipation.

In 2018, the FDA approved prucalopride for the treatment of chronic constipation. It is a highly selective serotonin 5-hydroxytryptamine 4 (5-HT4) receptor agonist that increases the release of serotonin (5-HT) by the enterochromaffin cells in the intestinal mucosa of the small bowel. It acts on neurons along the enteric nervous system. By releasing acetylcholine, it stimulates intestinal motility directly. In addition, it secretes fluid into the intestines, which has an additional prokinetic effect. Prucalopride at a dosage of 1 and 4 mg once daily was found to be superior to placebo in 4-week and 12-week trials. It was safe and well tolerated in patients 65 years of age or older.[42,43] In the United States, the recommended dose in adults is 2 mg once daily with a lower dose (1 mg daily) recommended for patients with kidney disease. Adverse events include abdominal pain, nausea, diarrhea, abdominal bloating, flatulence, headache, dizziness, and fatigue. Uncommon but potentially serious adverse events include exacerbation of depression and suicidality, warranting extreme caution in at-risk patients. Two 5-HT4 receptor agonists were approved for treatment of chronic constipation in the past (cisapride in 1993, tegaserod in 2002), but both were subsequently withdrawn from general use because of serious cardiovascular events, including cardiac ischemia, strokes, cardiac arrhythmias, and prolongation of the corrected QT interval. Tegaserod became available again in 2019 but is only recommended for patients between the ages of 18 and 65 years.[44] Prucalopride is a highly selective 5-HT4 receptor agonist that has not been associated with any cardiovascular adverse events.[45]

Tenapanor is a first-in-class agent, a selective sodium-hydrogen exchanger (NHE3) inhibitor that was approved in 2019 for the treatment of IBS-C.[46] It also is approved to treat hyperphosphatemia in patients with chronic kidney disease. It works by decreasing the absorption of sodium from the intestines, resulting in water secretion in the lumen, which in turn causes softer stool because of increased intestinal transit. In phase III double-blind, placebo controlled trials, tenapanor 50 mg twice daily met the combined primary end point of greater than or equal to 30% reduction in abdominal pain and an increase of greater than or equal to 1 completed spontaneous bowel movement in the same week for greater than or equal to 6 of 12 treatment weeks.[47,48] Chief side effects were diarrhea and abdominal distention.[46]

FECAL IMPACTION

If constipation continues to be an issue, awareness of the risk of fecal impaction must be present. Fecal impaction results from the person's inability to sense a stool in the rectum, and this impaired sensitivity fails to provide a signal for the bowel to evacuate. Risk factors include altered abnormal anatomy, such as an anal stricture or rectal mass, in addition to rectal sensorimotor dysfunction and decreased mobility, which are more common in institutionalized elderly.[49] Rectal examination is essential in the evaluation of constipation and may reveal a rectum full of hardened stool. The practitioner must also be aware that the impaction may occur above the rectum, in which case abdominal radiograph or cross-sectional imaging may be required for detection. Treatment of fecal impaction includes digital disimpaction with manual fragmentation followed by warm-water enemas. If this is ineffective, distal colonic cleansing using warm-water enemas with the aid of a sigmoidoscopic or use of water-soluble contrast media such as Gastrografin for both diagnostic and therapeutic purposes may be necessary.[50] In rare cases, if there is abdominal tenderness and a concern for ischemia or perforation, emergent imaging with CT and possible surgery may be required because a rare complication of fecal impaction is stercoral ulcer perforation.[51] Because recurrence of fecal impaction is common, it is important to treat constipation proactively with dietary measures, adequate fluids, and pharmacotherapies.

BIOFEEDBACK/VISCERAL MANIPULATION

Elderly patients who do not respond to medical therapy or who have had fecal impaction may also meet Rome IV criteria for a defecation disorder.[52] Defecation disorders result in impaired evacuation with inadequate or absent intrarectal propulsion and either paradoxic or inadequate anal sphincter relaxation during simulated defecation.

This important cause of chronic constipation is likely underdiagnosed because, in addition to clinical suspicion, physiologic testing such as anorectal manometry, balloon expulsion testing, colon transit study, or fluoroscopic or magnetic resonance defecography is required, but may not be readily available. If a defecation disorder without evidence of structural abnormality such as rectocele, enterocele, or prolapse is identified, biofeedback-aided pelvic floor therapy is the best management option. Even if those structural abnormalities are present, conservative biofeedback/pelvic floor rehabilitation by an experienced practitioner is still warranted if possible. Often, patients with a defecation disorder may also have an epiphenomenon or coexistent slow transit constipation, and treatments for these disorders may need to be combined.[53] With biofeedback, defecation disorders have been shown to be eliminated in 91% of patients, and 85% had confirmed improvement in the balloon expulsion test.[54] However, high-quality biofeedback may not be widely available. Furthermore, patients need to participate actively in this form of therapy and this may not be always possible if limitations in mobility or cognition are present. Medicare and Medicaid in most states in the United States now provide coverage of this effective treatment.

Another therapy for patients who fail biofeedback is visceral manipulation. Visceral manipulation is being taught by physical therapists, has commonly also been used by osteopaths, and can be used in patients who fail biofeedback.[55] There are no randomized controlled studies of this modality, but a small study in elderly patients with stroke showed that, compared with standard physical therapy, there were significant improvements in several intestinal symptoms, including abdominal pain/discomfort, frequency of bowel movements, and bloating.[56] An added advantage of this therapy is that it does not require the patient to be mobile, although studies suggest that physical activity does help with constipation.

SURGICAL INTERVENTIONS

Surgical interventions should be approached carefully in elderly patients, who may have comorbidities that increase risk. If a patient with severe slow transit constipation without global gut hypomotility and or defecation dysfunction is refractory to medical treatments, subtotal colectomy with ileorectal anastomosis could be considered.[57] Confidence that there is no element of defecation disorder and that the underlying cause is a motility delay is imperative to avoid poor postoperative outcomes. Alternatively, less invasive surgeries, such as percutaneous endoscopic cecostomy with insertion of an indwelling catheter or appendiceal conduit (Malone procedure), may be used to infuse water into proximal colon. These minimally invasive surgeries can be performed under local anesthesia with conscious sedation, making them less risky.[58] Potential postoperative intestinal complications include ileus, anastomotic leakage or bleeding, small bowel obstruction, and wound infection. Emergent endoscopy and subsequent surgery may be required for obstruction from a sigmoid or cecal volvulus (and bascule subtype), which may result from long-standing constipation and associated colonic redundancy.[59]

NOVEL TREATMENTS

Several small studies have evaluated sacral nerve stimulation (SNS) in chronic constipation but the results have been conflicting. A recent report showed that SNS has a 30% response in refractory constipation.[60] Bilateral transcutaneous tibial nerve stimulation was studied in a small number of geriatric patients (aged >65 years) with refractory chronic constipation and showed a reduction in both time spent on the toilet and stool softener use.[61] Neither of these treatments has been approved by the FDA at the time of this writing.

In addition, a vibrating capsule is also under investigation for the treatment of constipation (Vibrant capsule). It is made of biocompatible materials that stimulate the walls of the large intestine to increase peristalsis and generate spontaneous bowel movements.[62] There have been 2 double-blind sham-controlled phase II studies in patients with chronic constipation. The studies differed in the way the pulses were delivered from the capsules. Post hoc analyses of the 2 studies showed that, during and within 3 hours of the onset of vibrations, there was a significantly greater percentage of complete spontaneous bowel movements in the active group compared with the sham group, but overall responder rates were not different between the 2 groups. The only serious adverse event was an anxiety attack in 1 patient.

OPIOID-INDUCED CONSTIPATION

Opioid analgesic therapy is commonly used to treat chronic noncancer pain in adults, including elderly patients. Opioid-induced constipation (OIC) is the most common adverse effect, occurring at a rate of 41%.[63] Evidence suggests the risk of OIC increases with age.[64] Opioids cause constipation by blocking opioid receptors, including the μ-opioid receptor, and cause slowing of colonic transit and decreasing intestinal and colonic secretion.[65] Nonpharmacologic and pharmacologic treatments that are available for the management of OIC have not been well studied in the elderly, and treatment guidelines specifically for the management of elderly patients with OIC are not available. However, a review of the evidence in the literature for treatment of adult patients with OIC recommends nonpharmacologic interventions (eg, dietary measures, increased fluid ingestion, increased physical activity, biofeedback training), and use of over-the-counter laxatives as first-line therapy.[66] However, these initial measures are ineffective in more than 50% of patients. More recently, a new generation of therapeutic agents known as peripherally acting μ-opioid receptor antagonists (PAMORAs) has been tested in OIC, and some of these agents directly target opioid receptors in the gut. A recent American Gastroenterological Association Institute Technical Review on the Medical Management of

Table 5		
Peripherally acting μ-opioid receptor antagonists used in opioid-induced constipation		
Medication	**Dose**	**Side Effects**
Methylnaltrexone	450 mg daily orally Or 8 mg/0.6 mL SC daily Or 12 mg/0.6 mL SC daily	Abdominal pain Opioid withdrawal (rare) Renal/liver failure requires dose adjustment Bowel tear
Naldemedine	0.2 mg orally daily	Abdominal pain Nausea and vomiting Diarrhea Bowel tear
Naloxegol	12.5–25 mg orally daily[a]	Abdominal pain Diarrhea Opioid withdrawal (rare) Bowel tear

Abbreviation: SC, subcutaneous.
[a] Do not take with grapefruit juice.

OIC that focused on the efficacy of laxatives, PAMORAs (naldemedine, naloxegol, alvimopan, and methylnaltrexone), selective 5-HT agonists (prucalopride), and intestinal secretagogues (lubiprostone) concluded that there was indirect evidence (moderate quality) that supported the use of over-the-counter laxatives but there were insufficient data comparing the efficacy of laxatives versus prescription medications targeted to treat OIC.[67] The investigators also found that there was evidence to support the use of naldemedine (high-quality evidence), naloxegol (moderate quality), and methylnaltrexone (low quality) for OIC but limited evidence to support the use of lubiprostone (low quality) and prucalopride (low quality). The findings in this review are consistent with other recent systematic reviews of therapies for the management of OIC.[68,69] Of note, analysis of 3 phase 3 clinical trials in patients aged greater than or equal to 65 years showed that naldemedine was effective in OIC, 51.8% versus 37.6% in placebo, which was statistically significant. **Table 5** provides a listing of PAMORAs and doses used in OIC.

SUMMARY

Chronic constipation in the elderly is a common digestive symptom that adversely affects quality of life and health care costs. Its reported prevalence is high, especially for patients living in residential care. A comprehensive evaluation of historical factors unique to this demographic includes mobility assessment, access to food and hydration, coexistent conditions, and the medications used to treat them. Careful physical examination and physiologic testing if first-line interventions fail is key to managing elderly patients, who may have an overly robust response to catharsis and incontinence if diminished rectal sensorimotor dysfunction or sphincteric weakness is present, exacerbation of abdominal distress if a defecation disorder or fecal impaction is present, and coexistent physical limitations worsening symptoms. Diet and lifestyle modifications are often ineffective to manage constipation in the elderly and a multifactorial approach is suggested. Fiber supplementation, regimented bowel routines and behavior techniques, and osmotic laxatives are an effective first line of therapy for many patients. A consistent clinical history of issues with evacuation or inadequate or paradoxic response to standard initial therapy should prompt an assessment for a defecation disorder. If identified, and the patient is able to participate, biofeedback is the treatment of choice. Although data to support safety in this demographic are sparse, there is evidence to support safety and efficacy of pharmacotherapy, including secretagogues and the prokinetics linaclotide and prucalopride in the elderly. The prokinetic agent tegaserod should be avoided in patients 65 years of age or older because of the risk of cardiac and intestinal ischemia. Use of lactulose may be limited because of increased diarrhea if lactose intolerance is present, and magnesium-based cathartic agents may put patients with renal disease at risk of toxicity. Surgery is rarely indicated in the management of constipation. Novel treatments need to be explored in larger clinical trials. Additional attention to addressing therapy for constipation in the elderly is needed to tailor treatment in this complex population and to improve the quality of life of these patients while minimizing side effects of urgency, diarrhea, incontinence, and electrolyte derangements.

CLINICS CARE POINTS

- Clinicians must distinguish primary from secondary constipation in elderly individuals.

- Pelvic floor dysfunction significantly contributes to constipation in elderly individuals and rectal exam and anorectal manometry are important diagnostic tools
- Fecal seepage or incontinence do not rule out constipation and may reflect water around solid stool
- In patients with normal transit constipation increasing fiber supplementation and fluids is first line therapy
- Patients with slow transit constipation are not likely to benefit from fiber supplementation and may experience exacerbation of symptoms
- Treatment of pelvic floor dysfunction can improve CIC 20-50%.
- Linaclotide, Plecanatide, Lubiprostone and Prucalopride have all shown proven efficacy in treating chronic constipation
- Surgical treatment for constipation should primarily be considered only in severe slow transit constipation without serious co-morbidities
- For opioid induced constipation no studies have compared OTC laxative to PA-MORAs but moderate to high quality evidence exist for the use of naloxegol and naldemedine.

DISCLOSURE

S. Lucak: consultant for Abbie Vie, Allergan, and Ironwood; speaker's bureau for Abbie Vie, Alfasigma, and Ironwood. T.N. Lunsford: Biomerica InFoods IBS technology. L.A. Harris has done consulting for Allergan, Ironwood, Salix Pharmaceuticals, Takeda (formerly Shire), Commonwealth Laboratories, and the Rome Foundation.

REFERENCES

1. Suares NC, Ford AC. Prevalence and risk factors of chronic idiopathic constipation in the community: systematic review and meta-analysis. Am J Gastroenterol 2011;106:1582–91.
2. Gallegos-Orozco JF, Foxx-Orenstein AE, Sterler S, et al. Chronic constipation in the elderly. Am J Gastroenterol 2012;107:18–25.
3. Fleming V, Wade WE. A review of laxative therapies for treatment of chronic constipation in older adults. Am J Geriatr Pharmacother 2010;8:514–50.
4. Mearin F, Lacy BE, Chang L, et al. Bowel disorders. Gastroenterology 2016;150: 1393–407.
5. Yu SW, Rao SS. Anorectal physiology and pathophysiology in the elderly. Clin Geriatr Med 2014;30(1):95–106.
6. Wolf AMD, Fontham ETH, Church TR, et al. Colorectal cancer screening in average –risk adults: 2018 guideline update from the American Cancer Society. CA Cancer J Clin 2018;68(4):250–81.
7. Olson SH, Mignone L, Nakraseive C, et al. Symptoms of ovarian cancer. Obstet Gynecol 2001;98(2):212–7.
8. Rao SS, Singh S. Clinical utility of colonic and anorectal manometry in chronic constipation. J Clin Gastroenterol 2010;44(9):597–609.
9. Lee BE, Kim GH. How to perform and interpret balloon expulsion test. J Neurogastroenterol Motil 2014;20(3):407–9.
10. Bharucha AD, Phillips SF. Slow transit constipation. Gastroenterol Clin North Am 2001;30(1):77–95.
11. Rao SS, Paulson J, Saad R, et al. Assessment of colonic, whole gut and regional transit in elderly constipated and healthy subjects with novel wireless pH/pressure capsule (Smart Pill®). Gastroenterology 2009;136:A950.

12. O'Donnell L, Virjee J, Heaton KW. Detection of pseudodiarrhoea by simple clinical assessment of intestinal transit rate. BMJ 1990;300:439–40.

13. Storey M, Anderson P. Intake and race/ethnicity influence dietary fiber intake and vegetable consumption. Nutr Res 2014;34:844–50.

14. U.S. Department of Health and Human Services and U.S. Department of Agriculture. 2015 – 2020 dietary guidelines for Americans. 8th Edition. December 2015. Available at: http://health.gov/dietaryguidelines/2015/guidelines/. Accessed July 5, 2020.

15. Attaluri A, Donahoe R, Valestin J, et al. Randomised clinical trial: dried plums (prunes) vs. psyllium for constipation. Aliment Pharmacol Ther 2011;33(7):822–8.

16. Chang CC, Lin YT, Lu YT, et al. Kiwifruit improves bowel function in patients with irritable bowel syndrome with constipation. Asia Pac J Clin Nutr 2010;19(4):451–7.

17. Locke GR 3rd, Pemberton JH, Phillips SF. American Gastroenterological Association Medical Position Statement: guidelines on constipation. Gastroenterology 2000;119(6):1761–6.

18. Choung RS, Locke GR 3rd, Rey E, et al. Factors associated with persistent and nonpersistent chronic constipation, over 20 years. Clin Gastroenterol Hepatol 2012;10(5):494–500.

19. Vazquez Roque M, Bouras EP. Epidemiology and management of chronic constipation in elderly patients. Clin Interv Aging 2015;10:919–30.

20. Ditah I, Devaki P, Luma HN, et al. Prevalence, trends, and risk factors for fecal incontinence in United States adults, 2005-2010. Clin Gastroenterol Hepatol 2014;12(4):636–43.e2.

21. Leung FW, Rao SS. Approach to fecal incontinence and constipation in older hospitalized patients. Hosp Pract 2011;39(1):97–104.

22. Suares NC, Ford AC. Systematic review: the effects of fibre in the management of chronic idiopathic constipation. Aliment Pharmacol Ther 2011;33(8):895–901.

23. American College of Gastroenterology Chronic Constipation Task Force. An evidence-based approach to the management of chronic constipation in North America. Am J Gastroenterol 2005;100(Suppl 1):S1-S4.

24. Ramkumar D, Rao SS. Efficacy and safety of traditional medical therapies for chronic constipation: systematic review. Am J Gastroenterol 2005;100(4):936–71.

25. Schiller LR, Emmett M, Santa Ana CA, et al. Osmotic effects of polyethylene glycol. Gastroenterology 1988;94(4):933–41.

26. Di Palma JA, Cleveland MV, McGowan J, et al. A randomized, multicenter comparison of polyethylene glycol laxative and tegaserod in treatment of patients with chronic constipation. Am J Gastroenterol 2007;102(9):1964–71.

27. Corazziari E, Badiali D, Bazzocchi G, et al. Long term efficacy, safety, and tolerability of low daily doses of isosmotic polyethylene glycol electrolyte balanced solution (PMF-100) in the treatment of functional chronic constipation. Gut 2000;46(4):522–6.

28. Dupont C, Campagne A, Constant F. Efficacy and safety of a magnesium sulfate-rich natural mineral water for patients with functional constipation. Clin Gastroenterol Hepatol 2014;12(8):1280–7.

29. Nishikawa M, Shimada N, Kanzaki M, et al. The characteristics of patients with hypermagnesemia who underwent emergency hemodialysis. Acute Med Surg 2018;5(3):222–9.

30. Schiller LR. Review article: the therapy of constipation. Aliment Pharmacol Ther 2001;15(6):749–63.

31. Kienzle-Horn S, Vix JM, Schuijt C, et al. Efficacy and safety of bisacodyl in the acute treatment of constipation: a double-blind, randomized, placebo-controlled study. Aliment Pharmacol Ther 2006;23(10):1479–88.

32. Kiernan JA, Heinicke EA. Sennosides do not kill myenteric neurons in the colon of the rat or mouse. Neuroscience 1989;30(3):837–42.

33. Tack J, Müller-Lissner S, Stanghellini V, et al. Diagnosis and treatment of chronic constipation–a European perspective. Neurogastroenterol Motil 2011;23(8):697–710.

34. Bharucha AE, Wald A. Chronic constipation. Mayo Clin Proc 2019;94(11):2340–57.

35. Bass P, Dennis S. The laxative effects of lactulose in normal and constipated subjects. J Clin Gastroenterol 1981;3(Suppl 1):23–8.

36. Bryant AP, Busby RW, Bartolini WP, et al. Linaclotide is a potent and selective guanylate cyclase C agonist that elicits pharmacological effects locally in the gastrointestinal tract. Life Sci 2010;86(19–20):760–5.

37. Sharma A, Herekar AA, Bhagatwala J, et al. Profile of plecanatide in the treatment of chronic idiopathic constipation: design, development, and place in therapy. Clin Exp Gastroenterol 2019;12:31–6.

38. Lembo AJ, Kurtz CB, Macdougall JE, et al. Efficacy of linaclotide for patients with chronic constipation. Gastroenterology 2010;138(3):886–95.e1.

39. Miner PB Jr, Koltun WD, Wiener GJ, et al. A randomized phase III clinical trial of plecanatide, a uroguanylin analog, in patients with chronic idiopathic constipation. Am J Gastroenterol 2017;112(4):613-621.

40. Menees SB, Franklin H, Chey WD. Evaluation of plecanatide for the treatment of chronic idiopathic constipation and irritable bowel syndrome-constipation in patients aged 65 or older. Clin Ther 2020;42(7):1406–14.

41. Barish CF, Drossman D, Johanson JF, et al. Efficacy and safety of lubiprostone in patients with chronic constipation. Dig Dis Sci 2010;55(4):1090–7.

42. Quigley EM, Vandeplassche L, Kerstens R, et al. Clinical trial: the efficacy, impact on quality of life, and safety and tolerability of prucalopride in severe chronic constipation–a 12-week, randomized, double-blind, placebo-controlled study. Aliment Pharmacol Ther 2009;29(3):315–28.

43. Müller-Lissner S, Rykx A, Kerstens R, et al. A double-blind, placebo-controlled study of prucalopride in elderly patients with chronic constipation. Neurogastroenterol Motil 2010;22(9):991.e5.

44. In brief: tegaserod (Zelnorm) returns. Med Lett Drugs Ther 2019;61(1571):72.

45. Vijayvargiya P, Camilleri M. Use of prucalopride in adults with chronic idiopathic constipation. Expert Rev Clin Pharmacol 2019;12(7):579–89.

46. Markham A. Tepanor: first approval. Drugs 2019;79:1897–903.

47. Chey WD, Lembo AJ, Korner P, et al. Efficacy and safety of tenapanor in patients with constipation predominant irritable bowel syndrome: a 12 week, double-blind, placebo-controlled, randomized phase 3 trial. Am J Gastroenterol 2017;112(Suppl 1):S226 [Abstract: 421].

48. Chey WD, Lembo AJ, Yan A, et al. Efficacy and safety of tenapanor in patients with constipation predominant irritable bowel syndrome: a 6-month, double-blind, placebo-controlled phase 3 trial (T3mpo-2). Gastroenterology 2018;154(6 Suppl 1):S-1362 [Abstract: 885].

49. De Giorgio R, Ruggeri E, Stanghellini V, et al. Chronic constipation in the elderly: a primer for the gastroenterologist. BMC Gastroenterol 2015;15:130.

50. Hussain ZH, Whitehead DA, Lacy BE. Fecal impaction. Curr Gastroenterol Rep 2014;16(9):404.

51. Vijayakumar C, Balagurunathan K, Prabhu R, et al. Stercoral ulcer not always indolent: a rare complication of fecal impaction. Cureus 2018;10(5):e2613.

52. Simren M, Palsson OS, Whitehead WE. Update on Rome IV criteria for colorectal disorders: implications for clinical practice. Curr Gastroenterol Rep 2017; 19(4):15.

53. Aziz I, Whitehead WE, Palsson OS, et al. An approach to the diagnosis and management of Rome IV functional disorders of chronic constipation. Expert Rev Gastroenterol Hepatol 2020;14(1):39–46.

54. Chiarioni G, Salandini L, Whitehead WE. Biofeedback benefits only patients with outlet dysfunction, not patients with isolated slow transit constipation. Gastroenterology 2005;129(1):86–97.

55. Archambault-Ezenwa L, Brewer J, Markowski A. A comprehensive physical therapy approach including visceral manipulation after failed biofeedback therapy for constipation. Tech Coloproctol 2016;20(8):603–7.

56. Pasin Neto H, Borges RA. Visceral mobilization and functional constipation in stroke survivors: a randomized, controlled, double-blind, clinical trial. Cureus 2020;12(5):e8058.

57. Bharucha AE, Rao SSC, Shin AS. Surgical interventions and the Use of device-aided therapy for the treatment of fecal incontinence and defecatory disorders. Clin Gastroenterol Hepatol 2017;15(12):1844-1854.

58. Wilkinson-Smith V, Bharucha AE, Emmanuel A, et al. When all seems lost: management of refractory constipation-Surgery, rectal irrigation, percutaneous endoscopic colostomy, and more. Neurogastroenterol Motil 2018;30(5):e13352.

59. Perrot L, Fohlen A, Alves A, et al. Management of the colonic volvulus in 2016. J Visc Surg 2016;153(3):183–92.

60. Gortazar de Las Casas S, Rubio-Pérez I, Saavedra Ambrosy J, et al. Sacral nerve stimulation for constipation: long-term outcomes. Tech Coloproctol 2019;23(6): 559–64.

61. Gokce AH, Gokce FS. Effects of bilateral transcutaneous tibial nerve stimulation on constipation severity in geriatric patients: a prospective clinical study. Geriatr Gerontol Int 2020;20(2):101–5.

62. Rao SSC, Lembo A, Chey WD, et al. Effects of the vibrating capsule on colonic circadian rhythm and bowel symptoms in chronic idiopathic constipation [published online ahead of print, 2020 May 25]. Neurogastroenterol Motil 2020;e13890. https://doi.org/10.1111/nmo.13890.

63. Kalso E, Edwards JE, Moore RA, et al. Opioids in chronic non-cancer pain: systematic review of efficacy and safety. Pain 2004;112(3):372–80.

64. Rosti G, Gatti A, Costantini A, et al. Opioid-related bowel dysfunction: prevalence and identification of predictive factors in a large sample of Italian patients on chronic treatment. Eur Rev Med Pharmacol Sci 2010;14(12):1045–50.

65. Kurz A, Sessler DI. Opioid-induced bowel dysfunction: pathophysiology and potential new therapies. Drugs 2003;63(7):649–71.

66. Dorn S, Lembo A, Cremonini F. Opioid-induced bowel dysfunction: epidemiology, pathophysiology, diagnosis, and initial therapeutic approach. Am J Gastroenterol Suppl 2014;2(1):31–7.

67. Hanson B, Siddique SM, Scarlett Y, et al. American Gastroenterological association Institute clinical guidelines Committee. American Gastroenterological association Institute Technical review on the medical management of opioid-induced constipation. Gastroenterology 2019;156(1):229–53.e5.

68. Luthra P, Burr NE, Brenner DM, et al. Efficacy of pharmacological therapies for the treatment of opioid-induced constipation: systematic review and network meta-analysis. Gut 2019;68(3):434–44.

69. Nee J, Zakari M, Sugarman MA, et al. Efficacy of treatments for opioid-induced constipation: systematic review and meta-analysis. Clin Gastroenterol Hepatol 2018;16(10):1569–84.e2.

Common Diarrheal Illnesses in the Elderly

Enad Dawod, MD[a], Carl V. Crawford, MD[b],*

KEYWORDS

- Diarrhea • Elderly • Geriatrics • Infectious diarrhea • *Clostridioides difficile* infection
- Malabsorption • Osmotic diarrhea • Secretory diarrhea

KEY POINTS

- Diarrhea is a common problem among the elderly that can have a spectrum of disease severity.
- Certain physiologic processes and mechanisms are specific in common diarrheal conditions.
- Fluid, medicinal, and nutritional management should be tailored to address the physiologic consequences of specific diarrheal causes.
- Early and correct management of diarrhea can decrease the risk of morbidity and mortality in the elderly.

INTRODUCTION

Diarrhea in the elderly, although a common medical symptom, can range from a benign self-limited disease to a life-threatening condition. Diarrhea can be defined as 3 or more unformed bowel movements or stool weight greater than 200 g in 24 hours due to disruption of the secretion and absorption of water and electrolytes within the small or large intestine. Risk factors for diarrhea depend on the patient's exposures, physical condition, comorbidities, and their treatments. The frailty of older adults places them at higher risk for morbidity and mortality from electrolyte abnormalities and dehydration, even from short episodes of diarrhea. The duration of illness can be acute lasting up to 2 weeks or chronic lasting longer than a month, each requiring specific diagnostic evaluations. Classification of diarrhea can fall into several physiologic and mechanistic groups: infectious, osmotic, secretory, promotile, or inflammatory.[1] An approach to common diarrheal scenarios with these mechanisms in mind will link the correct diagnosis to treatment while minimizing complications in the elderly.

[a] Department of Medicine, Weill Cornell Medicine, New York Presbyterian Hospital, 1305 York Avenue, 4th Floor, New York, NY 10021, USA; [b] Division of Gastroenterology, Weill Cornell Medicine, New York Presbyterian Hospital, 1305 York Avenue, 4th Floor, New York, NY 10021, USA
* Corresponding author.
E-mail address: cvc9002@med.cornell.edu

Clin Geriatr Med 37 (2021) 103–117
https://doi.org/10.1016/j.cger.2020.08.008
0749-0690/21/© 2020 Elsevier Inc. All rights reserved.

INFECTIOUS DIARRHEA

The elderly are especially prone to infectious diarrhea and its complications because of age-related physiologic changes in the gastrointestinal tract. Acquisition of enteric pathogens occurs through fecal-oral exposure from potential reservoirs where the elderly may cohort such as hospitals, nursing homes, and skilled nursing facilities. Age-related decreases in gastric acid production compromise the stomach's barrier function against ingested pathogens. Immunosenescence results in the gradual decline in the production of secretory immunoglobulin A, the primary immune response of the gut mucosal surface, and increases the risk for gut-specific infections.[2] An increase in morbidity and mortality from enteric infections in the elderly stems from acute renal failure from intravascular volume depletion, arrhythmia from electrolyte abnormalities, or complications from other comorbid conditions. To prevent this, early recognition and prompt supportive treatment such as fluid and electrolyte repletion is vital. Traditional stool culture techniques are being supplanted by rapid molecular-based assays with high sensitivity and specificity that target the most common bacterial, viral, and protozoal agents.[3] Anti-infectives can help limit the duration and severity of infections but only in specific circumstances.[4] Given the high risk for horizontal transfer of infective agents in close quarters, prompt identification of infected individuals, environmental disinfection, isolation protocols, hand hygiene, and cohorting symptomatic patients are important to limit its spread.

Viruses dominate as the most common cause of infectious acute diarrhea. Norovirus, adenovirus, astrovirus, rotavirus, and sapovirus are encountered often with norovirus seen most frequently in adults.[5] Norovirus is associated with watery-diarrhea outbreaks in long-term residential facilities and has high virulence through fecal-oral and person-to-person transmission. Only 100 virions are needed to cause disease, yet infected individuals can shed billions of virions into the environment. This virus is important to recognize because 90% of norovirus-associated deaths occur in adults older than 65 years.[6] There are no current Food and Drug Administration–approved treatments for viral enteric pathogens but nitazoxanide, a parasiticidal agent, has been used off-label to treat refractory norovirus infections in the immunosuppressed population.[7] Its use as a therapeutic option in the elderly is still under investigation but worthy of consideration for those with refractory or severe disease. However, most enteric viral infections will resolve spontaneously in 1 to 2 weeks.

Bacterial enteropathogens can cause a range or mixture of physiologic types of diarrhea with approaches to management based on the organism and the severity of the disease.[3]

If diarrhea is severe or lasts longer than 1 week, stool testing either by culture or polymerase chain reaction (PCR)-based assays can guide specific antibiotic therapy. Empirical therapy is not usually recommended for community-acquired acute bacterial infections because risks include opportunistic Clostridioides difficile infection (CDI), Escherichia coli O157:H7–related hemolytic uremic syndrome, or prolonged shedding in salmonella infection. However, there are several scenarios where antibiotic therapy is acceptable. Antimicrobial therapy and hospitalization is indicated for those who have severe inflammatory disease defined as fever, volume depletion, or bloody diarrhea. In "traveler's diarrhea," where the common pathogens are usually known based on geographic exposure, specific antibiotics can be used for treatment.[8] CDI always requires immediate treatment because of its high risk of mortality. In all cases of infectious diarrhea, the mainstay of treatment is prompt and adequate rehydration with oral fluids containing salt and sugar such as sports drinks and soups.

Patients can then be advanced to a BRAT diet (bananas, rice, apple sauce, and toast) as tolerated.

CLOSTRIDIOIDES DIFFICILE INFECTION

CDI is a toxin-mediated inflammatory diarrhea that carries a high risk for morbidity and mortality in the elderly. Age-specific risk factors include frequent exposure to health care facilities, long courses of antibiotics, concomitant treatment with more than one antibiotic, hypoalbuminemia, and an increasing number of comorbidities.[9] The clinical spectrum of CDI ranges from mild inflammatory diarrhea to fulminant colitis and death.[9] It has a mortality rate of 5% for individuals aged 61 to 70 years and increases to more than 10% for people 80 years of age and older.[10] Because of its potential lethality, if CDI is identified by PCR amplification or immunoassay of one of its toxins (A or B) or if even highly suspected, it should be treated immediately, regardless of severity in the elderly.

The severity of CDI guides its antimicrobial and surgical treatment. Nonsevere and severe CDI should be treated with either vancomycin or fidaxomicin as first-line agents. Oral metronidazole is second line.[11] For fulminant CDI (shock/ileus, megacolon, pseudomembranous colitis, or end-organ damage) a combination of oral and rectal vancomycin with intravenous metronidazole is recommended. Total abdominal colectomy for patients with fulminant colitis should be considered early in their course, as those who benefit from surgery include those who are older than 65 years.[12] However, diverting loop ileostomy and direct vancomycin instillation through the stoma has been shown to carry less morbidity and mortality and allows for preservation of the colon.[13]

Recurrences of CDI (rCDI) can be as high as 60% in the elderly. Antibiotic treatments include fidaxomicin, vancomycin tapered over several weeks, or standard dose vancomycin followed by an oral "rifaximin chaser."[14–19] Nonantibiotic approaches include bezlotoxumab, a human monoclonal antibody directed against toxin B that provides passive immunity against CDI.[20] The other is fecal microbiota transfer (FMT), the transfer of stool from a healthy donor to a host, which has a cure rate as high as 90% in patients with rCDI. Although not FDA approved, FMT in the elderly seems to be efficacious on long-term follow-up.[21] Because of the disadvantage that the elderly have to develop rCDI, prevention is key. This can be through judicious use of antibiotics, stewardship programs, adherence to guideline-based therapy, and efforts to decrease horizontal transmission in long-term health care facilities and hospitals.

MEDICATIONS

Medications can be a frequent cause of diarrhea in the elderly (**Table 1**). Medications may lead to diarrhea through enhancement of osmotic drag, secretion, motility, or inflammation.[4] The treatment of all forms of medication-induced diarrhea is the removal of the offending agent. Symptomatic treatment can include antidiarrheals, but these are not without risks such as constipation, ileus, or altered mental status (see **Table 1**).

Osmotic drugs cause painless watery diarrhea by dragging water and ions into the intestinal lumen, increasing the water content of stool. Such drugs include added artificial sweeteners such as sugar alcohols (eg, sorbitol, mannitol) that are poorly absorbed and later fermented by gut bacteria. Some agents that contain sodium, magnesium, sulfate, or phosphate salts exploit this mechanism and are used intentionally as laxatives to treat constipation (**Table 2**).[4,22] Analysis of stool electrolytes

Table 1
Commonly used medications in the elderly stratified by prominent diarrheal mechanisms

Mechanism of Diarrhea	Osmotic	Inflammatory Diarrhea	Promotility	Secretory
Medications	Lactulose	NSAIDs	Acetylcholine esterase inhibitors	Bisacodyl
	Mg-based laxatives	Olmesartan	Thyroid hormone macrolides	Digoxin
	Polyethylene glycol	Chemotherapeutic agents	(clarithromycin/erythromycin)	Metformin misoprostol
	ACE inhibitors	(5-fluorouracil, methotrexate,		Caffeine carbamazepine
	Procainamide	irinotecan cisplatin,		Chemotherapeutic agents
	Quinidine	doxorubicin ipilimumab,		(epirubicin, docetaxel,
	Methyldopa	rituximab)		flucytosine)
	Sugar alcohols	SSRIs		Simvastatin
	(mannitol/sorbitol/xylitol)	antibiotics (clindamycin,		Theophylline
	Antibiotics (ampicillin,	amoxicillin, ampicillin,		Ticlopidine
	clindamycin)	cephalosporins)		

Abbreviations: ACE, angiotensin-converting enzyme; Mg, magnesium; NSAIDs, nonsteroidal antiinflammatory drugs; SSRI, selective serotonin reuptake inhibitor.
Data from Refs.[4,22,24,27,28,50,51]

Table 2
Antidiarrheal medications used in the treatment of acute, chronic, and inflammatory diarrheas

Drug Class/Agent	Mechanism of Action	Side Effects/Other Considerations
Opioid-like		
Loperamide	Stimulates μ-opioid receptor in the myenteric plexus	• Safe in inflammatory diarrhea • Associated with drowsiness, dizziness, nausea, and abdominal discomfort
Diphenoxylate-atropine	Inhibits intestinal prostaglandin and chloride secretion	• Avoid use in geriatric population as per Beers criteria[52] • Associated with sedation, dizziness, nausea, vomiting, dry mouth • Potential for withdrawal symptoms when stopped abruptly • Avoid if patient is on MOA (risk of hypertension and stoke)
Tincture of opium	Stimulates μ-opioid receptor in the myenteric plexus and also δ-opioid and κ-opioid receptors	• Associated with CNS depression, sedation, and altered mental status • Potential for hypotension or withdrawal symptoms when abruptly stopped
Eluxadoline	Mixed μ-opioid receptor agonist and δ-opioid antagonist	• Indicated for diarrhea predominant IBS (IBS-D) • Contraindicated in patients with pancreaticobiliary disease
Somatostatin Analogues		
Octreotide	Reduces the secretion of several pancreatic and GI hormones by acting directly on epithelial cells	• Used in severe secretory diarrhea • Risk for ileus, gallstones • Used in secretory diarrhea caused by VIP, serotonin, gastrin, secretin, and pancreatic polypeptide secreting tumors

(continued on next page)

Table 2
(continued)

Drug Class/Agent	Mechanism of Action	Side Effects/Other Considerations
Bile acid–binding resin		
Cholestyramine, colestipol, and colesevelam	Bile acid–binding resin/ sequestrant	• Chronic diarrhea due to bile acid malabsorption • Decrease fat soluble vitamins A, D, E, and K and folic acid absorption • Inactivation of other medications • Risk of hypertriglyceridemia • Chronic use associated with bleeding from vitamin K deficiency
Fiber supplements		
Polycarbophil, psyllium husk	Bulk-forming laxative	• Bloating, fecal impaction above strictures, fluid overload • Abdominal cramps, nausea, and vomiting
Pectin	Prebiotic	• Used to support bifidobacteria in IBS-D
5-HT3 receptor antagonists		
Alosetron	5-HT3 receptor antagonist	• Primarily used for IBS-D • Contraindicated if history of constipation, abnormal GI tract function, abnormal GI tract anatomy, or hypercoagulable states • Black box warning for ischemic colitis
Ondansetron	5-HT3 receptor antagonist	• Used in carcinoid syndrome–associated diarrhea • Rare Qtc prolongation risk • Rare risk for serotonin syndrome
Other		
Activated charcoal	Adsorbent agent for enterotoxins	• May cause black stool that can be confused with melena • May interfere with absorption of other medications

(continued on next page)

		Side Effects/Other
Drug Class/Agent	Mechanism of Action	Considerations
Bismuth subsalicylate	Inhibits intestinal prostaglandin and chloride secretion, exhibits antimicrobial effects, and binds to enterotoxins	• May stain the tongue and stool black (confused with melena) • Can decrease absorption of other medications • Caution should be used while taking aspirin or other salicylate-containing products • Should not be used long term due to bismuth encephalopathy

Table 2
(continued)

may reveal an increased stool osmotic gap[a] that suggests ingested exogenous ions as a cause for this form of diarrhea.[23]

Drugs can induce secretory diarrhea by decreasing absorption and/or increasing the secretion of fluid and electrolytes in the intestinal lumen (see **Table 2**). Secretagogues such as misoprostol, for example, cause diarrhea by increasing the level of cyclic AMP in the crypts of the small intestine leading to secretion of chloride and water into the lumen. Other drugs such as digoxin and colchicine impair fluid absorption from the villi of the small intestine by inhibiting cellular metabolism of ATP required for Na^+/K^+ exchange at the basolateral surface of the enterocyte.[4 4,24,25] A low stool osmolar gap can infer a secretory diarrhea and a deeper evaluation of the patient's medication list.

Other drugs increase the frequency of peristalsis (see **Table 2**). Rapid transit of fluid through the small intestine decreases the time for resorption of water that eventually exceeds the absorptive capacity of the colon leading to unformed stool. Stopping properistaltic agents will result in cessation of diarrhea. Paradoxically, drugs that slow peristalsis to treat diarrhea such as opioid-based agents[26] may result in small intestinal bacterial overgrowth (SIBO), which leads to an increase in deconjugated bile salts. These bile-salts will precipitate a secretory diarrhea in the colon[27,28] that in turn will respond best to bile acid–binding resins or SIBO-directed antibiotics.[29]

Drugs that cause inflammatory diarrhea do so by damaging the specialized cells of the small intestinal villi and colon (see **Table 2**). This leads to exudation of serum proteins, mucus, blood, and inflammatory cells that can result in a mixture of secretory and malabsorptive diarrhea. Colchicine and some chemotherapeutic agents inhibit microtubule polymerization and lead to inflammatory diarrhea.[30] This can be differentiated from other forms of diarrhea by testing for markers of inflammation in the stool such as fecal white blood cells and the proteins, lactoferrin and calprotectin. Cessation of offending medications leads to gradual resolution of symptoms. However,

---

[a] The formula for diarrheal stool osmolarity gap = 290 to 2[Na + K] where 290 mOsm represents normal stool osmolarity and 2 x [Na + K] represents the major measured stool cations and their corresponding anions. A normal osmolar gap is usually less than 50 mOsm. An osmotic cause for diarrhea will have an osmolar gap greater than 124 mOsm. A secretory cause will have an osmolar gap of less than 50 mOsm.

given that these medications may be required for a finite period of time, symptoms can be managed carefully with antidiarrheals until the treatment has been completed.[24]

Antibiotic-associated diarrhea (AAD) is a fairly common occurrence seen in approximately 5% to 30% of patients on antibiotics with age greater than 65 years being an important host-related factor.[31] AAD can begin at any time from initiation of almost any antibiotic to 2 months after. The pathophysiologic mechanism by which antibiotics cause diarrhea is multifactorial and includes impaired bile acid metabolism, carbohydrate malabsorption, and toxic or allergic effects on the intestinal epithelium, or promote increased motility.[32] Probiotics have been shown to be useful in preventing AAD. However, there are limited randomized clinical trials to recommend the correct strain, viability, dose, frequency, duration, and their safety in the elderly.[33] If possible, offending antibiotics should be discontinued as soon as it is feasible, as most cases will improve with time and with antidiarrheals for symptom relief.

ISCHEMIC COLITIS

Ischemic colitis presents as acute, inflammatory bloody diarrhea with localized abdominal pain, with 90% of cases seen in the sixth and seventh decade of life. Patients may typically have hypotension, thrombosis, constipation, vasculitis, or cancer as precipitants to the episode. The pathophysiology is related to a reperfusion injury after transient or persistent occlusive or nonocclusive disease of the mesenteric arterial supply to the watershed areas of the colon (splenic flexure or sigmoid). Although the diagnosis can be made clinically, one must exclude competing causes of inflammatory diarrhea in the elderly such as infectious diarrhea or inflammatory bowel disease (IBD). Medical management consists of intravenous hydration; optimization of hemodynamics; bowel rest; and withdrawal of offending agents with inflammatory, vasoconstrictive, or thrombotic effects.[34,35] In a minority of cases, signs of peritonitis or gangrenous ischemic colitis require segmental resection of the affected area and may carry a high risk for morbidity and mortality in the elderly.[35]

OVERFLOW DIARRHEA

Overflow diarrhea is a common yet frequently overlooked phenomenon of acute diarrhea in the elderly. Despite a patient's description of diarrhea, painless fecal incontinence, or encopresis, the underlying mechanism stems from severe constipation. The increased diameter of the rectosigmoid from affected stool triggers receptive relaxation of the anal sphincter and a secretory response in the proximal colon. This fosters seepage of fluid around the affected mass of hardened stool complicated by incontinence of watery stool. Unfortunately, patients with overflow diarrhea are often treated inappropriately with antidiarrheal agents that actually worsen the problem. This condition can be readily and easily diagnosed by rectal examination or a plain abdominal radiograph that shows significant stool burden.[36,37] Treatment of this condition relies on a combination of manual disimpaction, enemas, suppositories, and other laxatives to relieve fecal retention. Chronic management requires a maintenance bowel regimen to address risk factors for recurrent constipation.

MALABSORPTION

Impaired digestion and absorption of dietary carbohydrates and fats can lead to "malabsorption," a subtype of osmotic diarrhea. Over decades of life, there is a slow decline of gastrointestinal function, an increasing risk for developing digestive disorders, and increasing likelihood for surgery of the digestive tract. The main categories of malabsorption are therefore related to the following changes: (1) loss of enzymes required to hydrolyze carbohydrates and fats, (2) impaired delivery of biliary and pancreatic digestive products to the bowel lumen to emulsify fat, and (3) reduction in the effective absorptive surface area in the small intestine for carbohydrates and fats.

Lactose intolerance is the prototype of carbohydrate maldigestion and has a high prevalence in the elderly population up to 50%.[38] Age-related decline in lactase or other carbohydrate digesting enzymes allows for undigested sugars to act as osmotically active particles that drag water into the colon and fermented by gut bacteria to create gas and watery diarrhea. Replacement digestive enzymes exist for lactose and sucrose but are not available for all complex carbohydrates.[39] However, sugars that are difficult to digest can be identified through an exclusion diet low in fermentable oligosaccharides, disaccharides, monosaccharides, and polyols, known as a low FODMAPs diet and be avoided.[40]

Disruption of the hepatobiliary tract (eg, cholecystectomy) or pancreas (eg, Whipple or chronic pancreatitis) can lead to fat maldigestion. Symptoms range from bloating to fatty diarrhea (steatorrhea).[36] Lack of concentrated bile results in inability to emulsify fats in the diet and can be identified by finding free fatty acids (split fat) in the stool. However, a steady flow of bile can result in bile acid malabsorption (BAM), a secretory diarrhea of the colon. Inadequate lipase delivery to food results in impaired lipolysis of fat that can be detected on stool testing as neutral fat. Bile-related diarrhea is best managed with bile acid–binding resins, pancreatic insufficiency with lipase-containing enzymes, and a low fat diet with fat soluble vitamin supplementation for both.

Celiac disease and IBD are both conditions that decrease the effective absorptive surface area of the small intestine.[41] Because the liver and the pancreas are still able to digest and emulsify fats, stool tests may reveal unabsorbed split fat. The more extensive the disease, the worse the diarrhea and site-specific vitamin and mineral deficiencies such as vitamin B12, fat-soluble vitamins, and iron. Understanding these 2 malabsorptive conditions are important to effectively manage these symptoms in the elderly.

INFLAMMATORY BOWEL DISEASE

Ulcerative colitis and Crohn disease are chronic inflammatory diseases of the intestinal tract that have a bimodal peak with a new diagnosis assigned to 10% to 15% of patients older than 60 years.[42] This is distinct from IBD diagnosed at a younger age that carries into a higher age group over time. The overall prevalence of IBD in the elderly continues to increase, as IBD has a low mortality rate even when diagnosed at an early age. A high index of clinical suspicion, family history, and attention to red flags such as abdominal pain, weight loss, and bloody diarrhea may prompt imaging tests and biopsies of inflamed areas of the gastrointestinal (GI) tract. Treatment is aimed at inducing and maintaining remission with agents such as 5-aminosalicylates, steroids, immunomodulators, or biologics. Surgery is recommended for severe cases but may not always lead to cessation of diarrhea.[42]

Crohn disease can inflame any part of the GI tract, and surgeries of the small bowel can also result in diarrhea. In patients who have required extensive small bowel resections that result in diarrhea, the short-gut syndrome can be managed in different ways. Teduglutide, a glucagon-like peptide-2 analogue, stimulates hyperplasia and hypertrophy of enterocytes and promotes more water and electrolyte absorption.[43] The pathophysiology of diarrhea in those after terminal ileum resection is based on the length of bowel removed. Bile malabsorption occurs when less than 100 cm is removed and can be treated with bile acid–binding resins. A combination of fat malabsorption and BAM can occur when more than 100 cm is removed and can be treated with a combination of special low fat diets and bile acid–binding resins.

Patients with ulcerative colitis who have had curative colectomies with pouch creation may develop diarrhea for several reasons. The close proximity of the small intestine to the rectum with the loss of a true colonic reservoir to hold stool can lead to hyperdefecation that can be treated with antidiarrheals. Pouches may also develop noninfectious inflammation termed pouchitis that can be managed with antidiarrheals, probiotics, and antibiotics before considering immunosuppression.[44,45]

CELIAC DISEASE

Celiac disease is an immune inflammatory reaction to gluten, the water insoluble protein found in wheat. Exposure to gluten erodes the surface area provided by the small intestinal villi in patients with celiac disease. If only the proximal small bowel is involved, one may only see vague GI symptoms with isolated iron or folate deficiency. If the entire small bowel is involved then diarrhea, weight loss, vitamin deficiencies, and steatorrhea ensues. Given the variable mix of gastrointestinal symptoms, the diagnosis is often delayed. However, serologic markers to test for celiac disease include tissue transglutaminase antibodies, deamidated gliadin peptide antibodies, and genetic markers (human leukocyte antigens DQ2 and DQ8). Patients are at an increased risk for T-cell lymphoma if not strictly adherent to the only treatment—a gluten-free diet.[41] A gluten-free diet results in regeneration of the small intestinal villi and improvement in diarrhea symptoms.

MICROSCOPIC COLITIS

Microscopic colitis is a common cause of chronic mixed inflammatory and secretory diarrhea in the elderly. The incidence is 5 to 10 times higher in those older than 65 years. The 2 forms of microscopic colitis, collagenous and lymphocytic, seem normal on endoscopic examination; however, histologic examination shows increased intraepithelial lymphocytes in the colonic mucosa. Increased deposition of subepithelial collagen is the hallmark of collagenous colitis. In most of the cases, the watery diarrhea is self-limited and without complications of dehydration or abdominal pain, but symptoms can last indefinitely in some. Risk factors associated with microscopic colitis include female gender, autoimmune disorders, personal history of malignancy, and celiac disease. Several medications have also been associated with microscopic colitis, although their pathophysiological mechanisms are not clearly understood. Drugs with a high likelihood to cause microscopic colitis include acarbose, nonsteroidal anti-inflammatory drugs, aspirin, clozapine, phytochemicals, proton pump inhibitors, histamine 2 receptor antagonists, sertraline, and ticlopidine.[46,47] For most of the cases, treatment includes correcting underlying autoimmune disorders or withdrawal of offending medications. The anti-inflammatory medications, bismuth subsalicylate or 5-aminosalicylic acid, can be started early and tapered off for mild disease. Steroids such as budesonide or prednisone can be used in short courses for moderate disease. Immunomodulators, biologics, or surgery are reserved for refractory, severe cases.[48,49]

SUMMARY

Diarrhea is a common problem among the elderly that can range from minor alterations in quality of life from frequent loose stools to potentially lethal and catastrophic outcomes. Deaths related to diarrhea are well established among older adults living in both the community as well in nursing homes, so attention to the early onset of diarrhea and management should follow a thoughtful approach. Careful analysis should focus on etiologic and epidemiologic risk factors in the medical history, surgical history, travel history, food consumption, medications, and environmental exposures. Most episodes of acute diarrhea can be managed conservatively if they are mild to moderate, resolve within 48 hours, and are not accompanied by worrisome signs. An admission is indicated for those older than 65 years if symptoms are severe, prolonged, results in dehydration, the patient seems toxic, there is evidence of colitis or gross blood in the stool, severe abdominal pain, fever, or if empirical therapy has failed. Laboratory testing is usually not needed but blood tests can be used to assess for electrolyte disturbances, degree of dehydration, systemic infection, or amount of blood loss. Specific stool tests can categorize diarrhea (infectious, secretory, osmotic, malabsorptive, promotile, or inflammatory) to help guide therapy. Imaging is rarely necessary except to assess for severity of disease. Although antidiarrheals can provide symptom relief and typically have a low side-effect profile, they should be used with caution in the elderly, as these medications can worsen infectious diarrhea by promoting invasiveness of pathogens, delay addressing the underlying cause, or precipitate other complications. Management should always include oral rehydration and attempts at a BRAT diet but chronic or malabsorptive diarrhea often requires more involved nutritional support and vitamin supplementation. Understanding the physiologic process causing diarrhea can help identify a common clinical diagnosis that can be managed early and sufficiently to decrease the risk of morbidity and mortality in the elderly.

CLINICS CARE POINTS

- Diarrhea is a common illness in the elderly with a potential for higher morbidity and mortality compared to the general population due to electrolyte abnormalities and dehydration.
- For community-acquired acute bacterial infections, Empiric antibiotic therapy is not usually recommended with few exceptions.
- *Clostridioides difficile* infection requires prompt recognition, diagnosis and immediate treatment because of its high risk for mortality
- early recognition and prompt supportive treatment such as fluid and electrolyte repletion is vital regardless of cause of infectious diarrhea.
- removal of the offending agent is the mainstay treatment of medication associated diarrhea
- Ischemic colitis is a clinical diagnosis ,treatment includes intravenous hydration; optimization of hemodynamics; bowel rest; and withdrawal of offending agents with inflammatory, vasoconstrictive, or thrombotic effects.
- In overflow diarrhea, diagnosis can be easily made with a rectal exam and abdominal X-rays. Antidiarrheals medications should be avoided. Manual disimpaction, enemas, suppositories, and other laxatives are used to treat this condition
- Malabsorption occurs due impaired digestion and absorption of dietary carbohydrates and fats

- Lactose intolerance has high prevalence among the elderly population. Replacement digestive enzymes exist for lactose and sucrose. Other sugars can be identified and excluded through FODMAP.
- Disruption of the hepatobiliary tract by procedures such as cholecystectomy or pancreas such as Whipple lead to fat maldigestion. Bile-related diarrhea is best managed with bile acid–binding resins, pancreatic insufficiency with lipase containing enzymes, and a low fat diet with fat soluble vitamin supplementation for both.
- IBD is a common new diagnosis in the population older than 60. Treatment is aimed at inducing and maintaining remission with agents such as 5-aminosalicylates, steroids, immunomodulators, or biologics.
- Surgery is reserved for refractory cases of IBD, and may not cause relief of the diarrhea. Patients with extensive bowel resection can also develop diarrhea.
- A gluten-free diet results improvement in diarrhea symptoms. Non- adherence to gluten free diet increase risk of T-cell lymphomas.
- Microscopic colitis is a common cause of chronic diarrhea in elderly. Diagnosis is made histologically in a normal appearing mucosa on endoscopy.
- In the evaluation of diarrhea, once should take into account etiologic and epidemiologic risk factors in the medical history, surgical history, travel history, food consumption, medications, and environmental exposures.
- Indications for admission include : severe prolonged illness, resulting in dehydration, toxic appearing patient, evidence of colitis or gross blood in the stool, severe abdominal pain and tenderness, fever, or if empirical therapy has failed.
- antidiarrheals should be used with extreme caution in the elderly, as they can exacerbate infectious diarrhea by promoting invasiveness of pathogens, delay addressing the underlying cause and increase the risk of other complications.
- Management of diarrhea should always include oral rehydration and attempts at a BRAT diet
- Chronic or malabsorptive diarrhea often requires more involved nutritional support.

DISCLOSURE

C.V. Crawford: Speaker's bureau for Merck & Co., Inc, Site PI Ferring Pharmaceuticals, Site PI Finch Therapeutics, Site PI Summit Therapeutics, Site PI Artrugen Therapeutics and also a speaker for Romark Laboratories, LC. E. Dawod has nothing to disclose.

REFERENCES

1. Sherbaniuk RW. Symposium on inflammatory disease of the intestine. The physiology of diarrhea. Can Med Assoc J 1964;91(1):1–6.
2. Shintaro Sato HK, Fujihashi K. Mucosal immunosenescence in the gastrointestinal tract. Gerontology 2015;61(4):336–42.
3. Shane AL, Mody RK, Crump JA, et al. 2017 Infectious diseases society of America clinical practice guidelines for the diagnosis and management of infectious diarrhea. Clin Infect Dis 2017;65(12):e45–80.
4. Ratnaike RN, Jones TE. Mechanisms of drug-induced diarrhoea in the elderly. Drugs Aging 1998;13(3):245–53.
5. Zheng DP, Widdowson MA, Glass RI, et al. Molecular epidemiology of genogroup II-genotype 4 noroviruses in the United States between 1994 and 2006. J Clin Microbiol 2010;48(1):168–77.

6. Lisa Lindsay JW, De Coster I, Van Damme P, et al. A decade of norovirus disease risk among older adults in upper-middle and high income countries: a systematic review. BMC Infect Dis 2015;15:425.
7. Siddiq DM, Koo HL, Adachi JA, et al. Norovirus gastroenteritis successfully treated with nitazoxanide. J Infect 2011;63(5):394–7.
8. Riddle MS, DuPont HL, Connor BA. ACG clinical guideline: diagnosis, treatment, andprevention of acute diarrheal infections in adults. Am J Gastroenterol 2016; 111(5):602–22.
9. Jump RL. Clostridium difficile infection in older adults. Aging Health 2013;9(4): 403–14.
10. Asempa TE, Nicolau DP. Clostridium difficile infection in the elderly: an update on management. Clin Interv Aging 2017;12:1799–809.
11. Cornely OA, Nathwani D, Ivanescu C, et al. Clinical efficacy of fidaxomicin compared with vancomycin and metronidazole in Clostridium difficile infections: a meta-analysis and indirect treatment comparison. J Antimicrob Chemother 2014;69(11):2892–900.
12. Ferrada P, Velopulos CG, Sultan S, et al. Timing and type of surgical treatment of clostridium difficile-associated disease: a practice management guideline from the Eastern association for the surgery of trauma. J Trauma Acute Care Surg 2014;76(6):1484–93.
13. Neal MD, Alverdy JC, Hall DE, et al. Diverting loop ileostomy and colonic lavage: an alternative to total abdominal colectomy for the treatment of severe, complicated Clostridium difficile associated disease. Ann Surg 2011;254(3):423–7 [discussion: 427–9].
14. Garey KW, Jiang ZD, Bellard A, et al. Rifaximin in treatment of recurrent clostridium difficile-associated diarrhea: an uncontrolled pilot study. J Clin Gastroenterol 2009;43(1):91–3.
15. Johnson S, Schriever C, Galang M, et al. Interruption of recurrent clostridium difficile-associated diarrhea episodes by serial therapy with vancomycin and rifaximin. Clin Infect Dis 2007;44(6):846–8.
16. McFarland LV, Elmer GW, Surawicz CM. Breaking the cycle: treatment strategies for 163 cases of recurrent clostridium difficile disease. Am J Gastroenterol 2002; 97(7):1769–75.
17. Surawicz CM, McFarland LV, Greenberg RN, et al. The search for a better treatment for recurrent clostridium difficile disease: use of high-dose vancomycin combined with Saccharomyces boulardii. Clin Infect Dis 2000;31(4):1012–7.
18. Tedesco FJ, Gordon D, Fortson WC. Approach to patients with multiple relapses of antibiotic-associated pseudomembranous colitis. Am J Gastroenterol 1985; 80(11):867–8.
19. Louie TJ, Muller MA, Mullane KM, et al. Fidaxomicin versus vancomycin for Clostridium difficile infection. N Engl J Med 2011;364(5):422–31.
20. Gerding DN, Kelly CP, Rahav G, et al. Bezlotoxumab for prevention of recurrent clostridium difficile infection in patients at increased risk for recurrence. Clin Infect Dis 2018;67(5):649–56.
21. Girotra M, Gang S, Anand R, et al. Fecal microbiota transplantation for recurrent clostridium difficile infection in the elderly: long-term outcomes and microbiota changes. Dig Dis Sci 2016;61(10):3007–15.
22. Hammer HF, Santa Ana CA, Schiller LR, et al. Studies of osmotic diarrhea induced in normal subjects by ingestion of polyethylene glycol and lactulose. J Clin Invest 1989;84(4):1056–62.

23. Shiau YF, Feldman GM, Rensnick MA, et al. Stool electrolyte and osmolality measurements in the evaluation of diarrheal disorders. Ann Intern Med 1985;102(6): 773–5.

24. Philip NA, Ahmed N, Pitchumoni CS. Spectrum of drug-induced chronic diarrhea. J Clin Gastroenterol 2017;51(2):111–7.

25. Field M. Intestinal ion transport and the pathophysiology of diarrhea. J Clin Invest 2003;111(7):931–43.

26. Uday C, Ghoshal RS, Ghoshal U. Small intestinal bacterial overgrowth and irritable bowel syndrome: a bridge between functional organic dichotomy. Gut Liver 2017;11(2):196–208.

27. Abraham B, Sellin JH. Drug-induced diarrhea. Curr Gastroenterol Rep 2007;9(5): 365–72.

28. Chassany O, Michaux A, Bergmann JF. Drug-induced diarrhoea. Drug Saf 2000; 22(1):53–72.

29. Walters JR, Pattni SS. Managing bile acid diarrhoea. Therap Adv Gastroenterol 2010;3(6):349–57.

30. Skoufias DA, Wilson L. Mechanism of inhibition of microtubule polymerization by colchicine: inhibitory potencies of unliganded colchicine and tubulin-colchicine complexes. Biochemistry 1992;31(3):738–46.

31. McFarland LV. Antibiotic-associated diarrhea: epidemiology, trends and treatment. Future Microbiol 2008;3(5):563–78.

32. Bignardi GE. Risk factors for Clostridium difficile infection. J Hosp Infect 1998; 40(1):1–15.

33. Barbut F, Meynard JL. Managing antibiotic associated diarrhoea. BMJ 2002; 7350:324.

34. Koutroubakis IE. Ischemic colitis: clinical practice in diagnosis and treatment. World J Gastroenterol 2008;14(48):7302–8.

35. Fabiola De Vita RP. Gianfranco Amicucci, and Sergio Leardicorresponding author, Acute ischemic colitis in elderly: medical or surgical urgency? BMC Geriatr 2009;9:2009.

36. Holt PR. Diarrhea and malabsorption in the elderly. Gastroenterol Clin North Am 2001;30(2):427–44.

37. Kinnunen O, Jauhonen P, Salokannd J, et al. Diarrhea and fecal impaction in elderly long-stay patients. Z Gerontol 1989;22(6):321–3.

38. Kim R, Chang P, Riordan SM. Lactose intolerance in the older adult. Aging Health 2007;31(8):892–900.

39. Di Stefano M, Veneto G, Malservisi S, et al. Lactose malabsorption and intolerance in the elderly. Scand J Gastroenterol 2001;36(12):1274–8.

40. Hill P, Muir JG, Gibson PR. Controversies and recent developments of the low-FODMAP Diet. Gastroenterol Hepatol (N Y) 2017;13(1):36–45.

41. Kagnoff MF. Overview and pathogenesis of celiac disease. Gastroenterology 2005;128(4 Suppl 1):S10–8.

42. Taleban S, Colombel JF, Mohler MJ, et al. Inflammatory bowel disease and the elderly: a review. J Crohns Colitis 2015;9(6):507–15.

43. Wallis K, Walters JR, Gabe S. Short bowel syndrome: the role of GLP-2 on improving outcome. Curr Opin Clin Nutr Metab Care 2009;12(5):526–32.

44. Kedia S, Limdi JK, Ahuja V. Management of inflammatory bowel disease in older persons: evolving paradigms. Intest Res 2018;16(2):194–208.

45. Tran V, Limketkai NB, Sauk JS. IBD in the elderly: management challenges and therapeutic considerations. Curr Gastroenterol Rep 2019;21(11):60.

46. Pascua MF, Kedia P, Weiner MG, et al. Microscopic colitis and medication use. Clin Med Insights Gastroenterol 2011;3(11):11–9.
47. Lucendo AJ. Drug exposure and the risk of microscopic colitis: a critical update. Drugs R D 2017;17(1):79–81.
48. Ogundipe OA, Campbell A. Microscopic colitis impacts quality of life in older people. BMJ Case Rep 2019;12(6):e228092.
49. Pardi DS. Microscopic colitis. Clin Geriatr Med 2014;30(1):55–65.
50. Abraham BP, Sellin JH. Drug-induced, factitious, & idiopathic diarrhoea. Best Pract Res Clin Gastroenterol 2012;26(5):633–48.
51. Cappell MS. Colonic toxicity of administered drugs and chemicals. Am J Gastroenterol 2004;99(6):1175–90.
52. 2019 American Geriatrics Society Beers Criteria® Update Expert Panel. American geriatrics society 2019 updated AGS beers criteria® for potentially inappropriate medication use in older adults. J Am Geriatr Soc 2019;67(4):674–94.

Functional Bowel Disease

Aiya Aboubakr, MD[a], Michelle S. Cohen, MD[b],*

KEYWORDS

- Functional gastrointestinal disorders • Functional bowel disorders
- Irritable bowel syndrome

KEY POINTS

- Irritable bowel syndrome (IBS) is a common functional bowel disorder that affects individuals regardless of age and gender and can result in impaired quality of life and significant health care resource utilization.
- The diagnosis of IBS is based on clinical symptoms using the Rome IV criteria; laboratory or radiographic abnormalities suggest an alternate diagnosis.
- IBS is categorized into 4 subtypes based on the predominant bowel habit: constipation, diarrhea, mixed, or unclassified.
- The treatment of IBS is individually tailored based on subtype, predominant symptoms, symptom severity, age, and comorbidities.
- Therapeutic options for IBS include dietary and lifestyle modifications, pharmacotherapy that alter gut function, neuromodulators, and psychotherapy.

INTRODUCTION

Functional gastrointestinal disorders (FGIDs), also referred to as disorders of gut-brain interaction, are among the most commonly encountered diagnoses in gastroenterology.[1] Although these disorders can affect individuals regardless of age, gender, and race, they are more commonly diagnosed in women and at age 50 years or younger.[1–3] The symptoms range in severity and can result in impaired quality of life, absenteeism, and significant health care resource utilization.[4–6]

FGIDs exist in a separate clinical domain from organic or motility disorders and relate to an "illness experience."[1] The biopsychosocial conceptual model has been used to explain the gut-brain relationship in FGIDs, in which physiologic symptoms result from the connection between the central and enteric nervous systems.[1] Proposed alterations in the function and communication of the 2 nervous systems that result in the patient's symptom presentation include motility disturbance, visceral hypersensitivity, altered mucosal and immune function, altered gut microbiota, and/or altered central nervous system processing.[1]

[a] Department of Medicine, NewYork-Presbyterian Hospital/Weill Cornell Medical Center, 530 East 70th Street, M-507, New York, NY 10021, USA; [b] Division of Gastroenterology and Hepatology, Weill Cornell Medical College, 1305 York Avenue, 4th Floor, New York, NY 10021, USA
* Corresponding author.
E-mail address: mic9102@med.cornell.edu

Clin Geriatr Med 37 (2021) 119–129
https://doi.org/10.1016/j.cger.2020.08.009
0749-0690/21/© 2020 Elsevier Inc. All rights reserved.

geriatric.theclinics.com

The Rome IV (2016) is the current diagnostic standard for FGIDs.[1] It categorizes the disorders based on anatomic region and symptoms. It identifies 6 functional bowel disorders with symptoms attributable to the small and large intestine: irritable bowel syndrome (IBS), functional constipation, functional diarrhea, functional abdominal bloating/distention, unspecified functional bowel disorder, and opioid-induced constipation.[7,8] This article provides a framework for managing a patient with IBS, the most common of the functional bowel disorders, with special consideration to the management of the geriatric patient in whom IBS is suspected.

EPIDEMIOLOGY

The prevalence of IBS in the United States ranges between 8% and 17%.[9,10] A limited number of population studies have compared prevalence based on age, but most found that rate of IBS decreased with increased age without statistical significance.[2] Nonetheless, IBS was prevalent in up to 7.3% of individuals older than 60 years.[2]

Associated Conditions

Patients with IBS can be diagnosed with additional FGIDs, most commonly functional dyspepsia.[11] Significantly higher levels of anxiety and depression have been found in patients with IBS compared with healthy controls.[12,13] Associated extraintestinal conditions include fibromyalgia, chronic fatigue syndrome, chronic pelvic pain, and sleep disturbances.[13]

DEFINITION

The Rome IV diagnostic criteria for IBS is the presence of recurrent abdominal pain, on average, at least 1 day per week in the last 3 months, associated with 2 or more of the following criteria:

- Related to defecation
- Associated with a change in frequency of stool
- Associated with a change in form (appearance) of stool

Criteria must be fulfilled for the previous 3 months with symptom onset at least 6 months before diagnosis.[1]

Classification

IBS can be categorized into 4 subtypes based on the predominant bowel habit, using the Bristol Stool Form Scale (**Fig. 1**).[14] The scale, which has been validated for use in adults, ranges from 1 to 7 based on stool consistency: 1 and 2 correspond to hardened stools that may be difficult to pass (constipation), 3 to 5 correspond to normal consistency, and 6 to 7 to softer consistencies (diarrhea).[15] The current threshold for the predominant bowel type is 25% of bowel movements.

- IBS with constipation (IBS-C): greater than 25% of bowel movements are type 1 or 2 and less than 25% are type 6 or 7.
- IBS with diarrhea (IBS-D): greater than 25% of bowel movements are type 6 or 7 and less than 25% are type 1 or 2.
- IBS with mixed symptoms (IBS-M): greater than 25% of bowel movements are type 1 or 2 and greater than 25% are type 6 or 7.
- Unclassified IBS (IBS-U): meets the criteria for IBS as mentioned earlier, but the bowel habits are not accurately described by any of the aforementioned subtypes.

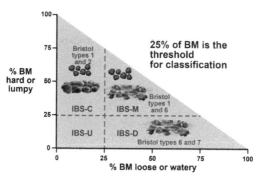

Fig. 1. IBS subtypes using 25% of bowel movement consistency for classification. (*From* Mearin F, Lacy BE, Chang L, et al. Bowel disorders. Gastroenterology 2016;150(6):1396; with permission.)

It is important to recognize that IBS subtype assigned to an individual patient may change over time.

Symptom Severity

In addition to classification by stool morphology, IBS can be categorized based on severity of symptoms into mild, moderate, and severe disease.[1] The severity is determined by psychosocial difficulties, number of additional symptoms, health care use, and activity or work restriction.[1] More severe symptoms tend to occur in women compared with men and in younger patients compared with elderly.[1] As detailed later in the Management section, severity can be used to guide treatment.

POSTINFECTIOUS IRRITABLE BOWEL SYNDROME

Postinfectious IBS (PI-IBS) refers to the development of new IBS symptoms after an acute gastrointestinal illness in a patient who did not previously meet criteria for IBS.[16,17] The incidence of PI-IBS ranges from 3.7% to 36%.[17] Proposed mechanisms to explain the pathophysiology of PI-IBS include mucosal injury and inflammation, mast cell hyperplasia, changes in enteric neuromodulation, and changes in the gut microbiome.[16,17] It tends to occur more frequently following bacterial infections associated with mucosal ulceration, for example, *Campylobacter jejuni* and *Escherichia coli* O157:H7.[17,18] Additional risk factors for developing PI-IBS include prolonged duration of initial illness, female gender, age younger than 60 years, and psychological stressors such as anxiety, depression, or an adverse life event preceding illness.[17,19,20] Management is similar to the treatment of IBS as detailed later. Most patients can expect their symptoms to gradually improve over time, whereas others will continue to experience persistent symptoms for years after diagnosis.[21]

DIAGNOSIS
Clinical Evaluation

A thorough history of a patient's presenting symptoms is integral to the diagnosis of IBS (**Table 1**). The goal is to understand the characteristics of the patient's abdominal pain and bowel habits, at baseline and when symptoms are active. The presence of alarm signs and symptoms should be part of the history, as their absence supports a diagnosis of IBS.[3,22]

Table 1
Evaluation of a patient with suspected irritable bowel syndrome

A Guided Approach to Interviewing the Patient with Suspected IBS
- Describe bowel habits (eg, frequency, consistency of stool, duration of bowel movements, degree of evacuation)
- Is abdominal pain associated with a change in bowel habits? If so, describe the pain
- How often do these symptoms occur?
- When did the symptoms start?
- Is there a previous diagnosis of IBS? If so, are these symptoms similar or different?
- Are there any associated symptoms (gastrointestinal and extraintestinal)?
- Are there any triggers or patterns to shift (eg, medications, foods, travel, mood)?
- List of current medications
- Was there a recent infection?
- Is there a family history of gastrointestinal disorders or diseases?

Alarm Signs and Symptoms*
- Onset of symptoms after 50 years or age
- Unintentional weight loss
- Family history of gastrointestinal malignancy in first-degree relative
- Gastrointestinal bleeding
- Iron-deficiency anemia
- Progressively worsening symptoms
- Nocturnal diarrhea

*The presence of any of these symptoms should warrant further evaluation.

Diagnostic Testing
- All patients should receive standard laboratory evaluation including complete blood count, basic metabolic panel, liver function testing, and age-appropriate colorectal cancer and gynecologic cancer screening. Additional testing can be tailored based on specific IBS subtype suspected

IBS-Constipation	IBS-Diarrhea/IBS-Mixed
• Thyroid function testing	• C-reactive protein
• Stool guaiac	• Thyroid function testing
• Colonoscopy	• Inflammatory markers (ESR, CRP)
• Motility testing	• Celiac serologies
• Anorectal manometry	• Fecal calprotectin or lactoferrin
	• Stool culture, ova and parasites
	• Breath Tests
	• Stool guaiac
	• Colonoscopy with biopsy

Data from Chey WD, Kurlander J, Eswaran S. Irritable bowel syndrome: a clinical review. JAMA. 2015;313(9):949–58; and Moayyedi P, Mearin F, Azpiroz F, et al. Irritable bowel syndrome diagnosis and management: A simplified algorithm for clinical practice. United European Gastroenterol J. 2017;5(6):773–88.

Physical Examination

The physical examination in patients with IBS is often unremarkable, although patients may report nonspecific tenderness on abdominal examination.[7] The presence of significant physical examination findings suggests alternative cause of the patient's symptoms.[8]

Laboratory Evaluation

The diagnosis of IBS is not made based on the presence of biomarkers. The decision to check certain laboratories and stool tests should be based on the predominant bowel pattern the patient reports at the time of evaluation and suspicion for alternative causes (see **Table 1**).[3,8,22] The presence of laboratory abnormalities in a patient with symptoms that suggest IBS should warrant further evaluation.

Imaging/Procedures

No radiographic abnormalities should be identified in a patient with IBS. Luminal evaluation (upper endoscopy, flexible sigmoidoscopy, colonoscopy) may be performed in selected cases.[8] Indications include age-appropriate screening, alarming signs or symptoms, positive family history of colorectal cancer or inflammatory bowel disease, and/or persistent diarrhea despite empirical treatment of IBS-D.[3,8,22] If a colonoscopy is pursued for evaluation of diarrhea, random biopsies should be taken to evaluate for microscopic colitis.[23] Testing for other suspected diagnoses, for example, hydrogen or urea breath test, can be considered based on clinical suspicion.[8]

Differential Diagnosis

The differential diagnosis for IBS includes organic causes (infection, inflammatory, autoimmune, structural, and malignancies) as well as motility disorders. Inflammatory bowel disease, celiac disease, lactose and fructose intolerances, microscopic colitis, and laxative abuse are examples of causes that can mimic IBS.[3,22] It is possible to have an overlap of both IBS and organic or motility disorders, and clinical judgment must be used to determine if further evaluation is warranted.

MANAGEMENT

The treatment of IBS is tailored on an individual basis based on IBS-subtype, predominant symptoms (eg, diarrhea, constipation, abdominal pain), symptom severity, age, and comorbidities. Therapeutic options range from dietary and lifestyle modifications, to over-the-counter and prescription pharmacotherapy to alter gut function, to neuromodulators and psychotherapy.[6,22] These agents target the proposed pathophysiology, including visceral hypersensitivity, motility, secretion, and the microbiome.[1]

When symptom severity is used as a framework for treatment, patients with mild symptoms can often be managed with diet, medication modifications, and over-the-counter options. As the symptoms progress from mild to moderate, additional prescription therapies can be used including neuromodulators. Patients with severe symptoms require the most intensive care and benefit from a multidisciplinary approach, including a psychiatrist. Psychotherapy that focuses on the brain-gut interaction (eg, cognitive behavioral therapy, hypnotherapy, mindfulness) can be beneficial at any symptom level but most often is introduced at the moderate level.[24]

The treatment options are divided into IBS-C and IBS-D. Because of their mixed bowel pattern, patients with IBS-M especially require a personalized approach and can include recommendations from both categories.

Management of Irritable Bowel Syndrome with Constipation

The initial management of IBS-C should begin with soluble fiber supplementation and over-the-counter laxatives. It is important to discuss and monitor adverse symptoms, including the potential to exacerbate bloating, flatulence, and abdominal discomfort.[3,12] Fiber may not be a good first-line option for a patient with IBS who reports bloating as a predominant symptom. Osmotic laxatives (polyethylene glycol and magnesium) have been shown to offer patients relief with their constipation but do not significantly affect abdominal pain and/or bloating.[25] Stimulant laxatives such as senna and bisacodyl are also available over the counter for constipation, but they can worsen abdominal cramping.

The next step in management of constipation in IBS-C includes Food and Drug Administration–approved pharmacologic options: prosecretory agents (intestinal secretagogues) and prokinetics (serotonin agonists).

- The prosecretory class includes *lubiprostone, linaclotide, and plecanatide.* These agents increase water secretion into the lumen of the colon to facilitate a decrease in colon transit time.[12] Lubiprostone activates secretion via chloride channels, whereas linaclotide and plecanatide work via stimulation of guanylate cyclase-C.[12,26] In addition to its effects on transit, linaclotide has been shown to improve abdominal pain by its effect on cyclic guanosine monophosphate.[12,27] The main adverse effect of lubiprostone is nausea, whereas diarrhea is the main side effect of linaclotide and plecanatide.
- The prokinetic class includes *prucalopride* and *tegaserod.* These agents activate serotonin 5-HT4 receptors in the gastrointestinal tract and increase colonic transit time.[12,28] Frequent adverse reactions include headache and abdominal pain.[12,28,29] Prucalopride requires altered dosing for renal impairment, and it is important to assess renal function in a geriatric patient before initiation.[28] It is also important to note that tegaserod is only approved for use in female patients younger than 65 years with low risk for cardiovascular ischemia,[29] but prucalopride has no similar restrictions.

Management of Irritable Bowel Syndrome with Diarrhea

The initial management of IBS-D should start with fiber, dietary modification, and over-the-counter antimotility agents such as loperamide. Similar to IBS-C, patients with mild IBS-D can benefit from water-soluble fiber as a bulking agent.[12,30] Loperamide is an μ-opioid receptor agonist that increases colonic transit time and decreases fluid secretion.[31] Although loperamide can improve diarrhea, it may not relieve abdominal pain and bloating.[31] It is important to counsel patients on appropriate use of this medication and set their expectations for symptomatic relief.

The next step in management of diarrhea in IBS-D is pharmaceutical options that include rifaximin, antimotility agents, and bile acid sequestrants.

- *Rifaximin* is a nonsystemic antibiotic whose mechanism of action in IBS-D is not fully understood, but proposed mechanisms include direct antibiotic effects, modulation of host inflammatory response, and modification of gut microbiota and gut motility.[32,33] Studies demonstrate rifaximin can offer short-term symptomatic relief for IBS-D,[34] and it is important to educate the patient on the expected duration of its effects. Patients can be considered for repeat treatment if symptoms recur.[35] It is safe and well tolerated, with no restrictions for use in elderly population.
- The antimotility agents are *eluxadoline* and *alosetron.* Eluxadoline is a mixed μ-opioid and κ-opioid receptor agonist and δ-opioid receptor antagonist in the enteric nervous system.[36] The mechanism of action is complex but includes decreased gastrointestinal motility and secretion and analgesic effects.[36] The most common side effects are nausea, constipation, or abdominal pain.[36] Because of reports of pancreatitis, eluxadoline is contraindicated in patients who had a cholecystectomy, have biliary disease (eg, sphincter of Oddi dysfunction), history of pancreatitis, chronic liver disease, and heavy alcohol use.[12] Alosetron is a selective 5-HT3 antagonist that also results in decreased colonic transit and reduced gastrointestinal secretion.[37,38] A low dose is currently approved only for women with severe IBS-D who have not had a response to conventional therapy.[37] It was previously approved at a higher dose for men and women but was withdrawn due to concerns for ischemic colitis and severe constipation.[39] There is no dose adjustment for age; however, elderly patients may be at greater risk for these complications.[39]

- Bile acid sequestrants include *cholestyramine, colestipol*, and *colesevelam*. It has been proposed that bile acid malabsorption may occur in a subset of patients with IBS-D.[22,40] Testing is currently limited in the United States; however, it is a treatment option to consider if other modalities have been unsuccessful.[8,41]

Management of Global Irritable Bowel Syndrome Symptoms

The following treatments can be used for all IBS subtypes to target global symptomatology, including abdominal pain, bloating, and flatulence.

- Antispasmodics refer to a group of medications that act as smooth muscle relaxants and can be used to address IBS symptoms.[12,42] In studies, they have been shown to improve stool consistency, stool frequency, and abdominal cramping. Anticholinergics (such as hyoscyamine or dicyclomine) are included in this category. Although generally well tolerated, these agents should be used with caution in elderly patients given their side-effect profiles.
- Peppermint oil, specifically its' L-menthol component, is safe and effective for the relief of abdominal pain and global IBS symptoms compared with placebo.[43] The proposed mechanism of action is antagonism of calcium channel receptors in smooth muscle cells, but it may also have antimicrobial, immunomodulation, and anesthetic properties.[43,44] It can improve pain, bloating, pain with evacuation, and urgency but does not affect bowel habits.[44]
- Probiotics are commonly used by patients with IBS. Multiple studies have had varying results on its efficacy, but probiotics may improve global symptoms, bloating, and flatulence.[12]
- Neuromodulators for use in IBS include tricyclic antidepressants (TCAs), serotonin and norepinephrine reuptake inhibitors (SNRIs), and selective serotonin reuptake inhibitors (SSRIs).[8,45] The decision to use a particular agent is based on IBS subtype and predominant symptoms. TCAs should be considered the first line for treating pain in patients with IBS and IBS-D, whereas SSRIs are favored for IBS-C. SNRIs can be used for both IBS-D and IBS-C.[45]
  - TCAs (*amitriptyline, imipramine, desipramine, nortriptyline*) inhibit the reuptake of serotonin and norepinephrine, which leads to slowed gastrointestinal transit that is advantageous in IBS-D.[45] Their use in the geriatric population is limited by their anticholinergic, antihistamine, and anti-alpha-adrenergic effects. In addition, TCAs are associated with an increased risk of arrhythmias and should be avoided in patients with prolonged QT intervals or bundle branch blocks.[45]
  - SSRIs (*fluoxetine, sertraline, citalopram, and escitalopram*) increase gut motility via their effect on serotonin release in the gastrointestinal tract and can be particularly useful in patients with IBS with anxiety.[45] Their use can be limited by their adverse side effect profile including nausea, insomnia, and sexual dysfunction and the length of time that is required before they have an effect.[3]
  - SNRIs (*duloxetine, venlafaxine*) share similar side-effect profiles with both SSRIs and TCAs; however, they cause less constipation compared with TCAs, thus are an option for patients with pain-predominant IBS-C.

Dietary Modification

Patients with IBS often note their symptoms are sensitive to food and many restrict their diet to modify their symptoms.[3,46] Dietary changes have been shown to provide relief in IBS symptoms, particularly in IBS-D/M, including the low FODMAP (fermentable oligo-di-monosaccharides and polyols) diet.[47,48] FODMAPs are short-chain carbohydrates commonly found in foods that are poorly absorbed in the gastrointes-tinal tract.[47] Their impaired digestion can cause abdominal pain, bloating, and alter-ations in bowel habits.[46] Although the low FODMAP diet (in which foods are restricted, reintroduced, and then personalized to avoid trigger foods) has been shown to effectively reduce symptoms in some patients with IBS, the quality of the evidence remains mixed and the approach may not be sustainable as a long-term therapeutic option.[12,48,49] Patients may benefit from working with a trained dietitian/nutritionist to find individualized dietary modifications based on food-symptom association.[46]

DISCUSSION

IBS is a common functional bowel disorder that requires a strong physician-patient relationship to manage given the complexity of its pathophysiology. It can be partic-ularly challenging to diagnose and manage IBS in the geriatric population, who often have multiple comorbidities, atypical symptom presentations, and higher suspicion to rule out organic pathologies. Multiple targets across the brain-gut interaction are avail-able to address IBS, based on the subtype, predominant symptoms, and severity of symptoms. It is recommended that management start with dietary and lifestyle mod-ifications and over-the-counter modalities before initiation of specialty pharmaco-therapy that alter gut function. In a geriatric patient, close attention must be paid to the adverse effects and drug-drug interactions of prescription medication.

CLINICS CARE POINTS

- The diagnosis of IBS is made using the Rome IV diagnostic criteria and is cate-gorized into four subtypes based on the predominant bowel habit.
- Evaluation for the patient with suspected IBS should include a thorough history. Testing (such as labs, breath tests, imaging, endoscopy/colonoscopy) can be obtained to rule out organic etiologies of symptoms based upon history and de-gree of suspicion for alternate diagnoses.
- The treatment of IBS is tailored on an individual basis based on disease subtype and predominant symptom(s), and includes lifestyle modifications, pharmaco-therapy to alter gut function, and psychotherapy.

DISCLOSURE

The authors have nothing to disclose.

REFERENCES

1. Drossman D. Functional GI and Rome IV. Gastroenterology 2016;150:1263–79.
2. Lovell RM, Ford AC. Global prevalence of, and risk factors for, irritable bowel syn-drome: a meta-analysis. Clin Gastroenterol Hepatol 2012;10:712–21.
3. Chey WD, Kurlander J, Eswaran S. Irritable bowel syndrome: a clinical review. JAMA 2015;313(9):949–58.
4. Leong SA, Barghout V, Birnbaum HG, et al. The economic consequences of irri-table bowel syndrome: a us employer perspective. Arch Intern Med 2003;163:929–35.
5. Sandler RS, Everhart JE, Donwitz M, et al. The burden of selected digestive dis-eases in the United States. Gastroenterology 2002;122:1500–11.
6. Levy RL, Von Korff M, Whitehead WE, et al. Costs of care for irritable bowel syn-drome patients in a health maintenance organization. Am J Gastroenterol 2001;96:3122–9.

7. Longstreth GF, Thompson WG, Chey WD, et al. Functional bowel disorders. Gastroenterology 2006;130:1480–91.

8. Lacy BE, Mearin F, Chang L, et al. Bowel disorders. Gastroenterology 2016;150: 1393–407.

9. Hungin AP, Chang L, Locke GR, et al. Irritable bowel syndrome in the United States: prevalence, symptom patterns and impact. Aliment Pharmacol Ther 2005;21:1365–75.

10. Saito YA, Schoenfeld P, Locke GR III. The epidemiology of irritable bowel syndrome in North America: a systematic review. Am J Gastroenterol 2002;97(8): 1910–5.

11. Agréus L, Svärdsudd K, Nyrén O, et al. Irritable bowel syndrome and dyspepsia in the general population: overlap and lack of stability over time. Gastroenterology 1995;109:671–80.

12. Ford AC, Moayyedi P, Chey WD, et al. American College of Gastroenterology monograph on management of irritable bowel syndrome. Am J Gastroenterol 2018;113(Suppl 2):1–18.

13. Sperber AD, Dekel R. Irritable bowel syndrome and co-morbid gastrointestinal and extra-gastrointestinal functional syndromes. J Neurogastroenterol Motil 2010;16:113–9.

14. Lewis SJ, Heaton KW. Stool form scale as a useful guide to intestinal transit time. Scand J Gastroenterol 1997;32:920–4.

15. Blake MR, Raker JM, Whelan K. Validity and reliability of the Bristol stool form scale in healthy adults and patients with diarrhoea-predominant irritable bowel syndrome. Aliment Pharmacol Ther 2016;44:693–703.

16. Dunlop SP, Jenkins D, Spiller RC. Distinctive clinical, psychological, and histological features of postinfective irritable bowel syndrome. Am J Gastroenterol 2003; 98:1578–83.

17. Spiller R, Garsed K. Postinfectious irritable bowel syndrome. Gastroenterology 2009;136:1979–88.

18. Spiller RC, Jenkins D, Thornley JP, et al. Increased rectal mucosal enteroendocrine cells, T-lymphocytes, and increased gut permeability following acute Campylobacter enteritis and in post-dysenteric irritable bowel syndrome. Gut 2000;47:804–11.

19. Neal KR, Hebden J, Spiller R. Prevalence of gastrointestinal symptoms six months after bacterial gastroenteritis and risk factors for development of the irritable bowel syndrome: postal survey of patients. Br Med J 1997;314:779–82.

20. Gwee KA, Leong YL, Graham C, et al. The role of psychological and biological factors in postinfective gut dysfunction. Gut 1000;44:400–0.

21. Neal KR, Barker L, Spiller RC. Prognosis in post-infective irritable bowel syndrome: a six year follow up study. Gut 2002;51:410–3.

22. Moayyedi P, Mearin F, Azpiroz F, et al. Irritable bowel syndrome diagnosis and management: a simplified algorithm for clinical practice. United European Gastroenterol J 2017;5(6):773–88.

23. Limsui D, Pardi DS, Camilleri M, et al. Symptomatic overlap between irritable bowel syndrome and micro- scopic colitis. Inflamm Bowel Dis 2007;13:175–81.

24. Ford AC, Quigley EM, Lacy BE, et al. Effect of antidepressants and psychological therapies, including hypnotherapy, in irritable bowel syndrome: systematic review and meta-analysis. Am J Gastroenterol 2014;109(9):1350–65.

25. Chapman RW, Stanghellini V, Geraint M, et al. Randomized clinical trial: macrogol/PEG 3350 plus electrolytes for treatment of patients with constipation associated with irritable bowel syndrome. Am J Gastroenterol 2013;108:1508–15.

26. Drossman DA, Chey WD, Johanson JF, et al. Clinical trial: lubiprostone in patients with constipation-associated irritable bowel syndrome - results of two randomized, placebo-controlled studies. Aliment Pharmacol Ther 2009;29:329–41.

27. Chey, Lembo JA, Lavins BJ, et al. Linaclotide for irritable bowel syndrome with constipation: a 26-week, randomized, double-blind, placebo-controlled trial to evaluate efficacy and safety. Am J Gastroenterol 2012;107:1702–12.

28. Omer A, Quigley EMM. An update on prucalopride in the treatment of chronic constipation. Therap Adv Gastroenterol 2017;10(11):877–87.

29. Madia VN, Messore A, Saccoliti F, et al. Tegaserod for the treatment of irritable bowel syndrome. Antiinflamm Antiallergy Agents Med Chem 2019;18:1.

30. Eswaran S, Muir J, Chey WD. Fiber and functional gastrointestinal disorders. Am J Gastroenterol 2013;108:718–27.

31. Hovdenak N. Loperamide treatment of the irritable bowel syndrome. Scand J Gastroenterol 1987;130:81–4.

32. Chang C. Short-course therapy for diarrhea-predominant irritable bowel syndrome: understanding the mechanism, impact on gut microbiota, and safety and tolerability of rifaximin. Clin Exp Gastroenterol 2018;11:335–45.

33. Pimentel M. Review article: potential mechanisms of action of rifaxamin in the management of irritable bowel syndrome with diarrhoea. Aliment Pharmacol Ther 2016;43(suppl 1):37–49.

34. Pimentel M, Lembo A, Chey WD, et al. Rifaximin therapy for patients with irritable bowel syndrome without constipation. N Engl J Med 2011;364:22–32.

35. Lembo A, Pimentel M, Rao SS, et al. Repeat treatment with rifaximin is safe and effective in patients with diarrhea-predominant irritable bowel syndrome. Gastroenterology 2016;151(6):1113–21.

36. Lembo AJ, Lacy BE, Zuckerman MJ, et al. Eluxadoline for irritable bowel syndrome with diarrhea. N Engl J Med 2016;374:242–53.

37. Mayer EA, Bradesi S. Alosetron and irritable bowel syndrome. Expert Opin Pharmacother 2003;4:2089–98.

38. Gershon MD, Tack J. The serotonin signaling system: from basic understanding to drug development for functional GI disorders. Gastroenterology 2007;132:397–414.

39. Miller DP, Alfredson T, Cook SF, et al. Incidence of colonic ischemia, hospitalized complications of constipation, and bowel surgery in relation to use of alosetron hydrochloride. Am J Gastroenterol 2003;98:1117–22.

40. Slattery SA, Niaz O, Aziz Q, et al. Systematic review with meta-analysis: the prevalence of bile acid malabsorption in the irritable bowel syndrome with diarrhoea. Aliment Pharmacol Ther 2015;42:3–11.

41. Sadowski DC, Camilleri M, Chey WD, et al. Canadian association of gastroenterology clinical practice guideline on the management of bile acid diarrhea. Clin Gastroenterol Hepatol 2020;18:24–41.

42. Annaházi A, Róka R, Rosztóczy A, et al. Role of antispasmodics in the treatment of irritable bowel syndrome. World J Gastroenterol 2014;20(20):6031–43.

43. Alammar N, Wang L, Saberi B, et al. The impact of peppermint oil on the irritable bowel syndrome: a meta-analysis of the pooled clinical data. BMC Complement Altern Med 2019;19(1):21.

44. Cash BD, Epstein MS, Shah SM. A novel delivery system of peppermint oil is an effective therapy for irritable bowel syndrome symptoms. Dig Dis Sci 2016;61(2):560–71.

45. Drossman DA, Tack J, Ford AC, et al. Neuromodulators for functional gastrointestinal disorders (disorders of gut-brain interaction): a Rome foundation working team report. Gastroenterology 2018;154:1140–71.e1.

46. Chey W. Food: the main course to wellness and illness in patients with irritable bowel syndrome. Am J Gastroenterol 2016;111(3):366–71.
47. Halmos EP, Power VA, Shepherd SJ, et al. A diet low in FODMAPs reduces symptoms of irritable bowel syndrome. Gastroenterology 2014;146:67–75.
48. Gibson PR, Shepherd SJ. Evidence-based dietary management of functional gastrointestinal symptoms: the FODMAP approach. J Gastroenterol Hepatol 2010;25:252–8.
49. Whelan K, Martin LD, Staudacher HM, et al. The low FODMAP diet in the management of irritable bowel syndrome: an evidence-based review of FODMAP restriction, reintroduction and personalisation in clinical practice. J Hum Nutr Diet 2018; 31:239–55.

Nutrition and Weight Management in the Elderly

Carolyn Newberry, MD[a],*, Gregory Dakin, MD[b]

KEYWORDS

- Digestion • Metabolism • Aging • Nutrition • Malnutrition • Obesity

KEY POINTS

- Changes in the digestive tract and metabolism occur throughout the life cycle and may alter swallowing function, digestive capabilities, and prevalence of gastrointestinal symptoms in elderly populations.
- These changes, coupled with alterations in oral intake, can predispose older persons to developing malnutrition, sarcopenia, and sarcopenic obesity.
- Physicians should recognize the complex nature of nutrition and weight management planning and screen early and often for malnutrition in this population.

INTRODUCTION

Aging changes the way the body digests food and absorbs nutrients as well as how it stores energy in the form of muscle and fat. The natural aging process is characterized by gradual loss of lean muscle mass with concomitant increase in adiposity, a process known as sarcopenia. This process can be exacerbated by other environmental pressures including alterations in dietary intake and physical activity in addition to inherent changes within the digestive tract itself (**Table 1**). The following is a review of these factors and how they are implicated in nutritional status and weight management in the elderly.

DIGESTION AND METABOLISM IN AGING
Deglutition

Swallowing is divided into 3 phases, which can all be affected by aging as well as concomitant medical conditions and medications. The oral phase of swallowing begins with food entering the mouth and is characterized by manipulating this food via mastication and salivary lubrication into a bolus that is transferred into the pharynx. Decreased jaw strength, changes in dentition, and reduction in salivary production

[a] Division of Gastroenterology, Weill Cornell Medical Center, 1305 York Avenue, 4th Floor, New York, NY 10021, USA; [b] Division of GI, Metabolic, & Bariatric Surgery, 525 East 68th Street, Box 294, New York, NY 10065, USA
* Corresponding author.
E-mail address: can9054@med.cornell.edu

Clin Geriatr Med 37 (2021) 131–140
https://doi.org/10.1016/j.cger.2020.08.010
0749-0690/21/© 2020 Elsevier Inc. All rights reserved.

Table 1
The effect of aging on the gastrointestinal tract and nutritional status

	Age-Related Changes	Effect on Oral Intake/Nutritional Status
Deglutition	Poor dentition, reduced muscular coordination and strength, decreased salivary production, reduced peristaltic pressures, increased esophageal sphincter tone	Poorer tolerance of certain food textures, increased time to feed, increased rates of dysphagia and aspiration
Digestion	Reduced gastric accommodation; reduced gastric, small intestinal, and colonic motility; alterations in pancreatic enzymes secretion; enhanced rates of small intestinal bacterial overgrowth	Increased gastrointestinal symptoms with oral intake, reduction in digestion and absorption of nutrients
Metabolism	Reduced total energy expenditure, decreased adaptability to changes in calorie intake, increased fat deposition	Excessive weight loss or gain with changes in oral intake, changes in body composition (sarcopenia, sarcopenic obesity)
Appetite	Reduced drive to eat, reduced pleasure associated with eating	Decreased overall intake
Social factors	Isolation, dementia, food availability, poor functional status	Increased food insecurity/ embarrassment during meals leading to decreased overall intake

can reduce the efficacy of the oral phase in older persons.[1] The second phase of swallowing, known as the pharyngeal phase, is involuntary and includes projection of the food bolus into the esophagus. This is where the involuntary esophageal phase of swallowing occurs, which includes propulsion of the bolus via peristalsis into the stomach.[2] Aging has been shown to lengthen the time of both the pharyngeal and esophageal phases.[3] Reduced peristaltic pressures and development of hiatal hernias may also occur, further limiting swallowing efficacy.[4]

This deterioration of the natural swallowing mechanism along all phases is associated with enhanced rates of dysphagia and aspiration in seniors. This phenomenon coupled with increased rates of neurologic and musculoskeletal disease leads to high rates of swallowing dysfunction in this population.[5] Epidemiologic studies have shown the prevalence of dysphagia in community dwelling individuals older than 50 years is between 15% and 22% and that this number increases to to 40% to 60% in nursing home and assisted living communities.[2] These rates are expected to increase with increasing numbers of persons older than 65 years in the general population. Because of their complicated nature and diverse origins, swallowing dysfunction may be insidious in onset and go unrecognized.[6] Swallowing abnormalities alter an individual's ability to eat by limiting the textures and quantities of food that can be consumed. Dysphagia diets are difficult to follow and associated with embarrassment regarding the need to change eating patterns in social settings. These factors can lead to isolation and further reduction in intake.[7] Proper management of swallowing dysfunction is imperative in both community dwelling and institutionalized persons. Compensatory management strategies include postural adjustments and alterations in swallowing maneuvers, which can be used before dietary modifications, which are less tolerated. Alternative feeding strategies including hand feeding may also be appropriate for patients who are unable to feed themselves.[8]

Digestion

In addition to swallowing dysfunction, the digestive process itself changes during aging. For example, in the healthy digestive tract, a set of stereotypical responses occur within the stomach after receiving a food bolus. These include accommodation of the bolus into the gastric fundus followed by mechanical mixing of the contents with gastric secretions such as stomach acid.[9] The ability for the stomach to accommodate decreases over time, with delays in emptying leading to enhancement of nausea and reflux in older individuals.[4] Although gastric acid secretion remains constant in elderly persons with healthy digestive tracts, concomitant medical conditions (including increased prevalence of pernicious anemia and *Helicobacter pylori* infection) may reduce secretion capabilities. Gastric acid secretion may also be affected by medications including antireflux drugs that are commonly prescribed.[10]

Beyond the stomach, foregut and intestinal motility as well as hepatobiliary digestive enzyme secretion may be altered. The normal small bowel receives partially digested food particles and continues to mix these with digestive enzymes to facilitate more distal absorption. Aging reduces small bowel motility, with reduction in migrating motor complexes and physiologic contractions after eating.[4] Reduction in motility can further enhance gastrointestinal distress and predispose patients to small intestinal bacterial overgrowth. Common complaints include bloating, distention, and diarrhea, which are most severe postprandially.[11] Pancreatic enzyme secretion decreases over time, leading to fat and carbohydrate malabsorption and loose stools. The gallbladder becomes less responsive to cholecystokinin, leading to reduced contractions and bile secretion and subsequent steatorrhea.[12] The mass of the liver decreases with aging due to decreased hepatic blood flow and hepatocyte degradation. Whether this leads to reduced liver function itself is controversial, although predisposes the elderly to liver injury secondary to ingestion of hepatotoxic medications or additional alterations in blood flow.[13]

In terms of colonic activity, although diarrhea is common due to previously stated foregut and hepatobiliary changes, abnormal bowel patterns may also be defined by constipation. Normally, the colon contracts segmentally resulting in propulsion of contents into the rectum for excretion.[14] Reduction in nerve endings with aging leads to reduced propulsions and stasis of stool.[15] Bowel habits in the elderly may fluctuate between diarrhea and constipation due to these physiologic changes as well as alterations in dietary intake to compensate.

Metabolism

Metabolism is altered in aging and may affect the ability of seniors to regulate overall energy intake. Total energy expenditure (TEE) decreases with time, with a large prospective cohort study using calorimetry noting a drop in TEE of 274 kcal/d over a 7-year time period in participants aged 70 to 79 years. Expected compensatory mechanisms to achieve weight and body composition homeostasis are also blunted. Metabolomic studies have demonstrated elderly volunteers are unable to adjust their resting energy expenditure levels to the same degree as younger participants in response to changes in caloric intake.[16] This inability to metabolically adapt can lead to enhanced weight fluctuations after times of altered calorie consumption.[17] Neurohormonal alterations are prevalent, affecting regulators of blood sugar levels and appetite.[16] Plasma insulin has been found to be correlative to adipocyte density and volume. Insulin insensitivity increases with aging and can lead to enhanced fat deposition. Effectiveness of satiety hormones including Leptin and neuropeptide Y is variable with aging and may alter hunger pathways. Coupled with alterations in previously mentioned gastrointestinal hormone secretion and physiologic adaptations, the elderly may have persistent changes in eating patterns that can lead to both inadequate and overconsumption of calories.[18]

NUTRITIONAL STATUS IN THE ELDERLY
Body Compositional Changes

Normal aging is associated with a gradual increase in adipose tissue with a concomitant reduction in muscle, a process termed "sarcopenia." Muscle is defined by both the amount (ie, mass) that is present and its associated function (ie, power).[19] Accelerated redistribution of these tissues can occur as a response to sedentary lifestyle, certain eating patterns (ie, western diet), and genetics.[20] This tissue redistribution and its functional change can also be enhanced by chronic disease processes. Although some degree of muscle loss and fat gain is expected in the setting of aging (ie, primary sarcopenia), accelerated states due to lifestyle, medications, and diseases is common and can lead to increased morbidity and mortality, a process termed "secondary sarcopenia."[21] Frailty, which corresponds to performance on the hand grip strength test and 6-minute walk test, considers muscle mass and performance.[22] The increased development of frailty and sarcopenia secondary to adoption of western lifestyles is of growing public health concern and is especially pertinent in the elderly. Sarcopenia has been found to be associated with increased risk of disability and mortality in older individuals.[19] Because of its relationship to these health outcomes, body composition has more recently been defined as a better marker of health than weight or body mass index (BMI) alone and may be used to assess vitality in elderly populations.[23]

In terms of protective measures against sarcopenia and frailty, diet quality and physical activity have been found to play a large role. This correlation has been analyzed in a systematic review of 23 studies, which reported the positive relationship between poor diet quality as defined by vegetable intake and enhanced rates of sarcopenia.[24] A common marker for diet quality is the Healthy Eating Index (HEI), which considers intake of vegetables, fruits, nuts, soy, white meat in comparison to red meat, cereal fiber, trans fat, polyunsaturated fatty acids in comparison to saturated fatty acids, multivitamin use, and alcohol.[25] Higher quality diets defined by the HEI have been shown to be protective against sarcopenia as well as overall mortality. In the same vein, physical activity in the setting of adequate protein intake enhances muscle mass and has positive metabolomic effects.[26] Lifestyle interventions in these populations is important to reduce morbidity associated with body compositional changes.

Nutritional Assessment

Conducting a nutritional assessment in elderly individuals includes anthropometrics (such as weight, height, waist, and hip measurements), dietary recall, and laboratory investigation (including total protein and albumin levels and inflammatory markers) (**Box 1**). Nutritional screening tools have also been developed, which risk stratify persons after assessment of current body weight and BMI, recent oral intake, feeding abilities, concomitant medical problems, and presence of acute illness.[27] The most validated nutrition screening tool in the elderly is the Mini Nutrition Assessment, which has both short and long forms. This survey considers both standard screening parameters (BMI, weight loss, recent oral intake, and presence of disease) as well as

---

Box 1
Basic tenets of nutritional screening in elderly patients

Limitations to oral feeding (structural, cognitive, accessibility)

Recent oral intake

Current BMI

Percentage of recent total body weight loss

Laboratory evaluation

Anthropometrics

Comorbid health conditions and medications

---

assessment of immobility and neuropsychological disease.[28] Screening identifies high-risk patients for further diagnostic testing and management.

Malnutrition and Nutritional Intervention Planning

Elderly persons often do not meet nutritional requirements as defined by nationally set Recommended Daily Allowances, which themselves may underestimate need in older individuals.[29,30] The most frequent changes in eating behavior in this population include reduction in overall intake and type of food consumed.[4] Fresh foods including fruits and vegetables may be consumed at lower frequencies, a result of accessibility and tolerance. This predisposes these persons, who already have high rates of medical comorbidities and medication use, to poorer nutrition statuses.[31] Elderly patients who are noted to be at high nutritional risk on malnutrition screening tools and/or clinical assessment should undergo a more comprehensive nutritional analysis. This includes a further investigation into underlying causes, individual food preferences, and limitations to normal eating patterns. Dietary intake can be monitored for several days after which intervention planning should take place.[27] A multidisciplinary team comprised of physicians, nurses, dietitians, and occupational therapists has been found to be the most effective in implementing nutritional protocols in both nursing home and home care persons and should be used when possible.[32] In terms of dietary approaches to increase oral intake, these are individualized. Important considerations for teams include the patient's underlying medical history, personal food preferences, allergies and sensitivities, food accessibility, living situation, and overall health status. Intervention options include augmentation of oral intake through dietary counseling, meal enrichment, and feeding protocols as well as formal nutritional support through feeding tubes and/or infusion.[33]

Obesity and Weight Management

Aging causes gradual loss of muscle mass with increased propensity to store excess energy as fat. Older individuals are less able to adapt metabolically to changes in caloric consumption. These factors, along with increasing life expectancy and prevalence of overweight and obese individuals in the population, necessitate discussion of obesity and sarcopenic obesity management in this population. In terms of defining obesity in the elderly, this proves challenging, as BMI cutoffs set by the World Health Organization do not differ by age despite known anthropometric changes over time. Normally, a BMI between 18.5 and 24.9 is considered healthy, 25 and 30 overweight, and greater than 30 obese; however, some geriatric literature suggests a normal BMI for persons older than 65 years is 24 to 29.[34] Notably the relationship between mortality and obesity in patients older than 65 years is also controversial with a well-reported "obesity paradox" that notes neutral or even improvement of length of life with obese status.[35]

In terms of weight management planning, efforts may concentrate more on weight maintenance, especially maintenance of muscle mass, than overall loss in contrast to younger individuals. Notably, large dietary and lifestyle fluctuations over time leading to weight cycling have been correlated with enhanced rates of sarcopenic obesity in aging populations, further highlighting the need for consistency of care.[36] In general, aggressive weight loss efforts are associated with reduction in both fat and lean body mass, which may be detrimental to older persons.[34] Emphasis on medical optimization including management of chronic conditions and, when possible, elimination of medications associated with weight gain is important. In terms of diet, limited research exists on optimal patterns to promote weight maintenance and/or loss in elderly populations, and this should by individualized based on preference and accessibility. A nutrient-rich isocaloric diet is generally the best approach, although moderate hypocaloric diets (no more than a 500-kcal deficit per day) can be considered. Ensuring adequate protein intake is important, with a recommendation of at least 1 g per kilogram of body weight per day in healthy individuals and higher amounts in those with acute or chronic illness.[33,37] Any reduction in caloric intake should be coupled with adequate physical activity to promote maintenance of lean muscle mass. Aerobic exercise including walking, cycling, and swimming is appropriate and has additional cardiovascular benefits.[34]

The role of medically supported weight loss through bariatric procedures in elderly populations is still unknown, although can be considered in select individuals. It is estimated that 20% of the elderly population are eligible for bariatric surgery. The National Institutes of Health guidelines for bariatric surgery established in 1991 initially limited the procedure to patients younger than or equal to 60 years but later lifted this restriction in 2006. Despite this change, procedures in the elderly remain controversial, and prospective, controlled, interventional trials comparing surgery to medical and dietary management do not exist. A large retrospective review of the National Surgical Quality Improvement Program (NSQIP) database analyzed 41,475 patients who underwent laparoscopic gastric bypass between 2011 and 2015 and compared the outcomes for patients older than 65 years to patients younger than 65 years. Elderly patients undergoing Roux-en-Y gastric bypass (RYGB) had a higher rate of serious early morbidity but similar 30-day mortality. Elderly patients undergoing sleeve gastrectomy had both higher serious morbidity and 30-day mortality. The average length of stay was prolonged regardless of procedure type. Although complications were increased, the overall rate remained very low (4% and 0.29%, respectively) leading the investigators to conclude that elderly patients should be counseled in their higher risk but should not be denied surgery based on age alone.[38] Similar findings and conclusions have published in later large meta-analyses that confirmed although there is a higher morbidity and mortality rate in older individuals undergoing these procedures, rates overall are low, especially when undergoing sleeve gastrectomy.[39,40] In terms of risk stratifying surgical candidates, a large study of patients in the American College of Surgeons National Surgical Quality Improvement database comparing those older than and younger than 70 years correlated higher complication rates with impaired functional status and the RYGB procedure.[41]

Weight loss data after surgery in the elderly population is similarly sparse. One study showed a 26.9% total body weight loss at 1-year follow-up, but this was significantly lower than that of the younger patient cohort.[42] Other studies have reported significant weight loss in elderly populations.[43,44] It is reasonable to conclude that older persons stand to gain substantially from the benefits that bariatric surgery may offer. However, this population is at higher risk for surgical complications, and thus each patient must be considered on an individual basis with attention not directed to age, but rather functional status and the presence of comorbid conditions.

SUMMARY

Elderly persons are at increased risk of malnutrition and changes in body composition including sarcopenia and sarcopenic obesity. This increased risk is secondary to alterations in deglutition, digestion, metabolism, and dietary patterns over time as well as higher prevalence of comorbid disease and medication use. Older individuals should be assessed early and often for malnutrition, with more formal assessment and nutritional planning in those who are deemed high risk. Although nutritional protocols should be individualized, basic tenets including promotion of high-quality foods, aerobic exercise, and early intervention guided treatment plans.

CLINICS CARE POINTS

- Aging can negatively affect swallowing function, digestion, and metabolism, which may lead to reduced oral intake, development of gastrointestinal symptoms, malabsorption, and alterations in weight homeostasis in elderly individuals.
- Elderly patients should be screened with the Mini Nutritional Assessment Tool on a regular basis to identify nutritional complications early and aid in care planning.
- Aggressive weight management programs are generally not recommended in persons >65 years old, however some patients may be able to pursue hypocaloric diets and even bariatric procedures with close medical supervision.

DISCLOSURE

The authors have nothing to disclose.

REFERENCES

1. Khan A, Carmona R, Traube M. Dysphagia in the elderly. Clin Geriatr Med 2014; 30(1):43–53. Available at: https://www.clinicalkey.es/playcontent/1-s2.0-S0749069013000918.
2. Aslam M, Vaezi MF. Dysphagia in the elderly. Gastroenterol Hepatol 2013;9(12): 784–95. Available at: https://www.ncbi.nlm.nih.gov/pubmed/24772045.
3. Namasivayam-MacDonald AM, Barbon CEA, Steele CM. A review of swallow timing in the elderly. Physiol Behav 2018;184:12–26. Available at: https://www.sciencedirect.com/science/article/pii/S0031938417303621.
4. Firth M, Prather CM. Gastrointestinal motility problems in the elderly patient. Gastroenterology 2002;122(6):1688–700. Available at: https://www.sciencedirect.com/science/article/pii/S0016508502706781.
5. Ergun GA, Miskovitz PF. Aging and the esophagus: common pathologic conditions and their effect upon swallowing in the geriatric population. Dysphagia 1992;7(2):58–63. Available at: https://www.ncbi.nlm.nih.gov/pubmed/1572228.
6. Schindler JS, Kelly JH. Swallowing disorders in the elderly. Laryngoscope 2002; 112:589–602. Available at: https://www.ncbi.nlm.nih.gov/pubmed/12150508.
7. Seshadri S, Sellers CR, Kearney MH. Balancing eating with breathing: community-dwelling older adults' experiences of dysphagia and texture-

modified diets. Gerontologist 2018;58(4):749–58. Available at: https://www.ncbi.nlm.nih.gov/pubmed/28082276.

8. Sura L, Madhavan A, Carnaby G, et al. Dysphagia in the elderly: management and nutritional considerations. Clin Interv Aging 2012;7:287–98. Available at: https://www.ncbi.nlm.nih.gov/pmc/articles/PMC3426263/.

9. Sanjeevi A. Gastric motility. Curr Opin Gastroenterol 2007;23(6):625–30. Available at: http://ovidsp.ovid.com/ovidweb.cgi?T=JS&NEWS=n&CSC=Y&PAGE=fulltext&D=ovft&AN=00001574-200711000-00007.

10. Feldman M, Cryer B, McArthur K, et al. Effects of aging and gastritis on gastric acid and pepsin secretion in humans: a prospective study. Gastroenterology 1996;110(4):1043–52. Available at: https://www.sciencedirect.com/science/article/pii/S0016508596001588.

11. Newberry C, Tierney A, Pickett-Blakely O. Lactulose hydrogen breath test result is associated with age and gender. Biomed Res Int 2016;2016:1064029.

12. Russell RM. Changes in gastrointestinal function attributed to aging. Am J Clin Nutr 1992;55(6 Suppl):1203S–7S. Available at: https://www.ncbi.nlm.nih.gov/pubmed/1590257.

13. Anantharaju A, Feller A, Chedid A. Aging liver. Gerontology 2002;48(6):343–53. Available at: https://www.karger.com/Article/Abstract/65506.

14. Treadway S, Hobson A. Gastric, small bowel and colonic motility and breath-testing. Medicine 2019;47(6):363–6.

15. Salles N. Basic mechanisms of the aging gastrointestinal tract. Dig Dis 2007;25(2):112–7. Available at: https://www.karger.com/Article/Abstract/99474.

16. Roberts SB, Fuss P, Dallal GE, et al. Effects of age on energy expenditure and substrate oxidation during experimental overfeeding in healthy men. J Gerontol A Biol Sci Med Sci 1996;51(2):B148–57. Available at: https://www.ncbi.nlm.nih.gov/pubmed/8612099.

17. Das SK, Moriguti JC, McCrory MA, et al. An underfeeding study in healthy men and women provides further evidence of impaired regulation of energy expenditure in old age. J Nutr 2001;131(6):1833–8. Available at: https://www.ncbi.nlm.nih.gov/pubmed/11385075.

18. Nutrition and aging: changes in the regulation of energy metabolism with aging. Physiol Rev 2006;86(2):651–67. Available at: https://search.proquest.com/docview/67844995.

19. Landi F, Cruz-Jentoft AJ, Liperoti R, et al. Sarcopenia and mortality risk in frail older persons aged 80 years and older: results from ilSIRENTE study. Age Ageing 2013;42(2):203–9. Available at: https://www.ncbi.nlm.nih.gov/pubmed/23321202.

20. Fried LP, Tangen CM, Walston J, et al. Frailty in older adults: evidence for a phenotype. J Gerontol A Biol Sci Med Sci 2001;56(3):M146–57. Available at: https://www.ncbi.nlm.nih.gov/pubmed/11253156.

21. Cruz-Jentoft AJ, Landi F. Sarcopenia. Clin Med (Lond) 2014;14(2):183–6. Available at: https://www.ncbi.nlm.nih.gov/pubmed/24715131.

22. Rodríguez-Mañas L, Féart C, Mann G, et al. Searching for an operational definition of frailty: a delphi method based consensus statement. the frailty operative definition-consensus conference project. J Gerontol A Biol Sci Med Sci 2013;68(1):62–7. Available at: https://www.ncbi.nlm.nih.gov/pubmed/22511289.

23. Kuczmarski RJ. Need for body composition information in elderly subjects. Am J Clin Nutr 1989;50:1150–7. Available at: https://www.ncbi.nlm.nih.gov/pubmed/2683723.

24. Hengeveld LM, Wijnhoven HAH, Olthof MR, et al. Prospective associations of diet quality with incident frailty in older adults: the health, aging, and body composition study. J Am Geriatr Soc 2019;67(9):1835–42. Available at: https://www. narcis.nl/publication/RecordID/oai:research.vu.nl:publications%2Fe2b1570e-7d44-4747-8c9c-de5a2f24e14f.

25. Akbaraly T, Ferrie J, Berr C, et al. Alternative healthy eating index and mortality over 18 y of follow-up: results from the whitehall II cohort. Am J Clin Nutr 2011; 94(1):247–53. Available at: https://www.hal.inserm.fr/inserm-00608593.

26. Pillard F, Laoudj-Chenivesse D, Carnac G, et al. Physical activity and sarcopenia. Clin Geriatr Med 2011;27(3):449–70. Available at: https://www.clinicalkey.es/playcontent/1-s2.0-S074906901100022X.

27. Vellas B, Lauque S, Andrieu S, et al. Nutrition assessment in the elderly. Curr Opin Clin Nutr Metab Care 2001;4(1):5–8. Available at: http://ovidsp.ovid.com/ovidweb.cgi?T=JS&NEWS=n&CSC=Y&PAGE=fulltext&D=ovft&AN=00075197-200101000-00002.

28. Vellas B, Guigoz Y, Garry PJ, et al. The mini nutritional assessment (MNA) and its use in grading the nutritional state of elderly patients. Nutrition 1999;15(2): 116–22.

29. Wolfe RR, Miller SL, Miller KB. Optimal protein intake in the elderly. Clin Nutr 2008; 27(5):675–84. Available at: https://www.clinicalkey.es/playcontent/1-s2.0-S0261561408001179.

30. Skully R. Essential nutrient requirements of the elderly. Nutrition and Dietary Supplements 2014;6:59–68. Available at: https://search.proquest.com/docview/2229321219.

31. Anderson AL, Harris TB, Tylavsky FA, et al. Dietary patterns and survival of older adults. J Am Diet Assoc 2011;111(1):84–91. Available at: https://www.clinicalkey.es/playcontent/1-s2.0-S0002822310016482.

32. Beck AM, Christensen AG, Hansen BS, et al. Multidisciplinary nutritional support for undernutrition in nursing home and home-care: a cluster randomized controlled trial. Nutrition 2016;32(2):199–205. Available at: https://www.clinicalkey.es/playcontent/1-s2.0-S0899900715003445.

33. Volkert D, Beck AM, Cederholm T, et al. ESPEN guideline on clinical nutrition and hydration in geriatrics. Clin Nutr 2019;38(1):10–47. https://doi.org/10.1016/j.clnu.2018.05.024. Available at:.

34. Chau D, Cho L, Jani P, et al. Individualizing recommendations for weight management in the elderly. Curr Opin Clin Nutr Metab Care 2008;11(1):27–31. Available at: http://ovidsp.ovid.com/ovidweb.cgi?T=JS&NEWS=n&CSC=Y&PAGE=fulltext&D=ovft&AN=00075197-200801000-00006.

35. Decaria JE, Sharp C, Petrella RJ. Scoping review report Obesity in older adults. Int J Obes (Lond) 2012;36:1141–50. Available at: https://www.nature.com/articles/ijo201229.

36. Lee JS, Visser M, Tylavsky FA, et al. Weight loss and regain and effects on body composition: the health, aging and body composition study. J Gerontol A Biol Sci Med Sci 2010;65A(1):78–83. Available at: https://www.narcis.nl/publication/RecordID/oai:research.vu.nl:publications%2Fa5fc6e12-dacb-4689-9508-2b223dfad58d.

37. Bloom I, Shand C, Cooper C, et al. Diet quality and sarcopenia in older adults: a systematic review. Nutrients 2018;10(3):308. Available at: https://www.ncbi.nlm.nih.gov/pubmed/29510572.

38. Koh CY, Inaba CS, Sujatha-Bhaskar S, et al. Outcomes of laparoscopic bariatric surgery in the elderly population. Am Surg 2018;84(10):1600–3. Available at: https://www.ncbi.nlm.nih.gov/pubmed/30747677.

39. Giordano S, Victorzon M. Laparoscopic Roux-En-Y gastric bypass in elderly patients (60 Years or older): a meta-analysis of comparative studies. Scand J Surg 2018;107(1):6–13. Available at: https://www.ncbi.nlm.nih.gov/pubmed/?term=28942708.

40. Giordano S, Salminen P. Laparoscopic sleeve gastrectomy is safe for patients over 60 years of age: a meta-analysis of comparative studies. J Laparoendosc Adv Surg Tech A 2020;30(1):12–9. Available at: https://www.ncbi.nlm.nih.gov/pubmed/?term=31855106.

41. Pechman DM, Muñoz Flores F, Kinkhabwala CM, et al. Bariatric surgery in the elderly: outcomes analysis of patients over 70 using the ACS-NSQIP database. Surg Obes Relat Dis 2019;15(11):1923–32. Available at: https://www.ncbi.nlm.nih.gov/pubmed/31611184.

42. Abbas M, Cumella L, Zhang Y, et al. Outcomes of laparoscopic sleeve gastrectomy and Roux-en-Y gastric bypass in patients older than 60. Obes Surg 2015;25(12):2251–6. Available at: https://www.ncbi.nlm.nih.gov/pubmed/?term=26001882.

43. Sugerman HJ, DeMaria EJ, Kellum JM, et al. Effects of bariatric surgery in older patients. Ann Surg 2004;240:243–7. Available at: https://www.ncbi.nlm.nih.gov/pubmed/?term=15273547.

44. Sosa JL, Pombo H, Pallavicini H, et al. Laparoscopic gastric bypass beyond age 60. Obes Surg 2004;14:1398–401. Available at: https://www.ncbi.nlm.nih.gov/pubmed/15603658.

Diverticulosis, Diverticulitis, and Diverticular Bleeding

David Wan, MD[a], Tibor Krisko, MD[b],*

KEYWORDS

- Diverticulosis • Diverticulitis • Diverticular disease • Diverticula • Abdominal pain
- Hemorrhage • Hematochezia • Microbiome

KEY POINTS

- Although diverticulosis is common, complications such as diverticulitis, diverticular bleeding, or symptoms of disease are rare.
- Although the role of dietary fiber in diverticulosis is unclear, there is a clear benefit of increased fiber, physical activity, and tobacco cessation in reducing diverticulosis complications.
- Consuming nuts and seeds has been shown to actually decrease, not increase, rates of diverticular disease.
- Diverticular bleeding is the most common cause of lower gastrointestinal bleeding but typically self-resolves, and emergent colonoscopy does not result in improved clinical outcomes.
- In select patients with uncomplicated diverticulitis, the use of antibiotics may not be required.

INTRODUCTION

Colonic diverticula are mucosal and submucosal herniations in the muscle layer through the colonic wall (**Fig. 1**). They are the most common anatomic alteration of the colon, and age-dependent prevalence results in up to 75% of people older than 75 years affected, although most are usually asymptomatic.[1] However, in a minority of patients it can lead to a host of clinically relevant conditions, collectively referred to as *diverticular diseases*, and include the following (**Fig. 2**):

- Diverticulitis

a Division of Gastroenterology and Hepatology, Joan & Sanford I. Weill Department of Medicine, Weill Cornell Medicine, 1305 York Avenue, 4th Floor, New York, NY 10021, USA; b Division of Gastroenterology and Hepatology, Joan & Sanford I. Weill Department of Medicine, Weill Cornell Medicine, 413 East 69th Street, BRB 650, New York, NY 10021, USA
* Corresponding author.
E-mail address: Tik9022@med.cornell.edu

Clin Geriatr Med 37 (2021) 141–154
https://doi.org/10.1016/j.cger.2020.08.011
0749-0690/21/© 2020 Elsevier Inc. All rights reserved.

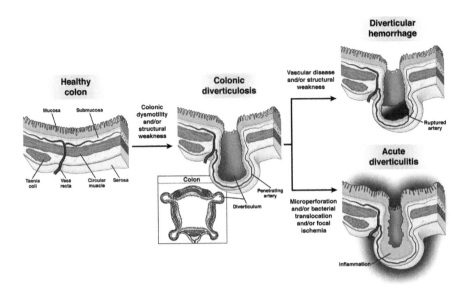

Fig. 1. Colonic diverticula form when mucosa and submucosa herniate through the envelope that surrounds the intramural vasa recta. Diverticular hemorrhage is an arterial bleed in an uninflamed diverticulum; acute diverticulitis is inflammation localized to a diverticulum and the surrounding mucosa triggered by microperforation or bacterial translocation or focal ischemia. (*From* Camilleri M, Sandler RS, Peery AF. Etiopathogenetic mechanisms in diverticular disease of the colon. Cell Mol Gastroenterol Hepatol. 2020;9(1):17; with permission.)

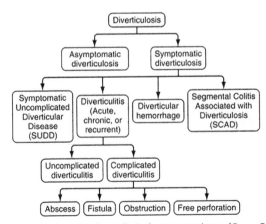

Fig. 2. Overview of diverticulosis and its clinical presentations. (*From* Bhuket TP, Stollman NH. Diverticular disease of the colon. In: Feldman M, Friedman LS, Brandt LJ, editors. Sleisenger and Fordtran's gastrointestinal and liver disease: pathophysiology/diagnosis/management. Philadelphia: Saunders/Elsevier; 2016. p. 2123-38; with permission.)

- Diverticular bleeding
- Segmental colitis associated with diverticula (SCAD)
- Symptomatic uncomplicated diverticular disease (SUDD)

Colonic diverticular diseases place a significant burden on the US health care system. They account for greater than 300,000 emergency department visits and more than 200,000 hospital admissions annually.[2] The management of these conditions continues to evolve as our understanding of these diseases is changing, and traditional ways of management are now being challenged.

EPIDEMIOLOGY

As noted, diverticulosis increases with age.[3] They are typically discovered incidentally on computed tomography (CT) scans or colonoscopies performed to evaluate various gastrointestinal complaints or for colorectal cancer screening, respectively (**Fig. 3**).

There are clear differences in the nature of diverticulosis in the East and Asia. In the West, diverticulosis is left sided, increases with age, and are pseudodiverticula, in which not all layers herniate through a defect in the muscularis. In Asia, diverticulosis is typically a true diverticulum, less prevalent, mainly right sided, appears earlier, and does not increase with time. However, after Asians immigrate to Western countries, the differences seem to dissipate with time, likely reflecting the influence of dietary changes.[4]

Diverticulitis is a spectrum of disease in which frank inflammation and infection develop amid a diverticulum, leading to microperforation and abdominal pain. Of the 10% to 15% of patients with diverticulosis who progress to symptomatic disease, one-third will develop diverticulitis,[5,6] which is the fourth most-common cause of acute abdominal pain in the elderly.[7] The vast majority (85%) will present with

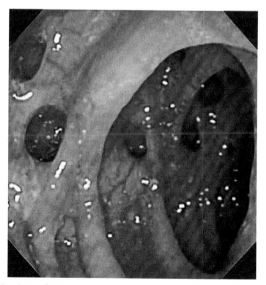

Fig. 3. Colonoscopic view of sigmoid diverticulosis. (*From* Bhuket TP, Stollman NH. Diverticular disease of the colon. In: Feldman M, Friedman LS, Brandt LJ, editors. Sleisenger and Fordtran's gastrointestinal and liver disease: pathophysiology/diagnosis/management. Philadelphia: Saunders/Elsevier; 2016. p. 2123-38; with permission.)

uncomplicated diverticulitis,[8] but a minority have a more complicated course, including abscesses, fistulas, obstruction, or frank perforation. Diverticulitis was the sixth ranked gastrointestinal diagnosis in US hospitals in 2014,[9] and although overall incidence is increasing, the rate of developing diverticulitis seems to decrease with increasing age.[5]

Diverticular bleeding is the main cause of acute lower gastrointestinal bleeding. In 2014, lower gastrointestinal bleeding accounted for more than 367,881 emergency room visits and 144,401 hospital admissions in the United States,[2] of which 30% to 65% were attributed to diverticular cause. The clinical picture of diverticular lower gastrointestinal bleeding can range from low-volume blood loss to substantial bleeding, causing hemodynamic instability and significant transfusion requirements.

PATHOPHYSIOLOGY
Diverticulosis and Diverticular Diseases

The traditional theory, proposed by Burkitt and Painter, was that low-fiber diet led to small-caliber, hard stools; increased intracolonic pressures; and resulted in formation of the small herniated colonic sacs at relative weak points of the wall where blood vessels penetrate.[10] This theory was based on observations that rural Africans had a lower diverticulosis burden than in the economically developed Western countries, which they attributed to lower dietary fiber intake in the West. However, neither fiber intake nor diverticulosis prevalence was measured.[11] It is now thought that diverticulosis and diverticular disease develops from complex factors that include (**Table 1**) altered colonic motility, visceral hypersensitivity, inflammation, genetic susceptibility, lifestyle (diet, tobacco smoking, medications), and gut microbiome imbalances.[12]

Enteric neuronal degeneration and *altered colonic motility* have been suggested to play a pathophysiologic role by studies showing decreased myenteric ganglia, glial cells, and interstitial cells of Cajal, the pacemaker cells of the gastrointestinal tract.[12] Enteric nerve dysregulation may also contribute to muscular hypertrophy and *visceral hypersensitivity* and is thought to lead to the symptoms of diverticular disease. The presence and role of *inflammation* in diverticula pathogenesis is unclear. In patients with asymptomatic diverticulosis, mucosal biopsies lacked evidence of inflammation.[13] However, studies of patients with symptomatic diverticular disease have shown increased neutrophilic or chronic lymphocytic infiltration.[12]

Genetic factors seem to play a role. In addition to aforementioned observations of phenotypic variation between East and West, a Swedish twin study suggested that the odds ratio of one twin with diverticular disease having an affected sibling was 7-fold in monozygotic as compared with 3-fold for dizygotic twins.[14] Recent studies have identified loci involved in neuromuscular regulation, vascular, and mesenchymal functions.[15]

Lifestyle factors such as vigorous physical activity seem to reduce the risk of diverticular disease, whereas obesity is associated with an increased risk.[16] Various *medications*, especially nonsteroidal antiinflammatory drugs, steroids, and opiates, are associated with diverticular bleeding and severity of diverticulitis.[17]

Diverticulitis

Diverticulitis has traditionally been attributed to obstruction of individual diverticula by fecaliths,[18] with subsequent local mechanical irritation and inflammation that progresses to ischemia and microperforation (see **Fig. 1**). Similar to diverticulosis in general, it is now recognized that genetics,[19] obesity,[20] physical inactivity, and tobacco[21] all play important roles in the pathophysiology of diverticulitis.

Table 1
Factors associated with diverticulosis and diverticular diseases

	Diverticulosis	Diverticular Diseases
Demographics		
Age	++	++
Race/ethnicity		
African-American	+	+
Hispanic or Caucasian	−	−
Female gender	−	−
Lifestyle/Environmental		
Diet		
Western diet (ie, high fat, red meat)	Unknown	+
High-fiber	+/−[a]	− −
Nuts, seeds	Unknown	−
Alcohol use	+	+
Smoking	Unknown	+
Vigorous physical activity	Unknown	−
Obesity	Unknown	+
Diabetes mellitus	Unknown	+
Ultraviolet light exposure	Unknown	−
Vitamin D levels	Unknown	−
Drugs		
Aspirin	Unknown	+
NSAIDs	Unknown	++
Corticosteroids	Unknown	+
Menopausal hormone therapy	Unknown	+
Opioids	Unknown	+
Genetic Susceptibility Variants		
Altered smooth muscle/nerve function	+	+
Epithelial function	+	+
Altered connective tissue	+	+
Visceral Hypersensitivity	N/A	+
Gut Microbiome Alterations	Unknown	+
Inflammation	N/A	+

Abbreviations: NSAID, nonsteroidal antiinflammatory drug; +, weak positive association; ++, strong positive association; −, weak negative correlation; − −, strong negative correlation.
[a] Studies have shown both lower and higher diverticular incidence with higher-fiber intake.

There has been particular debate regarding diet, with a longstanding belief that patients with diverticulosis should avoid consumption of nuts, popcorn, and seeds. However, this is not supported by recent studies including one of 47,228 men in which consumption of these foods *decreased* the incidence of diverticulitis.[22] Further analyses in that cohort linked a typical Western diet[23] and higher quantities of unprocessed red meat[24] to diverticulitis. A 2019 analysis of the Nurses' Health Study suggested that a higher intake of dietary fiber was protective for diverticulitis, with particular benefit from insoluble fiber and whole fruits.[25] Similar benefits from fiber were seen in 2 large Swedish cohorts.[26]

There has been significant interest in the role of the gut microbiome in diverticulitis, in particular for its ability to modulate inflammation and immunity,[27] which is suggested by the response of patients to antibiotics[28] and the fact that fiber's benefits may be mediated in part through fermentation into short-chain fatty acids.[26] However, much of the current data are descriptive and even conflicting, and further research is required.[29,30]

Diverticular Bleeding

Diverticular bleeding is thought to arise from the exposed vasa recta over the dome of the diverticulum as it herniates. The arterial vessel is superficially located in the neck or base of the diverticulum, and with progressive weakening of the artery and mechanical trauma, it can rupture into the lumen (see **Fig. 1**). It has been proposed that vascular disease or mechanical weakness could increase susceptibility to trauma from inspissated stool. Notably, diverticular bleeding is not related to inflammation, and significant bleeding rarely occurs in diverticulitis.

PRESENTATION, DIAGNOSIS, AND MANAGEMENT
Diverticulitis

Presentation and diagnosis

Patients with acute diverticulitis *typically present with* localized abdominal pain (most commonly left lower quadrant), altered bowel function, and fever. In the 15% to 30% of patients who have a more complicated course, guarding, peritonitis, and sepsis can be associated with abscesses, fistulae, obstruction, and perforation.[31,32] (**Box 1**). Elderly individuals can have atypical presentations with increased morbidity and mortality.[7,33]

The *differential diagnosis* of acute diverticulitis is broad and should include acute cholecystitis,[7,34] ischemic colitis, appendicitis, malignancy, urinary tract infection, nephrolithiasis, ovarian torsion,[35] inflammatory bowel disease, and bowel obstruction.[36] More mild or atypical presentations may be confused with irritable bowel syndrome (IBS), SUDD, or SCAD.[29]

Basic laboratories and lactate and urinalysis allow measurement of white blood cell count, assessment for alternate diagnoses (urinary tract infections, ischemia, gastrointestinal bleed, hepatobiliary disease), and markers of end organ damage.[9] Although nonspecific, C-reactive protein (CRP) may be useful. The nonspecific clinical presentation of acute diverticulitis has contributed to rates of misdiagnosis ranging from 34% to 68%[32,35] and has led to liberal use of imaging, particularly in elderly patients. Plain

---

Box 1
Hinchey classification of diverticulitis

1a	Pericolonic phlegmon and inflammation, no fluid collection
1b	Pericolonic abscess <4 cm
2	Pelvic or interloop abscess OR abscess >4 cm
3	Purulent peritonitis
4	Feculent peritonitis

Contributed by Stephanie Carr DO. *From* Colon diverticulitis. StatPearls Publishing LLC; 2020. This book is distributed under the terms of the Creative Commons Attribution 4.0 International License (http://creativecommons.org/licenses/by/4.0/), which permits use, duplication, adaptation, distribution, and reproduction in any medium or format, as long as you give appropriate credit to the original author(s) and the source, a link is provided to the Creative Commons license, and any changes made are indicated.

film abdominal radiographs provide rapid evaluation for perforation (free air) or alternate diagnoses (obstruction). More commonly, abdominal/pelvic CT scanning confirms the presence of diverticula as well as findings of inflammation, bowel wall thickening, "pericolic fat stranding, and corresponding complications (**Fig. 4**)."[32] Oral and intravenous contrast, as tolerated, improve diagnostic accuracy, and findings can be combined with the Hinchey classification system (see **Box 1**) to describe the extent of disease.

Although CT imaging has a clear role in the diagnosis of diverticulitis, particularly in patients older than 80 years,[36] recognition of associated costs and risks has led to efforts to develop alternatives. Ultrasound (US) has the benefits of avoidance of radiation and its rapid point-of-care use, and an investigational but promising strategy consists of using US as first-line imaging, with CT scanning reserved for negative or inconclusive studies.[21] In addition, studies to develop clinical decision rules have led to combining CRP and typical clinical features (*absence of vomiting, focal left lower-quadrant tenderness*) to yield adequate diagnostic certainty of acute left-sided diverticulitis without CT imaging, particularly in younger patients.[37] Finally, fecal calprotectin can be measured in stool as a marker of inflammation and may help distinguish uncomplicated diverticulitis from IBS.[38]

Medical management

Uncomplicated acute diverticulitis ± localized abscess is usually managed with conservative treatment[39] including fluids, analgesics, and diet as tolerated. Inpatient observation, particularly for the elderly, may be warranted.[40]

Antibiotics, both oral and parenteral, have been a traditional mainstay of medical treatment, although based mostly on expert opinion and nonrandomized trials.[41] When antibiotics are warranted, including most cases of complicated diverticulitis, common regimens include ciprofloxacin combined with metronidazole, amoxicillin-clavulanic acid, or clindamycin or metronidazole combined with trimethoprim/sulfamethoxazole or gentamicin.[21]

However, increased awareness of the risks of antibiotics and lack of supporting data have led to multicenter trials suggesting that antibiotics did not accelerate recovery or improve outcomes in uncomplicated diverticulitis.[42,43] A 11-year follow-up showed remarkable equivalence of the 2 approaches, providing additional evidence

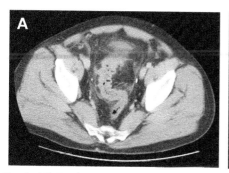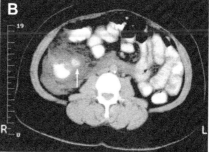

Fig. 4. (*A*) CT of a patient with acute uncomplicated diverticulitis showing colon wall thickening and stranding of the pericolic fat. (*B*) CT of a patient with a right lower quadrant abscess (*arrow*). (*From* Bhuket TP, Stollman NH. Diverticular disease of the colon. In: Feldman M, Friedman LS, Brandt LJ, editors. Sleisenger and Fordtran's gastrointestinal and liver disease: pathophysiology/diagnosis/management. Philadelphia: Saunders/Elsevier; 2016. p. 2123-38; with permission.)

that at least in a first episode of uncomplicated left-sided acute diverticulitis, it may be reasonable to defer antibiotics.[41] This approach is best limited to younger patients with mild disease (Hinchey 1a) and may benefit from shared decision-making.[44] Accordingly, guidelines suggest that "antibiotics be used *selectively* in cases of uncomplicated diverticulitis and on an individual basis rather than routinely."[30]

Surgery

Surgery should be reserved for more severe presentations of acute diverticulitis with peritonitis or perforation,[45] as rates of readmission for treatment failure following medical management of uncomplicated diverticulitis are only 6.6%.[46]

In the 20% of patients who require emergent surgery,[47] this traditionally consisted of open laparotomy, resection with diversion colostomy, and Hartmann pouch. Advances such as minimally invasive laparoscopy and lavage and resection with primary anastomosis can result in more rapid healing and less postsurgical complications,[48,49] provided patients are hemodynamically stable and local expertise permits this approach.[45,50]

Patient evaluation is critical in the *elderly when considering risks and benefits of surgical options*. Using a "multidimensional, comprehensive geriatric assessment," an unstable septic elderly patient will likely require prompt intervention, whereas a more healthy and stable older individual can often be treated surgically in a manner similar to a younger patient, potentially including resection and primary anastomosis, although further research is needed.[51]

Patients who lack peritonitis or evidence of perforation may nonetheless develop complications such as abscess or fistulae with a variable time course (**Fig. 3**B). Abscesses are commonly decompressed by the percutaneous route with CT guidance. Pelvic abscesses are associated with a higher rate of complications that may lead to interval sigmoid resection,[52] although evolving guidelines suggest that surgery is not always required, especially if they can be drained percutaneously.[6,53] Fistulae, including colovesicular, are typically managed surgically, often following initial antibiotic therapy.

Prognosis and prevention

Patients with acute uncomplicated diverticulitis typically improve over weeks. In addition to late presentations of aforementioned complications, a primary concern is recurrence. Accordingly, traditional practice included surgical referral following the second or third episode to consider elective prophylactic colectomy.[51] However, elective colonic resection following uncomplicated diverticulitis should *not* be routinely recommended, and rather should be an individualized patient-centered consideration, particularly in older individuals with increased risk of postsurgical complications.[30] This is supported by retrospective studies in which diverticulitis recurred in just 13.3% of patients, with only 3.9% having a second recurrence.[47] However, consideration of elective surgery is warranted in patients with "ongoing symptoms, pelvic abscesses" and those "at high risk of perforation during future episodes," for example, immunosuppressed patients.[52]

Diverticular Bleeding

Presentation and diagnosis

Diverticular bleeding typically presents with bright red blood per rectum. The differential diagnosis includes ischemic colitis, hemorrhoids, colorectal polyps or neoplasms, angioectasias, postpolypectomy bleeding, inflammatory bowel disease, infectious colitis, stercoral ulceration, colorectal varices, radiation proctopathy, nonsteroidal antiinflammatory drug-induced colopathy, and Dieula-foy lesions. Patients typically do not experience significant pain, but sometimes report mild cramping. In contrast to the scant amounts of red blood observed with hemorrhoidal bleeding, patients with diverticular bleeding report large volume red or maroon blood with or without clots. Sometimes the bleeding can be severe and cause hemodynamic instability. There have been various risk factors associated with worse outcomes, which include age, comorbidities, hypotension, tachycardia, and initial hematocritat presentation. Various risk stratification systems have incorporated these factors such as the Oakland, Strate, Sengupta, and AIM65 score.[54]

Management

The management of diverticular bleeding depends on the severity of the presentation. If a patient is stable, then the standard approach is to perform a colonoscopy.[55] Nonetheless, 80% of diverticular bleeding episodes self-resolve with low overall mortality and a rate of therapeutic endoscopic interventions of only 4.6%.[56] Although previous studies have demonstrated that emergent colonoscopy following rapid bowel purge increases colonoscopic therapeutic intervention rates, randomized controlled trials have shown that urgent, as compared with nonurgent, colonoscopy does not improve clinical outcomes.[55,57] In these studies, urgent colonoscopy had variable definitions, ranging from within 8 to 24 hours, whereas control groups ranged from 8 to 96 hours. Notably, urgent colonoscopy requires a rapid purge prep in which patients ingest up to 6 L of bowel preparation within 3 to 4 hours to produce clear rectal effluent and mobilization of an endoscopy team with 24-hour availability to promptly perform the colonoscopy. Consequently, urgent colonoscopy is difficult to achieve and in practice colonoscopies are customarily performed within 24 to 48 hours. In light of this, it is unclear if colonoscopies in context of diverticular bleeding confer any significant clinical benefit other than making a presumptive diagnosis or ruling out alternative causes such as angioectasia or colorectal cancer. Some even suggest that select low-risk patients can even be safely discharged from the emergency room.[58]

If a patient is tachycardic and/or hypotensive, some studies and guidelines have suggested the initial use of CT angiography to help localize the bleeding source.[58] CT angiography provides a fast, noninvasive means of locating the bleeding source and does not require a bowel preparation. If the CT angiography is positive, then interventional radiologists, gastroenterologists, and surgeons can better target the suspected lesion and develop a coordinated therapeutic plan. In rare cases when patients are too unstable for endoscopy or radiology, a surgical consultation is necessary for consideration of colectomy.

SEGMENTAL COLITIS ASSOCIATED WITH DIVERTICULOSIS

SCAD is defined as chronic inflammation in an area of colonic diverticulosis, and it may or may not include the diverticular orifice. However, there is wide variability in its clinical, endoscopic, and histologic presentation. The symptoms can include bleeding, diarrhea, or abdominal pain. The endoscopic appearance can include erythema, friability, and erosions. In general, the approach to treatment is similar to that in inflammatory bowel disease, with mild cases managed with probiotics, antibiotics, and/or 5-aminosalicylates, whereas more severe cases require steroids or even antitumor necrosis factor agents.

SYMPTOMATIC UNCOMPLICATED DIVERTICULAR DISEASE

SUDD is characterized by nonspecific abdominal pain in the absence of severe or overt inflammation. The pain is typically colicky, but can be constant, usually relieved with defecation, and can be associated with bloating and altered bowel habits. On examination, there may be left lower quadrant tenderness or fullness. Given the similarity in presentation, SUDD can be difficult to distinguish from IBS. It is possible that SUDD may even represent IBS in a patient with coincident, unrelated diverticulosis, although differences in cytokine and microbiome signatures between the two entities may exist.[38]

Nevertheless, the current treatment approach to SUDD is very similar to IBS, with initial efforts aimed at increasing fiber intake through diet or supplementation, with equal efficacy between soluble or insoluble forms. Three randomized controlled trials have been conducted and although heterogeneity limits conclusions, therapy with fiber seemed to improve symptoms.[12] Antibiotics such as the nonabsorbable, gut lumen–acting rifaximin have shown symptom reduction.[59] Other possible treatments include mesalamine, probiotics, and antispasmodics; however, the data underlying these are heterogeneous and thus it is difficult to make firm recommendations.[12] If lifestyle modifications and these initial treatments do not yield improvement, referral to a gastroenterologist is appropriate.

SUMMARY

Diverticulosis increases with age and may in fact be a normal part of aging. A minority of individuals with diverticulosis can develop diverticulitis, diverticular bleeding, and other symptomatic subtypes, collectively known as *diverticular disease*. The underlying pathophysiology includes genetic, lifestyle, and microbiome factors. *Diverticulitis* is characterized by abdominal pain and fever, and imaging is typically required to confirm the diagnosis. Antibiotics are part of traditional medical management, with surgery reserved for complicated disease. Recent research suggests that changes to "traditional management" may allow patients to forego CT scans or defer routine use of antibiotics. A variety of preventive interventions, particularly lifestyle modifications, can lessen the chance of recurrence. *Diverticular bleeding* presents with painless, large volume blood per rectum, and can be life-threatening but typically resolves spontaneously. Imaging can play a role in determining the source, but colonoscopy has traditionally been recommended. Recent investigations are refining the role and timing of these diagnostic studies. These diseases can present atypically in *elderly individuals*, requiring careful evaluation, liberal use of imaging, and careful weighing of risks and benefits of treatment options. Although much work remains to fully understand the pathophysiology and optimal treatment of diverticular diseases, attention to critical lifestyle factors such as diet, exercise, tobacco abstinence, and increased physical activity may reduce symptomatic diverticular disease while improving overall cardiometabolic health of our patients.

CLINICS CARE POINTS

- In patients with diverticulosis, high dietary fiber intake is associated with less diverticulitis, and should be encouraged. This also is true regarding the increased consumption of nuts, popcorns, and seeds, and discontinuation of these foods should be discouraged.
- In patients with uncomplicated diverticulitis, the benefit of traditional approaches centered on antibiotics and pursuit of surgery after recurrent episodes is no

longer clear. In patients with complicated diverticulitis, surgery is often necessary, but risks of surgery can be significant in elderly patients or those with significant co-morbidities. Thus, given varying patient ages, co-morbidities, presentations, and local expertise, shared-decision making is essential.
- In most patients with diverticular bleeding, the bleeding spontaneously stops and urgent colonoscopy within 24 hours does not improve clinical outcomes.

DISCLOSURE

The authors have nothing to disclose.

REFERENCES

1. Delvaux M. Diverticular disease of the colon in Europe: epidemiology, impact on citizen health and prevention. Aliment Pharmacol Ther 2003;18(Suppl 3):71–4.
2. Peery AF, Crockett SD, Murphy CC, et al. Burden and cost of gastrointestinal, liver, and pancreatic diseases in the United States: update 2018. Gastroenterology 2019;156(1):254–72.e1.
3. Everhart JE, Ruhl CE. Burden of digestive diseases in the United States part II: lower gastrointestinal diseases. Gastroenterology 2009;136(3):741–54.
4. Zullo A, Gatta L, Vassallo R, et al. Paradigm shift: the Copernican revolution in diverticular disease. Ann Gastroenterol 2019;32(6):541–53.
5. Shahedi K, Fuller G, Bolus R, et al. Long-term risk of acute diverticulitis among patients with incidental diverticulosis found during colonoscopy. Clin Gastroenterol Hepatol 2013;11(12):1609–13.
6. Strate LL, Morris AM. Epidemiology, pathophysiology, and treatment of diverticulitis. Gastroenterology 2019;156(5):1282–98.e1.
7. Perez-Hernandez JL, Teuffer-Carrion LT, Diaz-Aldana EV, et al. Acute abdominal pain in elderly patients evaluated in the emergency department at a tertiary level. Rev Gastroenterol Mex 2010;75(3):261–6.
8. Ambrosetti P, Chautems R, Soravia C, et al. Long-term outcome of mesocolic and pelvic diverticular abscesses of the left colon: a prospective study of 73 cases. Dis Colon Rectum 2005;48(4):787–91.
9. Rezapour M, Stollman N. Diverticular disease in the elderly. Curr Gastroenterol Rep 2019;21(9):46.
10. Painter NS. Diverticular disease of the colon–a disease of the century. Lancet 1969;2(7620):586–8.
11. Painter NS, Burkitt DP. Diverticular disease of the colon: a deficiency disease of western civilization. Br Med J 1971;2(5759):450–4.
12. Tursi A, Papa A, Danese S. Review article: the pathophysiology and medical management of diverticulosis and diverticular disease of the colon. Aliment Pharmacol Ther 2015;42(6):664–84.
13. Peery AF, Keku TO, Addamo C, et al. Colonic diverticula are not associated with mucosal inflammation or chronic gastrointestinal symptoms. Clin Gastroenterol Hepatol 2018;16(6):884–91.e1.
14. Granlund J, Svensson T, Olen O, et al. The genetic influence on diverticular disease a twin study. Aliment Pharmacol Ther 2012;35(9):1103–7.
15. Camilleri M, Sandler RS, Peery AF. Etiopathogenetic mechanisms in diverticular disease of the colon. Cell Mol Gastroenterol Hepatol 2020;9(1):15–32.
16. Hjern F, Wolk A, Hakansson N. Obesity, physical inactivity, and colonic diverticular disease requiring hospitalization in women: a prospective cohort study. Am J Gastroenterol 2012;107(2):296–302.

17. Strate LL, Liu YL, Huang ES, et al. Use of aspirin or nonsteroidal anti-inflammatory drugs increases risk for diverticulitis and diverticular bleeding. Gastroenterology 2011;140(5):1427–33.

18. Peery AF, Sandler RS. Diverticular disease: reconsidering conventional wisdom. Clin Gastroenterol Hepatol 2013;11(12):1532–7.

19. Reichert MC, Kupcinskas J, Schulz A, et al. Common variation in FAM155A is associated with diverticulitis but not diverticulosis. Sci Rep 2020;10(1):1658.

20. Patel K, Krishna SG, Porter K, et al. Diverticulitis in morbidly obese adults: a rise in hospitalizations with worse outcomes according to national US data. Dig Dis Sci 2020;65(9):2644–53.

21. Carabotti M, Annibale B. Treatment of diverticular disease: an update on latest evidence and clinical implications. Drugs Context 2018;7:212526.

22. Strate LL, Liu YL, Syngal S, et al. Nut, corn, and popcorn consumption and the incidence of diverticular disease. JAMA 2008;300(8):907–14.

23. Strate LL, Keeley BR, Cao Y, et al. Western dietary pattern increases, and prudent dietary pattern decreases, risk of incident diverticulitis in a prospective cohort study. Gastroenterology 2017;152(5):1023–30.e2.

24. Cao Y, Strate LL, Keeley BR, et al. Meat intake and risk of diverticulitis among men. Gut 2018;67(3):466–72.

25. Ma W, Nguyen LH, Song M, et al. Intake of dietary fiber, fruits, and vegetables and risk of diverticulitis. Am J Gastroenterol 2019;114(9):1531–8.

26. Mahmood MW, Abraham-Nordling M, Hakansson N, et al. High intake of dietary fibre from fruit and vegetables reduces the risk of hospitalisation for diverticular disease. Eur J Nutr 2019;58(6):2393–400.

27. Gueimonde M, Ouwehand A, Huhtinen H, et al. Qualitative and quantitative analyses of the bifidobacterial microbiota in the colonic mucosa of patients with colorectal cancer, diverticulitis and inflammatory bowel disease. World J Gastroenterol 2007;13(29):3985–9.

28. Lamiki P, Tsuchiya J, Pathak S, et al. Probiotics in diverticular disease of the colon: an open label study. J Gastrointestin Liver Dis 2010;19(1):31–6.

29. Tursi A. Current and evolving concepts on the pathogenesis of diverticular disease. J Gastrointestin Liver Dis 2019;28:225–35.

30. Stollman N, Smalley W, Hirano I, et al. American gastroenterological association institute guideline on the management of acute diverticulitis. Gastroenterology 2015;149(7):1944–9.

31. Eberhardt F, Crichton M, Dahl C, et al. Role of dietary fibre in older adults with asymptomatic (AS) or symptomatic uncomplicated diverticular disease (SUDD): systematic review and meta-analysis. Maturitas 2019;130:57–67.

32. Frickenstein AN, Jones MA, Behkam B, et al. Imaging inflammation and infection in the gastrointestinal tract. Int J Mol Sci 2019;21(1):243.

33. Magidson PD, Martinez JP. Abdominal pain in the geriatric patient. Emerg Med Clin North Am 2016;34(3):559–74.

34. Gonzalez-Urquijo M, Baca-Arzaga A, Lozano-Balderas G. Acute diverticulitis of the hepatic flexure mimicking acute cholecystitis. Rev Gastroenterol Mex 2020. S0375-0906(19)30170-3.

35. Andeweg CS, Knobben L, Hendriks JC, et al. How to diagnose acute left-sided colonic diverticulitis: proposal for a clinical scoring system. Ann Surg 2011;253(5):940–6.

36. Gardner CS, Jaffe TA, Nelson RC. Impact of CT in elderly patients presenting to the emergency department with acute abdominal pain. Abdom Imaging 2015;40(7):2877–82.

37. Lameris W, van Randen A, van Gulik TM, et al. A clinical decision rule to establish the diagnosis of acute diverticulitis at the emergency department. Dis Colon Rectum 2010;53(6):896–904.
38. Tursi A, Brandimarte G, Elisei W, et al. Faecal calprotectin in colonic diverticular disease: a case-control study. Int J Colorectal Dis 2009;24(1):49–55.
39. Ogino T, Mizushima T, Matsuda C, et al. Essential updates 2018/2019: colorectal (benign): recent updates (2018-2019) in the surgical treatment of benign colorectal diseases. Ann Gastroenterol Surg 2020;4(1):30–8.
40. Amato A, Mataloni F, Bruzzone M, et al. Hospital admission for complicated diverticulitis is increasing in Italy, especially in younger patients: a national database study. Tech Coloproctol 2020;24(3):237–45.
41. Isacson D, Smedh K, Nikberg M, et al. Long-term follow-up of the AVOD randomized trial of antibiotic avoidance in uncomplicated diverticulitis. Br J Surg 2019; 106(11):1542–8.
42. Chabok A, Pahlman L, Hjern F, et al. Randomized clinical trial of antibiotics in acute uncomplicated diverticulitis. Br J Surg 2012;99(4):532–9.
43. Daniels L, Unlu C, de Korte N, et al. Randomized clinical trial of observational versus antibiotic treatment for a first episode of CT-proven uncomplicated acute diverticulitis. Br J Surg 2017;104(1):52–61.
44. Eglinton TW. Randomized clinical trial of antibiotics in acute uncomplicated diverticulitis (Br J Surg 2012; 99: 532-539). Br J Surg 2012;99(4):540.
45. Pellino G, Podda M, Wheeler J, et al. Laparoscopy and resection with primary anastomosis for perforated diverticulitis: challenging old dogmas. Updates Surg 2020;72(1):21–8.
46. Al-Masrouri S, Garfinkle R, Al-Rashid F, et al. Readmission for treatment failure after nonoperative management of acute diverticulitis: a nationwide readmissions database analysis. Dis Colon Rectum 2020;63(2):217–25.
47. Broderick-Villa G, Burchette RJ, Collins JC, et al. Hospitalization for acute diverticulitis does not mandate routine elective colectomy. Arch Surg 2005;140(6): 576–81 [discussion: 581–73].
48. Binda GA, Papa A, Persiani R, et al. Hot topics in surgical management of acute diverticulitis. J Gastrointestin Liver Dis 2019;28(suppl. 4):29–34.
49. Baldock TE, Brown LR, McLean RC. Perforated diverticulitis in the North of England: trends in patient outcomes, management approach and the influence of subspecialisation. Ann R Coll Surg Engl 2019;101(8):563–70.
50. Zoog E, Giles WH, Maxwell RA. An update on the current management of perforated diverticulitis. Am Surg 2017;83(12):1321–8.
51. Cirocchi R, Nascimbeni R, Binda GA, et al. Surgical treatment of acute complicated diverticulitis in the elderly. Minerva Chir 2019;74(6):465–71.
52. Welbourn HL, Hartley JE. Management of acute diverticulitis and its complications. Indian J Surg 2014;76(6):429–35.
53. Strassle PD, Kinlaw AC, Chaumont N, et al. Rates of Elective colectomy for diverticulitis continued to increase after 2006 guideline change. Gastroenterology 2019;157(6):1679–81.e1.
54. Tapaskar N, Jones B, Mei S, et al. Comparison of clinical prediction tools and identification of risk factors for adverse outcomes in acute lower GI bleeding. Gastrointest Endosc 2019;89(5):1005–13.e2.
55. Strate LL, Gralnek IM. ACG clinical guideline: management of patients with acute lower gastrointestinal bleeding. Am J Gastroenterol 2016;111(5):755.
56. Ron-Tal Fisher O, Gralnek IM, Eisen GM, et al. Endoscopic hemostasis is rarely used for hematochezia: a population-based study from the clinical outcomes

research initiative national endoscopic database. Gastrointest Endosc 2014; 79(2):317–25.

57. Niikura R, Nagata N, Yamada A, et al. Efficacy and safety of early vs elective colonoscopy for acute lower gastrointestinal bleeding. Gastroenterology 2020; 158(1):168–75.e6.

58. Oakland K, Chadwick G, East JE, et al. Diagnosis and management of acute lower gastrointestinal bleeding: guidelines from the British society of gastroenterology. Gut 2019;68(5):776–89.

59. Bianchi M, Festa V, Moretti A, et al. Meta-analysis: long-term therapy with rifaximin in the management of uncomplicated diverticular disease. Aliment Pharmacol Ther 2011;33(8):902–10.

Upper Gastrointestinal Bleeding

Nicholas J. Costable, MD[a], David A. Greenwald, MD[b],*

KEYWORDS

- Gastrointestinal bleeding • Peptic Ulcer Disease • Hematemesis • Melena
- Hematochezia • NSAIDs • Aspirin • Warfarin

KEY POINTS

- It is prudent for providers caring for geriatric patients to have a sound understanding of upper gastrointestinal (GI) bleeding, because several age-related processes contribute to the increased incidence, morbidity, and mortality in this population.
- Providers caring for older adults should address modifiable risk factors for upper GI bleeding, including reducing the use of aspirin and NSAIDs (whenever possible) as well as coprescribing proton pump inhibitors (PPIs) in patients who will be initiated on long-term NSAID therapy.
- Management begins with assessment of airway protection (and intubation if indicated), placement of large-bore intravenous (IV) catheters, administration of isotonic crystalloid solution and/or blood products, and administration of IV PPI.

INTRODUCTION

Upper gastrointestinal (GI) tract hemorrhage is defined as GI bleeding that occurs proximal to the ligament of Treitz, the anatomic division between the duodenum and jejunum (**Figs. 1–6, Tables 1–3**). The annual incidence of hospitalization for acute upper GI bleeding is approximately 100 per 100,000 individuals,[1] with about 70% of cases of upper GI bleeding occurring in patients more than 60 years of age.[2] The incidence, morbidity, and mortality of upper GI bleeding all increase with age,[3] and therefore it is essential that all providers caring for older adults have a profound understanding of its presentation and management.

RISK FACTORS FOR UPPER GASTROINTESTINAL BLEEDING

Age, smoking, alcohol intake, history of peptic ulcer disease, portal hypertension, and certain medications have all been associated with a greater risk of upper GI bleeding.

[a] Department of Medicine, Icahn School of Medicine at Mount Sinai, 1 Gustav L Levy Place, New York, NY 10029, USA; [b] Division of Gastroenterology, Icahn School of Medicine at Mount Sinai, 5 East 98th Street, 11th Floor, New York, NY 10029, USA
* Corresponding author.
E-mail address: David.greenwald@mountsinai.org

Clin Geriatr Med 37 (2021) 155–172
https://doi.org/10.1016/j.cger.2020.09.001
0749-0690/21/© 2020 Elsevier Inc. All rights reserved.

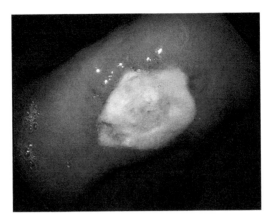

Fig. 1. Peptic ulcer.

Several studies have shown age to be an independent risk factor for upper GI hemorrhage,[4] which is likely caused by both physiologic alterations of the aging GI tract and the development of other age-related comorbidities that increase the risk of GI bleeding.

The parietal cells of the stomach produce about 2 L of hydrochloric acid per day, creating an intragastric pH of around 1 to 2.[5] This acidic environment is imperative for digestion, as well as providing an antimicrobial barrier from the outside world. The epithelial lining of the stomach would not be able to tolerate the high acidity of the stomach were it not for the production of a bicarbonate-rich mucosal layer that serves as a protective barrier. These protective and destructive factors normally exist in equilibrium and prevent mucosal destruction while permitting the early stages of digestion. In elderly patients, this equilibrium tends to be disrupted primarily by decreased gastric mucus production caused by/cause of the use of nonspecific cyclo-oxygenase (COX) inhibitors such as aspirin and other nonsteroidal antiinflammatory drugs (NSAIDs). COXs are enzymes involved in the production of prostaglandins, a group of lipid compounds that are involved in both inflammatory response (primarily via COX-2) and vasodilation to promote blood flow to splanchnic organs (primarily

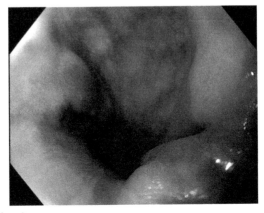

Fig. 2. Esophageal varices.

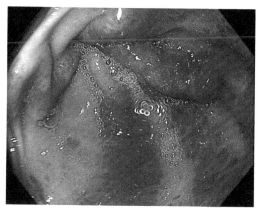

Fig. 3. Gastric antral vascular ectasia.

via COX-1). Medications that inhibit the synthesis of these prostaglandins lead to decreased submucosal blood flow and mucus production and leave the mucosa prone to injury.

Aspirin is one of the most commonly recommended medications among elderly adults. It is primarily used in secondary prophylaxis of coronary artery disease, peripheral vascular disease, and nonembolic stroke. However, it is estimated that approximately 25% of all adults in the United States more than 40 years of age without known cardiovascular disease take a daily aspirin without the recommendation of a physician.[6] Recent data have suggested that aspirin as primary prophylaxis in low-risk patients without known cardiovascular disease may be more harmful than beneficial. A large randomized controlled trial evaluating healthy adults more than 70 years of age with no prior cardiovascular history found that, at 5 years, patients taking aspirin for primary cardiovascular prophylaxis had no overall survival benefit but had a 38% relative risk increase of major hemorrhage compared with placebo.[7] In addition, a large multicenter trial showed that, in patients with moderate cardiovascular disease risk with no prior history of coronary artery disease, aspirin was not shown to decrease

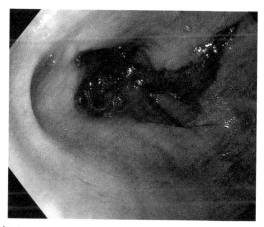

Fig. 4. Mallory-Weiss tear.

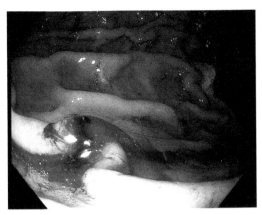

Fig. 5. Dieulafoy lesion.

the rate of cardiovascular ischemic events but was associated with a higher rate of GI bleeding.[8] Taken together, these studies suggest that the use of aspirin for primary prophylaxis of cardiovascular disease in older adults may be of limited utility and may be harmful. The decision to continue aspirin for primary prophylaxis in this group should be made on an individual basis in a patient-centered manner.

NSAIDs are also a class of COX inhibitors and are among the most prescribed and used medications in the United States. They are frequently prescribed as analgesics and antiinflammatory agents for conditions commonly associated with older age,

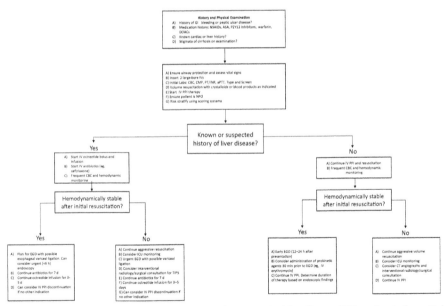

Fig. 6. Approach to patients with suspected upper GI bleeding. aPTT, activated partial thromboplastin time; ASA, aspirin; CBC, complete blood count; CMP, comprehensive metabolic panel; CT, computed tomography; DOAC, direct-acting oral anticoagulant; EGD, esophagogastroduodenoscopy; ICU, intensive care unit; INR, International Normalized Ratio; IV, intravenous; NPO, nil per os; NSAID, nonsteroidal antiinflammatory drug; PPI, proton pump inhibitor; PT, prothrombin time; TIPS, transjugular intrahepatic portosystemic shunt.

Table 1
Glasgow-Blatchford bleeding score

	Score Value
Blood Urea (mmol/L)	
6.5–7.9	2
8.0–9.9	3
10.0–25.0	4
>25.0	6
Hemoglobin for Men (g/dL)	
12.0–12.9	1
10.0–11.9	3
<10.0	6
Hemoglobin for Women (g/dL)	
10.0–11.9	1
<10.0	6
Other Markers	
Pulse ≥100 beats/min	1
Melena	1
Syncope	2
Liver disease	2
Heart failure	2

such as osteoarthritis, making them an important risk factor for upper GI bleeding in these patients. An estimated 1.2% of the population reports taking an NSAID at least once daily, and about 7.3% of patients more than 60 years of age report filling at least 1 NSAID prescription within the past year.[9] Approximately 2% to 4% of chronic NSAID users experience at least 1 major GI complication related to their NSAID use.[10] In the late 1990s, specific COX-2 inhibitors were introduced as potential GI-sparing antiinflammatory agents, owing to the lack of COX-1 inhibition. However, use of these agents has been shown to be associated with increased risk of myocardial infarction compared with nonselective COX inhibitors in patients with preexisting cardiovascular disease.[11] Therefore, their use warrants careful consideration in this patient population.

Patients who will be prescribed long-term NSAIDs should be evaluated for other risk factors for development of peptic ulcer disease, such as the presence of Helicobacter pylori, to minimize risk of GI bleeding. A 2005 meta-analysis studying H pylori eradication before starting chronic NSAID therapy showed a 57% risk reduction in development of peptic ulcer disease.[12] The effect on patients who are already on NSAID therapy is less well defined. Guidelines suggest patients at high risk for peptic ulcer disease who will be initiated on chronic NSAID therapy (age>64 years, corticosteroid use, antiplatelet agent use, previous history of peptic ulcer disease) should be coprescribed prophylactic agents to prevent NSAID-induced GI toxicity.[13] Randomized trials have shown that coadministration of either a proton pump inhibitor (PPI)[14] or misoprostol[15] (a prostaglandin E analogue) reduces rates of symptomatic peptic ulcer development. Histamine-2 (H2) receptor antagonist use has not been shown to be beneficial in prevention of peptic ulcer disease in these patients; however, their use can be considered in patients who are intolerant or have contraindications to PPIs or misoprostol.[16]

Table 2
Causes of upper gastrointestinal bleeding

Causes of Upper GI Bleeding	Comments
Peptic ulcer disease	Most common cause of upper GI bleeding in hospitalized patients. Risk factors include *Helicobacter pylori* infection and NSAID use
Erosive gastroeso-phagitis	Occurs as a part of long-standing gastroesophageal reflux and/or NSAID use. Rarely causes major bleeding
Esophageal/gastric varices	Can occur with diseases that cause increased risk of portal venous pressure, including cirrhosis and portal venous thrombosis
Mallory-Weiss tear	Mucosal tear near esophagogastric junction usually as a result of repetitive vomiting/retching. Predominant symptom is hematemesis
Dieulafoy lesion	Abnormally dilated submucosal arterial bleed. Can cause severe hemodynamic compromise given arterial nature
Arteriovenous malformations	Abnormal connection between arteries and veins. Mainly seen in distal small bowel, but may be present in upper GI tract
Gastric antral vascular ectasia	Abnormal dilatation of gastric veins associated with cirrhosis and chronic kidney disease
Portal hypertensive gastropathy	Result of submucosal congestion in diseases that increase portal pressure
Malignancy	Rare cause of overt upper GI bleeding
Aortoenteric fistula	Rare, but potentially fatal cause of upper GI bleeding. Should be considered in patients with aortic disease or recent aortic surgery

Abbreviations: GI, gastrointestinal; NSAID, nonsteroidal antiinflammatory drug.

The use of $P2Y_{12}$ inhibitors, such as clopidogrel, prasugrel, and ticagrelor, is also an important risk factor for GI bleeding. The $P2Y_{12}$ ADP receptor expressed on the surface of platelets plays a significant role in promoting platelet aggregation. Medications that competitively inhibit this receptor lead to impaired clot formation and thus higher risk of bleeding. $P2Y_{12}$ inhibitors are commonly prescribed for conditions that increase in prevalence with advancing age, such as secondary stroke prevention, acute coronary syndrome, and peripheral vascular disease. Although the increased risk for GI bleeding is a class effect of these medications, the rates of bleeding differ between the agents.[17] A meta-analysis of more than 60,000 patients showed that prasugrel, one of the third-generation $P2Y_{12}$ inhibitors, had a significantly higher rate of GI bleeding compared with clopidogrel.[17]

Warfarin is a commonly used anticoagulant that inhibits the synthesis of vitamin K–dependent factors II, VII, IX, and X as well as proteins C and S. It is used primarily for embolic stroke prevention in patients with atrial fibrillation, a condition affecting approximately 9% of patients more than 65 years of age, venous thromboembolism (VTE) prophylaxis, and anticoagulation after mechanical heart valve replacement.[18] It is well established that warfarin use is associated with an increased risk of GI hemorrhage.[19] Recently, warfarin use has declined because of the development of newer anticoagulants that do not require coagulation monitoring and have fewer drug-drug interactions.

Direct-acting oral anticoagulants (DOACs) are a class of relatively new anticoagulants that include dabigatran, rivaroxaban, apixaban, and edoxaban. These agents exert their effect by directly inhibiting different coagulation factors, leading to

	Table 3		
	Forrest classification of peptic ulcer bleeding		
Forrest Grade	**Endoscopic Findings**		**Rate of Rebleeding (%)[a]**
I	Active hemorrhage		—
Ia	Active pulsatile bleeding		55
Ib	Active nonpulsatile (oozing) bleeding		—
II	Stigmata of recent bleeding		—
IIa	Visible, nonbleeding vessel		50
IIb	Adherent clot		22
IIc	Hematin coated lesion		10
III	Clean-based ulcer		5

[a] Rate of rebleeding when endoscopic therapy is not performed.

Data from Laine L, Peterson WL. Bleeding peptic ulcer. New England Journal of Medicine. 1994;331(11):717–27.

impaired clot stabilization. Similar to warfarin, DOACs are primarily used in prevention of stroke in atrial fibrillation and VTE prophylaxis, but, unlike warfarin, they are not approved for anticoagulation after heart valve replacement. The landmark trials investigating the efficacy of these agents showed that the rates of GI bleeding were comparable with rates seen with warfarin.[20–22] However, in 1 study, dabigatran was shown to have a 50% relative risk increase in the rates of GI bleeding compared with warfarin.[20] A large population-based study investigating the risk of GI bleeding among patients using these agents found that apixaban had the most favorable GI safety profile, whereas rivaroxaban had the most unfavorable profile.[23] The study also found that, regardless of the agent used, patients aged 75 years or older had the highest risk of GI bleeding.[23]

PRESENTATION

Upper GI bleeding can vary greatly in clinical presentation from occult bleeding to life-threatening hemorrhage. The initial evaluation of a patient with suspected upper GI bleeding should always begin with a careful history and thorough physical examination. The history should focus on establishing the onset of symptoms, prior history of peptic ulcer disease or GI bleeding, prior endoscopy, use of high-risk medications (NSAIDs, aspirin, DOACs, $P2Y_{12}$ inhibitors, corticosteroids), alcohol use, and known diagnosis of liver disease or cirrhosis.

The most common presenting symptoms for an upper GI bleed are melena (black, tarry stool) and hematemesis. Melena occurs when the ferrous iron (Fe^{2+}) in hemoglobin is oxidized to the ferric (Fe^{3+}) form, which is where melena derives its distinct color. It suggests that the blood has spent typically greater than 4 to 6 hours in the GI tract and implies a more proximal source of bleeding. About 90% of cases of melena are caused by a GI bleed proximal to the ligament of Treitz, although it also may originate from the nasopharynx, small bowel, or right colon depending on gut transit time.[24] Large-volume upper GI bleeding may also present as hematochezia (bright red blood per rectum) caused by the more rapid transit of blood and less iron oxidation and is usually accompanied by hemodynamic instability.

Hematemesis refers to the presence of bright red blood in vomited material. Hematin-colored material in vomit is sometimes referred to as coffee-ground emesis for its resemblance to ground coffee. Coffee-ground emesis generally implies that blood in the stomach has been acted on by acid over time, whereas hematemesis can suggest a larger-volume bleed. Other symptoms that are less specific for upper GI bleeding that may be present include nausea, abdominal pain (primarily epigastric), lightheadedness, syncope, dyspnea, and fatigue.

CAUSES

The differential diagnosis of upper GI hemorrhage may be categorized into causes associated with portal hypertension and cirrhosis versus causes not associated with portal hypertension (**Table 2**). The most common causes of upper GI bleeding not attributed to portal hypertension are peptic ulcer disease and erosive gastritis/esophagitis. Peptic ulcer disease is the most common cause of upper GI bleeding and is discussed later. Erosive esophagitis and gastritis typically arise as a result of chronic acid reflux, adverse effects of medications (including NSAIDs, bisphosphonates, and tetracyclines), or infection (eg, candida species, cytomegalovirus, herpes simplex virus). Long-standing acid reflux tends to affect elderly patients more commonly and these patients are more likely to experience consequences such as erosive esophagitis compared with younger patients.[25] Medication-induced esophagitis is also an important consideration because several causal medications are more commonly prescribed for older adults. Bisphosphonates, in particular, are a class of medications well recognized as causing erosive esophagitis, perhaps in as many as 26% of patients.[26] Patients taking bisphosphonates should be advised to take the pill with 180 to 240 mL (6–8 oz) of water and remain upright for at least 30 minutes after swallowing to minimize the likelihood of esophageal injury.[26] Patients with erosive gastritis/esophagitis tend to present with hematemesis more commonly than melena, and the overall clinical course is generally more benign compared with bleeding from other causes.[25,27]

Mallory-Weiss tears are longitudinal mucosal lacerations at the gastroesophageal junction (GEJ) that occur with repeated episodes of retching or vomiting (**Fig. 4**).[28] These lacerations can lead to bleeding from submucosal blood vessels. Classically, these tears present in patients who have repeated episodes of emesis that are initially clear and progress to hematemesis.[29] Arteriovenous malformations (AVMs) are the most common vascular abnormalities associated with upper GI bleeding and are more common with increasing age.[30] The abnormal blood vessels dilate and erode through the overlying mucosa and lead to venous bleeding. They typically are present in the small bowel, but rarely also can be seen in the stomach. Patients with chronic renal dysfunction are at increased risk of developing AVMs. GI bleeding from AVMs also can be seen in patients with aortic stenosis in a triad known as Heyde syndrome. In contrast, Dieulafoy lesions are abnormally dilated submucosal arteries that erode overlying mucosa and may cause brisk arterial bleeding (**Fig. 5**). Because of the arterial nature of the bleeding, they have a greater propensity to cause significant hemodynamic instability as opposed to more benign bleeding from AVMs. Aortoenteric fistulas are a rare, but potentially devastating, cause of upper GI bleeding. They may either arise as de novo fistulas (primary) or as a result of aortic reconstruction (secondary), most commonly between the aorta and the duodenum.[31] They typically present first with a sentinel bleed, which may occur hours or days before a later massive hemorrhage. Because of the high mortality of aortoenteric fistulas, patients with known history of aortic disease who are being investigated for GI bleeding should be evaluated radiographically and endoscopically and undergo emergent surgical repair if a fistula is detected.

Esophageal variceal rupture is the most serious manifestation of upper GI bleeding because of portal hypertension. Portal hypertension is most often caused by cirrhosis, but it also can be caused by portal venous thrombus, hepatic vein thrombus (Budd-Chiari syndrome), or heart disease. Cirrhosis leads to portal hypertension via 2 distinct mechanisms: increased resistance to portal venous outflow caused by the fibrosed liver and increased production of splanchnic arterial vasodilators such as nitric oxide and endothelial-like growth factor.[32] This condition leads to shunting of portal blood into tributary veins and formation of thin-walled varices that are susceptible to rupture. The most common site of variceal formation is the distal esophagus (**Fig. 2**), but they can be found in the stomach and other parts of the GI tract as well. The annual rate of bleeding from varices is 5% and 15% among small and large varices respectively[33]. Portal hypertensive gastropathy (PHG) is another, usually less severe, cause of upper GI bleeding caused by portal hypertension. PHG refers to increased mucosal friability and edema as a result of portal hypertension. Gastric antral vascular ectasia (GAVE) may occur in patients with portal hypertension as a result of ectatic (dilated) gastric mucosal veins. Because of its appearance on endoscopy, GAVE is sometimes referred to as watermelon stomach (**Fig. 3**).

PEPTIC ULCER DISEASE AND *HELICOBACTER PYLORI*

Peptic ulcer disease is by far the most common cause of upper GI bleeding, accounting for approximately 60% of all presentations of upper GI bleeding.[1] A peptic ulcer is a defect in the gastric or duodenal mucosa that extends beyond the muscularis mucosa into the deeper layers of the GI wall (**Fig. 1**).[34] Ulcers can manifest anywhere on a spectrum from asymptomatic to life-threatening GI perforation. The most common causes of peptic ulcer disease are *H pylori* infection and chronic NSAID use (as described earlier).

H pylori is a spiral, urease-producing, gram-negative bacterium that is among the most common bacterial infections in the world.[35] The worldwide prevalence of *H pylori* infection is estimated to be around 50%, and prevalence increases with age. Studies have shown that *H pylori* is found in more than 50% of people more than 60 years of age in developed countries, such as the United States, and as many as 80% in underdeveloped countries.[36] The exact method of transmission is still unknown; however, studies have shown that children of parents infected with *H pylori* have higher rates of *H pylori* detection than children of uninfected parents, suggesting person-to-person and fecal-oral transmission early in life.

On entry into the GI tract, *H pylori* uses its flagella to travel toward the mucosal epithelium and move toward areas of high urea using chemotaxis.[37] The bacterium is able to adhere to foveolar cells in the mucosa and secrete virulence factors important for bacterial survival and proliferation. Urease is one of the most important virulence factors for *H pylori* survival because it cleaves urea into ammonia, which is used to buffer the highly acidic gastric environment. *H pylori* secretes other virulence factors that induce mucosal epithelial cell damage and weaken mucosal integrity leading to development of gastroduodenitis and peptic ulcers. Chronic gastritis as a result of *H pylori* infection leads to an increased risk of developing gastric adenocarcinoma or mucosal-associated lymphoid tissue lymphoma.

In most patients, *H pylori* infection is asymptomatic. However, in those with symptoms, disease may range from mild gastritis to severe peptic ulcer disease, which can lead to gastroduodenal perforations. Common presenting complaints may include postprandial epigastric pain or discomfort, usually starting within a few hours of eating, that can radiate toward the back.[38] Patients who develop ulcers along the gastric antrum near the pylorus may present with symptoms of gastric outlet obstruction, including early satiety, bloating, nausea, or vomiting.

Diagnosis of *H pylori* infection can be performed either through endoscopic biopsy, stool antigen testing, or urease breath testing.[39] Endoscopic biopsy with urease staining is one of the most sensitive and specific means of diagnosing *H pylori*, with a sensitivity and specificity of 90% and 95% respectively; however, it is also the most invasive and most expensive of all of the diagnostic tests. Urea breath testing (UBT) is a noninvasive test that may be used to detect *H pylori* presence. Patients are given a solution containing urea with a labeled carbon isotope (either C^{13} or C^{14}), which in the presence of *H pylori* is metabolized to ammonia and radiolabeled CO_2. The radiolabeled CO_2 is detected by machine; high levels of radiolabeled CO_2 implies the presence of *H pylori*. The sensitivity and specificity of UBT ranges from 88% to 95% and 95% to 100% respectively.[40] However, there is a high false-negative rate in patients using PPIs, bismuth, or antibiotics. One study of false-negative rates in patients taking PPIs showed a 33% false-negative rate in subsequent breath tests in patients who were taking PPIs.[41] Patients should be instructed to stop taking their PPIs at least 14 days before UBT because studies have shown that detection rates return to those of non-PPI users.[41] Stool antigen testing is another noninvasive diagnostic option that carries a sensitivity and specificity of 94% and 97% respectively.[40] As with UBT, stool antigen sensitivity is decreased in patients taking PPIs, bismuth, and antibiotics. Serologic tests for *H pylori* exist, but they do not reliably predict active infection from previous exposure, limiting their use.

Treatment of *H pylori* infection requires multidrug therapy because of the high rates of antibiotic resistance, often related to regional antibiotic usage. Current guidelines suggest 14 days of clarithromycin-based triple therapy, consisting of clarithromycin, amoxicillin, and PPI, as the first-line treatment of *H pylori* infection.[39] In patients who are allergic to penicillin, metronidazole may be substituted for amoxicillin. It is of note that eradication rates with triple therapy typically are less than 80%, mainly because of increasing clarithromycin resistance.[39] Guidelines suggest that patients with any prior macrolide exposure or patients in areas with known high rates of clarithromycin resistance should be initiated on bismuth-based quadruple therapy consisting of bismuth sulfate, metronidazole, tetracycline, and a PPI for 10 to 14 days.[39] It is therefore imperative that all patients beginning treatment of *H pylori* should be asked about prior antibiotic exposure, with particular attention paid to macrolide exposure.

All patients who undergo treatment of *H pylori* should be tested for cure, usually with UBT or stool antigen testing.[39] Patients should be off antibiotics for 4 weeks before stool antigen testing and PPIs for at least 2 weeks to decrease rates of false-negative results.[39]

INITIAL EVALUATION

Initial diagnostic evaluation should always begin with a thorough history and physical examination. Careful attention should be paid to the patient's mental status as well as for any signs of respiratory distress or difficulty protecting the airway. Patients should be evaluated for stigmata of chronic liver disease, including scleral icterus, jaundice, splenomegaly, ascites, spider angiomata, and palmar erythema. Every patient presenting with concern for upper GI bleeding should undergo digital rectal examination to evaluate for melanotic stool. A meta-analysis comparing presentation of upper versus lower GI bleeding found that patient-reported melena was associated with a likelihood ratio (LR) of 5.1 to 5.9 in favor of upper GI bleeding, whereas the presence of melena on digital rectal examination was associated with an LR of 25, showing the diagnostic importance of a rectal examination in suspected upper GI bleeding.[42] Nasogastric lavage is no longer recommended as part of the initial evaluation, because it has not been shown to reduce mortality in upper GI bleeding.[43]

Laboratory tests, including complete blood count, comprehensive metabolic panel, coagulation factors, and a type and screen, should be done in all patients as part of the initial evaluation. Blood urea nitrogen (BUN)/creatinine ratio of greater than 30 can suggest an upper GI source of bleeding and has been associated with an LR of 7.5.[42] Liver test abnormalities, thrombocytopenia, and coagulopathy that are otherwise not explained can suggest undiagnosed cirrhosis and prompt consideration of variceal hemorrhage as a possible cause.

Several predictive models using demographic information as well as laboratory values have been developed to help stratify patients with higher-risk GI bleeding from those with less high-risk bleeding. Among these predictive models, 2 of the most commonly used are the AIM65 score and the Glasgow-Blatchford score. The AIMS65 score uses preendoscopy data to predict in-hospital mortality for patients presenting with upper GI bleeding.[44] The score was derived from a large, multicenter database of more than 22,000 patients hospitalized for upper GI bleed. The study found that the following factors were associated with increased inpatient mortality: albumin level less than 3.0 g/dL, International Normalized Ratio (INR) greater than 1.5, altered mental status, systolic blood pressure less than 90 mm Hg at presentation, and age greater than 65 years. Mortality ranged from 0.3% in patients with zero of these risk factors to 25% in patients with all 5 risk factors present.[44] The Glasgow-Blatchford score was developed to help predict patients who are at high risk for requiring urgent endoscopic intervention for management of upper GI bleeding (**Table 1**). The score is based on BUN, hemoglobin, systolic blood pressure, heart rate, and the presence of melena, syncope, liver disease, and/or heart failure.[45] The score ranges from zero to 23 and the risk of urgent endoscopy increases with increasing score. Scores less than or equal to 1 have been associated with a low risk for needing urgent endoscopic intervention and these patients can be considered for outpatient evaluation.[46]

MANAGEMENT

Management of upper GI bleeding can be considered in terms of management of non-variceal hemorrhage versus management of variceal hemorrhage (**Fig. 6**). Regardless of cause, assessment of patients with suspected upper GI bleeding should always begin with evaluating the patient's ABCs (airway, breathing, circulation) and vital signs. Patients who are unable to protect their airways because of ongoing large-volume emesis or altered mental status should be intubated. All patients should have 2 large-bore intravenous (IV) catheters placed for volume resuscitation and possible transfusion of blood products. It is not recommended to use central venous catheters for volume resuscitation because the greater catheter length increases resistance and hinders flow of IV fluids and blood products.[47]

With regard to nonvariceal hemorrhage, all patients should be made nil per os (NPO) and immediately started on IV PPI therapy. PPIs help increase gastric pH, which in turn stabilizes blood clots and helps reduce rates of rebleeding.[12,48,49] A meta-analysis of 13 randomized trials published in 2014 comparing intermittent PPI therapy twice daily with continuous PPI infusion sought to compare rates of rebleeding. Intermittent PPI dosing was associated with a 28% relative risk reduction of rebleeding and was non-inferior to continuous PPI dosing.[50] The use of intermittent PPI dosing also allows increased accessibility to IV access, often needed for administration of fluids and/or blood products. Administration of prokinetic agents such as IV metoclopramide or erythromycin given 30 to 90 minutes before endoscopy may help with visualization of bleeding lesions during endoscopy and has been shown to reduce the rate of second-look endoscopy.[51]

Patients with known or suspected cirrhosis and upper GI bleeding should be administered a high-dose PPI, a vasoactive somatostatin analogue, and initiated on antibiotic prophylaxis for prevention of spontaneous bacterial peritonitis (SBP). Somatostatin analogues promote splanchnic vasoconstriction, which in turn helps to counteract the overproduction of vasodilatory compounds caused by cirrhosis.[52] This treatment helps to decrease forward flow into the portal venous system, thereby decreasing blood loss through bleeding varices. The use of vasoactive medications has been shown to improve rates of hemostasis and decreases mortality in patients with variceal hemorrhage.[52,53] Octreotide is the only available somatostatin analogue in the United States, and should be administered as a 50-µg IV bolus, followed by a continuous 50-µg/h infusion for 3 to 5 days. Antibiotic prophylaxis (with either ceftriaxone or norfloxacin) should be administered to all patients with suspected or known cirrhosis admitted for upper GI bleeding. A meta-analysis published in 2012 showed that antibiotic prophylaxis reduces the rate of bacterial infection (including SBP) and decreases mortality.[54] A trial comparing norfloxacin with ceftriaxone showed that ceftriaxone was superior to norfloxacin in prophylaxis of bacterial infections, making it the antibiotic of choice.[55] Patients should be treated for a total of 7 days and can be transitioned to oral antibiotics once the patient is able to tolerate liquids and solids by mouth.[53]

Patients should be transfused packed red blood cells when the hemoglobin level is 7.0 g/dL, with a goal hemoglobin of greater than or equal to 7.0 g/dL. A trial comparing restrictive (goal hemoglobin ≥7.0 g/dL) versus liberal (hemoglobin ≥10.0 g/dL) transfusion in patients hospitalized for acute upper GI bleeding found that the restrictive transfusion protocol was associated with a lower 45-day mortality.[56] Patients with thrombocytopenia, defined as having platelet count less than 50,000/µL, should be transfused with the goal being more than 50,000/µL. Patients with an INR greater than 2.0 not secondary to cirrhosis should be transfused with fresh frozen plasma. The management of coagulopathy in patients with cirrhosis is more challenging because the INR is not a reliable indication of coagulation status in cirrhosis.[53]

Endoscopic management is the mainstay of treatment both for patients with nonvariceal upper GI bleeding as well as patients with variceal hemorrhage. Current guidelines suggest that early endoscopy (defined as endoscopy within 24 hours of presentation) should be performed on patients presenting with nonvariceal GI bleeding, because it has been shown to reduce hospital length of stay and in-hospital mortality.[57] Urgent endoscopy (earlier than 12 hours of presentation) in patients with nonvariceal bleeding has been associated with higher risks of rebleeding and in-hospital mortality.[58] This finding is likely caused by inadequate resuscitation and emphasizes the importance of early recognition and management of upper GI bleeding. For peptic ulcers with visible bleeding or stigmata of recent bleeding, endoscopic therapy usually entails injection of the bleeding site with epinephrine along with a second means of obtaining hemostasis (such as placement of hemostatic clips, thermal coaptive coagulation, argon plasma coagulation, or fibrin sealant) [**Table 3**].[59] AVMs with visible bleeding can be treated with thermic therapy, such as argon plasma coagulation.[60]

In contrast, guidelines suggest that patients presenting with suspected variceal bleeding should undergo urgent endoscopy (within 12 hours of presentation).[53] Esophageal varices typically are managed with esophageal variceal ligation (ie, banding), which has been proved superior to endoscopic sclerotherapy in terms of rebleeding and eradication of varices.[61] All patients who undergo esophageal variceal ligation should have a follow-up endoscopy within 2 weeks to ensure obliteration of varices.[53] Those with persistent varices at 2 weeks should undergo biweekly endoscopy until complete variceal eradication is achieved.[53]

Despite the high efficacy of variceal ligation, up to 20% of patients' variceal hemorrhages may be refractory to standard endoscopic therapy, and this is associated with a high mortality.[53] For variceal bleeding that cannot be controlled with endoscopic therapy, treatment options include emergent placement of a transjugular intrahepatic portosystemic shunt (TIPS) or surgery. TIPS is generally preferred to surgery because it has a high success rate and a much lower mortality compared with surgery.[62] Patients hospitalized with esophageal variceal bleeding should be started on a nonselective β-blocker before discharge, because the combination of endoscopic therapy and nonselective beta-blockade has been shown to be superior to either therapy alone in secondary prevention of variceal bleeding.[63]

MANAGEMENT OF ANTICOAGULATION IN ACUTE UPPER GASTROINTESTINAL BLEEDING

The decision regarding the management of anticoagulation in the setting of acute upper GI bleeding largely depends on the amount of bleeding, the risk of thrombosis while discontinuing anticoagulation, and the indication for anticoagulation.[64]

Patients taking antiplatelet agents who are at especially high risk for thrombotic events with cessation of these antithrombotic agents include patients within 90 days of acute coronary syndrome (ACS), recent coronary stent placement (<1 year for drug eluting stents or <1 month for bare metal stents), patients with multiple stents, and those with a prior history of stent occlusion. The most significant complication of cessation of antiplatelet agents for these patients is stent thrombosis. Up to 6% of patients who have had a stent occlusion in the past develop a second stent occlusion within 1 year and have a much higher rate of cardiovascular death.[64] In addition, approximately 2.3% of patients hospitalized with ACS develop GI bleeding during the index hospitalization,[65] and these patients have a significantly higher in-hospital mortality compared with patients hospitalized with ACS who do not develop GI bleeding.[66] Guidelines recommend a multidisciplinary approach with the cardiology consultation before discontinuing antiplatelet agents in these high-risk patients because the risk of adverse cardiac events may exceed the risk of bleeding.[64]

Management of patients on warfarin presenting with upper GI bleeding depends on the severity of the bleeding and the indication for warfarin use. Patients with minor bleeding sometimes can be observed off warfarin without the administration of reversal agents.[64] Patients with supratherapeutic INR and life-threatening hemorrhage should be given either prothrombin complex concentrates (PCC) or fresh frozen plasma (FFP) to correct the coagulopathy.[64] Patients should be transfused to a goal INR of less than or equal to 2.5, because studies have shown comparable rates of successful hemostasis between patients with INRs of 1.5 to 2.5 and nonanticoagulated patients.[64] Therefore, it is recommended that endoscopic therapy should not be delayed in patients with serious GI bleeding and an INR less than 2.5. Vitamin K is less useful in the acute setting of hemorrhage because production of vitamin K–dependent factors can take several days. One study showed an absolute risk of embolism of about 1% in patients who had warfarin held for 4 to 7 days.[67] Patients with mechanical heart valves (especially patients with mitral valve replacement) are at particularly high risk of developing thrombotic complications from cessation of warfarin and INR reversal.[68] Clinicians should strongly consider cardiology consultation before reversal or cessation of warfarin in patients with mechanical valve replacement given the high mortality of prosthetic valve thrombus.[68] Reinitiation of warfarin after a procedure depends on the thromboembolic risk of the patient as well as risk of rebleeding.[64] A randomized trial published in 2015 showed that bridging with heparin in low-risk patients with atrial fibrillation during the periprocedural period did not decrease the risk of thromboembolic events but did result in a statistically increased risk of bleeding.[69] It is therefore recommended that low-risk patients start warfarin once adequate hemostasis is achieved, and not be bridged with heparin.[70] However, patients with high thromboembolic risk do benefit from bridging with heparin while awaiting a therapeutic INR after restarting warfarin.[70]

Few guidelines exist for the management of patients taking DOACs who present with upper GI bleeding. The most important principle is that DOACs have rapid onset of action (most within 1–4 hours of onset) and relatively rapid offset (usually within 12–24 hours). Drug clearance depends on the patient's creatinine clearance, which declines with age, and therefore patients with decreased renal function have impaired clearance of the drug.[71] Patients taking DOACs presenting with minor upper GI bleeding should have their next dose of DOAC held if the benefit of hemostasis is outweighed by the risk of thrombosis. For patients with moderate to severe GI bleeding who are hemodynamically stable, anticoagulation should be held, and endoscopic evaluation should be deferred for 12 to 24 hours to allow normal coagulation to return.[64] It is reasonable to consider administration of PCC or FFP along with urgent endoscopy in patients who have hemodynamically compromising bleeds. In addition, there are 2 available US Food and Drug Administration–approved reversal agents (idarucizumab for dabigatran; and andexanet alpha for rivaroxaban, apixaban, and edoxaban) that can be used in life-threatening hemorrhage.[64,72,73] Reinitiation of DOACs should be deferred until adequate hemostasis is ensured given the rapidity of onset of these agents.[64]

CLINICS CARE POINTS

- Scoring systems, including the Glasgow-Blatchford and AIMS65 scores, can help predict patients at higher risk for complications and in-hospital mortality.
- Patients with non-variceal upper gastrointestinal bleeding benefit from early endoscopic evaluation (within 24 hours of presentation), but inadequate resuscitation prior to endoscopy can lead to increased risk of adverse outcomes.
- Presence of melena on digital rectal exam is associated with a likelihood ratio of 25 of upper gastrointestinal bleeding and should be performed on all patients with suspected upper GI bleeding.

REFERENCES

1. Longstreth GF. Epidemiology of hospitalization for acute upper gastrointestinal hemorrhage: a population–based study. Am J Gastroenterol 1995;90:2.
2. Van Leerdam ME, Vreeburg E, Rauws EM, et al. Acute upper GI bleeding: did anything change?: time trend analysis of incidence and outcome of acute upper

GI bleeding between 1993/1994 and 2000. Am J Gastroenterol 2003;98(7): 1494–9.

3. Rockall TA, Logan RF, Devlin A, et al. Incidence of and mortality from acute upper gastrointestinal haemorrhage in the United Kingdom. BMJ 1995;311(6999): 222–6.

4. Kaplan RC, Heckbert SR, Koepsell TD, et al. Risk factors for gastrointestinal bleeding among older patients. Cardiovascular Health Study Investigators. J Am Geriatr Soc 2001;49(2):126–33.

5. Leung PS, editor. The gastrointestinal system: gastrointestinal, nutritional and hepatobiliary physiology. Netherlands: Springer Science & Business; 2014.

6. O'Brien, Colin W, Juraschek SP, et al. Prevalence of aspirin use for primary prevention of cardiovascular disease in the United States: results from the 2017 national health interview survey. Ann Intern Med 2019;171(8):596–8.

7. McNeil JJ, Woods RL, Nelson MR, et al. Effect of aspirin on disability-free survival in the healthy elderly. N Engl J Med 2018;379(16):1499–508.

8. Gaziano JM, Woods RL, Nelson MR, et al. Use of aspirin to reduce risk of initial vascular events in patients at moderate risk of cardiovascular disease (ARRIVE): a randomised, double-blind, placebo-controlled trial. Lancet 2018;392(10152): 1036–46.

9. Wongrakpanich S, Wongrakpanich A, Melhado K, et al. A comprehensive review of non-steroidal anti-inflammatory drug use in the elderly. Aging Dis 2018; 9(1):143.

10. Straus WL, Ofman JJ. Gastrointestinal toxicity associated with nonsteroidal anti-inflammatory drugs: epidemiologic and economic issues. Gastroenterol Clin 2001;30(4):895–920.

11. Claire B, Laine L, Reicin A, et al. Comparison of upper gastrointestinal toxicity of rofecoxib and naproxen in patients with rheumatoid arthritis. N Engl J Med 2000; 343(21):1520–8.

12. Leontiadis GI, Sharma VK, Howden CW. Systematic review and meta-analysis of proton pump inhibitor therapy in peptic ulcer bleeding. BMJ 2005;330(7491):568.

13. Bhatt DL, James S, Neena SA, et al. ACCF/ACG/AHA 2008 expert consensus document on reducing the gastrointestinal risks of antiplatelet therapy and NSAID use: a report of the American College of Cardiology Foundation Task Force on Clinical Expert Consensus Documents. J Am Coll Cardiol 2008; 52(18):1502–17.

14. Cullen D, Bardhan KD, Eisner M, et al. Primary gastroduodenal prophylaxis with omeprazole for non-steroidal anti-inflammatory drug users. Aliment Pharmacol Ther 1998;12(2):135–40.

15. Raskin JB, Richard HW, Joseph EJ, et al. Misoprostol dosage in the prevention of nonsteroidal anti-inflammatory drug-induced gastric and duodenal ulcers: a comparison of three regimens. Ann Intern Med 1995;123(5):344–50.

16. Hooper L, Brown TJ, Elliott R, et al. The effectiveness of five strategies for the prevention of gastrointestinal toxicity induced by non-steroidal anti-inflammatory drugs: systematic review. BMJ 2004;329(7472):948.

17. Guo C-G, Chen L, Chan EW, et al. Systematic review with meta-analysis: the risk of gastrointestinal bleeding in patients taking third-generation P2Y12 inhibitors compared with clopidogrel. Aliment Pharmacol Ther 2019;49(1):7–19.

18. January CT, Wann LS, Alpert JS, et al. 2014 AHA/ACC/HRS guideline for the management of patients with atrial fibrillation: a report of the American College of cardiology/American heart association Task Force on practice guidelines and the heart Rhythm Society. J Am Coll Cardiol 2014;64(21):e1–76.

19. Chen W-C, Chen YH, Hsu PI, et al. Gastrointestinal hemorrhage in warfarin anti-coagulated patients: incidence, risk factor, management, and outcome. Biomed Res Int 2014;2014:463767.
20. Connolly SJ, Ezekowitz MD, Yusuf S, et al. Dabigatran versus warfarin in patients with atrial fibrillation. N Engl J Med 2009;361(12):1139–51.
21. Granger CB, Alexander JH, McMurray JJ, et al. Apixaban versus warfarin in patients with atrial fibrillation. N Engl J Med 2011;365(11):981–92.
22. Patel MR, Mahaffey KW, Garg J, et al. Rivaroxaban versus warfarin in nonvalvular atrial fibrillation. N Engl J Med 2011;365(10):883–91.
23. Abraham NS, Noseworthy PA, Yao X, et al. Gastrointestinal safety of direct oral anticoagulants: a large population-based study. Gastroenterology 2017;152(5):1014–22.
24. Cappell MS, Friedel D. Initial management of acute upper gastrointestinal bleeding: from initial evaluation up to gastrointestinal endoscopy. Med Clin North Am 2008;92(3):491–509.
25. Chait MM. Gastroesophageal reflux disease: important considerations for the older patients. World J Gastrointest Endosc 2010;2(12):388.
26. De Groen, Piet C, et al. Esophagitis associated with the use of alendronate. N Engl J Med 1996;335(14):1016–21.
27. Guntipalli P, Chason R, Elliott A, et al. Upper gastrointestinal bleeding caused by severe esophagitis: a unique clinical syndrome. Dig Dis Sci 2014;59(12):2997–3003.
28. Mallory GKt. Hemorrhages from lacerations of the cardiac orifice of stomach due to vomiting. Am J Med Sci 1929;178:506–15.
29. Harris JM, DiPalma JA. Clinical significance of Mallory-Weiss tears. Am J Gastroenterol 1993;88:12.
30. Foutch PG. Angiodysplasia of the gastrointestinal tract. Am J Gastroenterol 1993;88:6.
31. O'Mara C, Imbembo AL. Paraprosthetic-enteric fistula. Surgery 1977;81(5):556–66.
32. García-Pagán JC, Gracia-Sancho J, Bosch J. Functional aspects on the pathophysiology of portal hypertension in cirrhosis. J Hepatol 2012;57(2):458–61.
33. North Italian Endoscopic Club for the Study and Treatment of Esophageal Varices. Prediction of the first variceal hemorrhage in patients with cirrhosis of the liver and esophageal varices. N Engl J Med 1988;319(15):983–9.
34. Vakil NB, Feldman M, Grover S. Peptic ulcer disease: clinical manifestations and diagnosis. UpToDate; 2016. p. 2016.
35. Cave DR. Transmission and epidemiology of Helicobacter pylori. Am J Med 1996;100:12S–8S.
36. Pounder RE, Ng D. The prevalence of Helicobacter pylori infection in different countries. Aliment Pharmacol Ther 1995;9:33–9.
37. Yoshiyama H, Nakazawa T. Unique mechanism of Helicobacter pylori for colonizing the gastric mucus. Microbes Infect 2000;2(1):55–60.
38. Barkun A, Leontiadis G. Systematic review of the symptom burden, quality of life impairment and costs associated with peptic ulcer disease. Am J Med 2010;123(4):358–66.
39. Chey WD, Leontiadis GI, Howden CW, et al. ACG clinical guideline: treatment of Helicobacter pylori infection. Am J Gastroenterol 2017;112(2):212–39.
40. Crowe SE, Feldman M, Ginsburg CH. Indications and diagnostic tests for Helicobacter pylori infection. Uptodate Wellesley 2010;17:3.

41. Laine L, Estrada R, Trujillo M, et al. Effect of proton-pump inhibitor therapy on diagnostic testing for Helicobacter pylori. Ann Intern Med 1998;129(7):547–50.
42. Srygley FD, Gerardo CJ, Tran T, et al. Does this patient have a severe upper gastrointestinal bleed? JAMA 2012;307(10):1072–9.
43. Huang ES, Karsan S, Kanwal F, et al. Impact of nasogastric lavage on outcomes in acute GI bleeding. Gastrointest Endosc 2011;74(5):971–80.
44. Saltzman JR, Tabak YP, Hyett BH, et al. A simple risk score accurately predicts in-hospital mortality, length of stay, and cost in acute upper GI bleeding. Gastrointest Endosc 2011;74(6):1215–24.
45. Blatchford O, Murray WR, Blatchford M. A risk score to predict need for treatment for upper gastrointestinal haemorrhage. Lancet 2000;356(9238):1318–21.
46. Stanley AJ, et al. Comparison of risk scoring systems for patients presenting with upper gastrointestinal bleeding: international multicentre prospective study. BMJ 2017;356:i6432.
47. Reddick AD, Ronald J, Morrison WG. Intravenous fluid resuscitation: was Poiseuille right? Emerg Med J 2011;28(3):201–2.
48. Kaviani MJ, Hashemi MR, Kazemifar AR, et al. Effect of oral omeprazole in reducing re-bleeding in bleeding peptic ulcers: a prospective, double-blind, randomized, clinical trial. Aliment Pharmacol Ther 2003;17(2):211–6.
49. Green FW, et al. Effect of acid and pepsin on blood coagulation and platelet aggregation: a possible contributor to prolonged gastroduodenal mucosal hemorrhage. Gastroenterology 1978;74(1):38–43.
50. Sachar H, Vaidya K, Laine L. Intermittent vs continuous proton pump inhibitor therapy for high-risk bleeding ulcers: a systematic review and meta-analysis. JAMA Intern Med 2014;174(11):1755–62.
51. Rahman R, Nguyen DL, Sohail U, et al. Pre-endoscopic erythromycin administration in upper gastrointestinal bleeding: an updated meta-analysis and systematic review. Ann Gastroenterol 2016;29(3):312.
52. Wells M, Chande N, Adams P, et al. Meta-analysis: vasoactive medications for the management of acute variceal bleeds. Aliment Pharmacol Ther 2012;35(11):1267–78.
53. Garcia-Tsao G, Abraldes JG, Berzigotti A, et al. Portal hypertensive bleeding in cirrhosis: risk stratification, diagnosis, and management: 2016 practice guidance by the American Association for the study of liver diseases. Hepatology 2017;65(1):310–35.
54. Chavez-Tapia NC, et al. Meta-analysis: antibiotic prophylaxis for cirrhotic patients with upper gastrointestinal bleeding–an updated Cochrane review. Aliment Pharmacol Ther 2011;34(5):509–18.
55. Fernández J, Del Arbol LR, Gómez C, et al. Norfloxacin vs ceftriaxone in the prophylaxis of infections in patients with advanced cirrhosis and hemorrhage. Gastroenterology 2006;131(4):1049–56.
56. Villanueva C, Colomo A, Bosch A, et al. Transfusion strategies for acute upper gastrointestinal bleeding. N Engl J Med 2013;368(1):11–21.
57. Garg SK, Anugwom C, Campbell J, et al. Early esophagogastroduodenoscopy is associated with better outcomes in upper gastrointestinal bleeding: a nationwide study. Endosc Int Open 2017;5(05):E376–86.
58. Kumar NL, et al. Timing of upper endoscopy influences outcomes in patients with acute nonvariceal upper GI bleeding. Gastrointest Endosc 2017;85(5):945–52.
59. Laine L, Jensen DM. Management of patients with ulcer bleeding. Am J Gastroenterol 2012;107(3):345–60.

60. Gerson LB, Fidler JL, Cave DR, et al. ACG clinical guideline: diagnosis and management of small bowel bleeding. Am J Gastroenterol 2015;110(9):1265–87.
61. Dai C, et al. Endoscopic variceal ligation compared with endoscopic injection sclerotherapy for treatment of esophageal variceal hemorrhage: a meta-analysis. World J Gastroenterol 2015;21(8):2534.
62. Sanyal B. Methods to achieve hemostasis in patients with acute variceal hemorrhage. Pleasanton (CA): Baishideng Publishing Group; UpToDate; 2014.
63. Thiele M, Krag A, Rohde U, et al. Meta-analysis: banding ligation and medical interventions for the prevention of rebleeding from oesophageal varices. Aliment Pharmacol Ther 2012;35(10):1155–65.
64. Acosta RD, Abraham NS, Chandrasekhara V, et al. The management of antithrombotic agents for patients undergoing GI endoscopy. Gastrointest Endosc 2016;83(1):3–16.
65. Abbas AE, Brodie B, Dixon S, et al. Incidence and prognostic impact of gastrointestinal bleeding after percutaneous coronary intervention for acute myocardial infarction. Am J Cardiol 2005;96(2):173–6.
66. Al-Mallah M, Bazari RN, Jankowski M, et al. Predictors and outcomes associated with gastrointestinal bleeding in patients with acute coronary syndromes. J Thromb Thrombolysis 2007;23(1):51–5.
67. Garcia DA, et al. Risk of thromboembolism with short-term interruption of warfarin therapy. Arch Intern Med 2008;168(1):63–9.
68. Roudaut R, Karim S, Lafitte S. Thrombosis of prosthetic heart valves: diagnosis and therapeutic considerations. Heart 2007;93(1):137–42.
69. Douketis JD, Spyropoulos AC, Kaatz S, et al. Perioperative bridging anticoagulation in patients with atrial fibrillation. N Engl J Med 2015;373(9):823–33.
70. Doherty JU, et al. 2017 ACC expert consensus decision pathway for periprocedural management of anticoagulation in patients with nonvalvular atrial fibrillation: a report of the American College of Cardiology Clinical Expert Consensus Document Task Force. J Am Coll Cardiol 2017;69(7):871–98.
71. Lutz J, Jurk K, Schinzel H. Direct oral anticoagulants in patients with chronic kidney disease: patient selection and special considerations. Int J Nephrol Renovasc Dis 2017;10:135.
72. Pollack JR, Charles V, et al. Idarucizumab for dabigatran reversal—full cohort analysis. N Engl J Med 2017;377(5):431–41.
73. Connolly SJ, et al. Full study report of andexanet alfa for bleeding associated with factor Xa inhibitors. N Engl J Med 2019;380(14):1326–35.

Colorectal Cancer Screening in the Elderly

Andrea L. Betesh, MD[a],*, Felice H. Schnoll-Sussman, MD[b]

KEYWORDS

- Colorectal cancer • Colon cancer • Colonoscopy • Screening • Elderly
- Shared decision-making

KEY POINTS

- Colorectal cancer (CRC) is common, and incidence increases with age. However, routine screening guidelines recommend careful consideration of individual patient factors when determining appropriateness of CRC screening after age 75 years.
- With increasing age and comorbidities, the long-term benefits of CRC screening begin to diminish, and the risk of adverse events increases.
- Engaging elderly patients in an open dialogue about the pros and cons of ongoing CRC screening, overall functional status, and their health priorities is essential in order to ensure screening in this age group is done only on appropriate patients.

INTRODUCTION

It is widely accepted that cancer screening tests should be done in appropriate patient populations, as the benefits of screening and the resultant cancer prevention and early detection are great, and the risks of screening are generally low. Colorectal cancer (CRC) is very common, and the incidence increases with age. The downstream preventative benefit of CRC screening follows a decade or more after the chosen screening test is performed, whereas the risks of the screening test occur at the time of testing. Therefore, as individuals age and grow closer to end of life, eventually the risk-to-benefit ratio of ongoing CRC screening can no longer be justified. Understanding this as clinicians and conveying this to patients in a logical yet sensitive manner can be challenging. Clinical guidelines do provide some direction, with most suggesting discontinuation of screening once a certain age is reached or life expectancy becomes less than a specific threshold. However, chronologic age is merely one factor to consider, as comorbid conditions impart substantial physiologic heterogeneity between individuals of the same numeric age. Predicting life expectancy and

[a] Department of Gastroenterology and Hepatology, New York-Presbyterian Hospital/Weill Cornell Medicine, 1305 York Avenue, 4th Floor, New York, NY 10021, USA; [b] Department of Gastroenterology and Hepatology, New York-Presbyterian Hospital/Weill Cornell Medicine, 1315 York Avenue, Ground Floor, New York, NY 10021, USA
* Corresponding author.
E-mail address: anb9279@med.cornell.edu

Clin Geriatr Med 37 (2021) 173–183
https://doi.org/10.1016/j.cger.2020.08.012
0749-0690/21/© 2020 Elsevier Inc. All rights reserved.

geriatric.theclinics.com

conveying this to patients is also problematic, and clinicians should seek to frame the conversation about ongoing cancer screening versus cessation of screening in a thoughtful and empathetic manner. Here the authors review pertinent data to consider when making recommendations to elderly patients about CRC screening.

EPIDEMIOLOGY

CRC is common and carries a high mortality rate, especially when diagnosed at late stage. It is the third most frequently diagnosed cancer in both men and women in the United States, and it is expected to account for more than 50,000 US cancer-related deaths in the year 2020.[1] The likelihood of being diagnosed with CRC increases with age. For example, for men aged 50 to 54 years CRC incidence is 67.9 per 100,000. However, for men aged 75 to 79 years CRC incidence jumps substantially to 226.6 per 100,000.[2]

COLORECTAL CANCER SCREENING GUIDELINES

The United States Preventative Services Task Force (USPSTF) recommends CRC screening for average risk individuals aged 50 to 75 years, citing a high certainty that this intervention provides overall net benefit to patients with minimal potential harms.[3] In order to be considered "average risk" there must be no personal history of colon polyps or CRC or family history of CRC in first-degree relatives. The USPSTF does not advocate for any specific CRC screening test, naming the lack of head-to-head studies demonstrating that any one test is superior to the others.[3] The United States Multi-Society Task Force (USMSTF), which represents the American College of Gastroenterology, the American Gastroenterological Association, and the American Society for Gastrointestinal Endoscopy, also recommends CRC screening in individuals aged 50 to 75 years, but in contrast to the USPSTF, the USMSTF has ranked the various CRC screening tests into 3 tiers based on performance features, costs, and practical considerations.[4]

When it comes to recommendations regarding cessation of screening, the data are less robust. The USPSTF states that the age at which the potential harms of CRC screening may begin to outweigh the benefits depends on multiple factors, including prior screening status, comorbid conditions, health status, and life expectancy.[3,5] Although there are no randomized control data, modeling studies have shown that few additional life years are gained relative to the increase in colonoscopy burden when CRC screening is extended beyond age 75 years in average-risk individuals with negative prior screening.[6] The USMSTF states that discontinuation of screening should be considered when patients who are up to date with screening and have had no prior positive screening tests reach age 75 years or when the life expectancy is less than 10 years; however, this is a weak recommendation with low quality of evidence.[4] For elderly individuals with no prior screening, microsimulation modeling suggests that one-time CRC screening may be cost-effective up to age 86 years.[7]

What about the elderly patient in whom there is already a history of prior colorectal neoplasia? There is little guidance on when to discontinue CRC surveillance for these patients. Given that individuals with a history of adenomas, especially high-risk adenomas, are at higher risk for developing CRC, the potential benefit for surveillance in elderly patients with a history of neoplasia likely exceeds the benefits for elderly patients engaged in average-risk screening. The USMSTF states that for individuals aged 75 to 85 years, this group may be more likely to benefit from surveillance depending on life-expectancy, and the decision to proceed with ongoing surveillance should be personalized.[8]

COLORECTAL CANCER SCREENING MODALITIES

A variety of tests are available for CRC screening (see **Table 1**[3,4]). The tests exist on a continuum of invasiveness and frequency, with stool-based tests occurring as frequently as annually on the noninvasive end of the spectrum, radiologic tests occurring every 5 years in the middle, and endoscopic tests with screening intervals as long as every 10 years on the invasive end of the spectrum. In short, the more invasive the test, the less frequent the screening is needed; the less invasive the test, the more frequent the screening interval. If a noncolonoscopy screening test is found to be positive, the patient is advised to have a follow-up colonoscopy to further evaluate the

Table 1
Colorectal cancer screening modalities

Screening Test	Testing Interval	Pros	Cons
Stool-based tests			
gFOBT	Every 1 y	• RCT data with mortality endpoints. • Does not require bowel preparation, anesthesia. • Test performed at home.	• Frequent testing interval. • Requires dietary modification in advance of testing. • Requires follow-up colonoscopy if positive. • Requires 3 specimens.
FIT	Every 1 y	• Improved accuracy compared with gFOBT. • Can be done with a single specimen. • Does not require bowel preparation, anesthesia. • Test performed at home.	• Frequent testing interval. • Requires follow-up colonoscopy if positive.
FIT-DNA	Every 3 y	• Higher sensitivity than FIT. • Can be done with a single specimen. • Does not require bowel preparation, anesthesia. • Test performed at home.	• Requires follow-up colonoscopy if positive. • Specificity is lower than FIT (resulting in higher rate of false positives and subsequent colonoscopies). • Insufficient evidence about appropriate long-term follow-up of abnormal test after a negative diagnostic colonoscopy.
Nonendoscopic direct-visualization tests			
CT colonography	Every 5 y	• Does not require sedation.	• Requires bowel preparation. • Requires follow-up colonoscopy if positive, which may not occur same day, thus necessitating bowel preparation twice.

Abbreviations: gFBOT, Guaiac fecal occult blood test; RCT, randomized controlled trial.

positive test. As mentioned earlier, the USPSTF does not give preference to any single test[3]; however, the USMSTF ranks colonoscopy every 10 years and fecal immuno-chemical testing (FIT) annually as the preferred tier 1 tests.[4]

Colonoscopy has several advantages over the other screening modalities, which include the capability to both diagnose and remove premalignant lesions at the time of the examination, making it both diagnostic and therapeutic, as well as the long allowable interval between negative screening examinations, and the ability to detect both cancerous and a variety of premalignant lesions other than CRC.[4] However, colonoscopy does require the patient to undertake a bowel preparation, is substantially more invasive, and carries more procedure and sedation-related risks than nonendo-scopic screening tests. It is important to point out that no randomized controlled trials for colonoscopy have been completed; however, multiple cohort studies, most notably the National Polyp Study, demonstrate reduction in CRC incidence and mortality due to colonoscopy and polypectomy.[9–11] For patients who value the highest-sensitivity screening modality and are willing to undergo an invasive test, colonoscopy is a reasonable choice.[4]

For individuals who prefer a noninvasive test that does not require bowel preparation or a procedure with sedation, FIT is a high-performing low-cost option. According to a meta-analysis, FIT has a one-time sensitivity for cancer of 79% and sensitivity for advanced adenomas of approximately 30%.[12] It is low cost (approximately $20).[4] Drawbacks include the need to repeat the test annually, the need to ensure that positive tests are followed-up with a diagnostic colonoscopy, and low sensitivity for serrated colonic lesions.[4] It is worth mentioning that serrated lesions typically exist in the proximal colon and are more difficult to detect endoscopically compared with adenomatous lesions. The prevalence of serrated lesions does increase with age: one study found a prevalence of serrated lesions to be 10% in patients aged 20 to 29 years (identified during examination not performed for CRC screening) and 16.4% in those older than 70 years.[13] In the elderly, cytologic dysplasia and molecular alterations are more frequently detected in serrated lesions compared with serrated lesions in younger patients.[14] So although FIT may be a good choice for elderly patients who prefer less invasive CRC screening tests, the limitations of the test in the elderly must be kept in mind.

A multitude of other screening tests exist and are delineated in more detail in **Table 1**.

COLORECTAL CANCER SCREENING IN THE ELDERLY
Defining the Elderly

In 2010, more than 40 million people in the United States were older than 65 years, and 5.5 million people were older than 85 years. The older-than-85-years group is a fast-growing segment of the population, and by the year 2030 20% of the US population is expected to be older than 65 years.[15] Historically, "elderly" has been defined as older than 65 years and "very elderly" is often defined as older than 75 years. However, there are significant limitations in defining elderly by chronologic age only. Among patients of the same chronologic age, but with different comorbidities and functional status, there exists considerable physiologic heterogeneity.[16]

Measuring Risk-to-Benefit of Screening in the Elderly

A key principle of cancer screening is that the benefits of screening ought to outweigh the risks. Therefore, it is important to be able to measure the risks and benefits in a given group to help determine if the test is warranted. Investigators have sought to objectively measure the risk-to-benefit ratio of CRC screening in the elderly. To examine risk difference of screening individuals in their early 70s compared with those in their late 70s, one group looked prospectively at more than 1.3 million Medicare beneficiaries aged 70 to 79 years. All patients included in this study had not undergone any CRC screening in the 5 years before inclusion in the study. Individuals were followed-up for more than 8 years to determine the 8-year risk of CRC in those who did and did not undergo CRC screening. In individuals aged 70 to 74 years, the 8-year risk for CRC was 2.19% in the group that did undergo screening colonoscopy group and 2.62% in the group that did not undergo screening, giving an absolute risk difference of −0.42%. Among those aged 75 to 79 years, the 8-year risk for CRC was 2.84% in the screening colonoscopy group and 2.97% in the no-screening group, with an absolute risk difference of −0.14%[17]; this demonstrates that as individuals progress through their 70s, the relative benefit of screening colonoscopy decreases.

In a cross-sectional study of 1244 patients undergoing screening colonoscopy at a single academic center, investigators sought to estimate the number of life years saved by undergoing screening colonoscopy, stratified by age group. Despite higher prevalence of adenomatous colon polyps in elderly patients (28.6% in the patients older than 80 years vs 13.8% in the 50- to 54-year-old group and 26.5% in the 75- to 79-year-old group), mean extension in life expectancy was much lower in the group aged 80 years or older compared with the 50- to 54-year-old group (0.13 years vs 0.85 years). Stated differently, even though prevalence of precancerous colon polyps increases with age, screening colonoscopy in those aged 80 years or older results in only 15% of the expected gain in life expectancy of younger patients[18] because of the long lag time between the detection of an adenomatous polyp and the time at which this precancerous polyp would be expected to turn into CRC. In very elderly patients, death may occur due to other comorbidities before the development of an adenomatous polyp into a frank cancer.

Inherent to the discussion of whether or not to proceed with screening is the decision of which test to choose. Some elderly patients may not be willing to undergo colonoscopy as a screening test, but they would be amenable to noninvasive stool–based screening tests. However, it is important to recognize the potential drawbacks of stool-based testing. In addition to poor sensitivity for serrated lesions,[4] there is also a risk of false-positive results with stool-based tests, which would prompt a recommendation for colonoscopy. Physicians and patients should discuss this possibility before proceeding with fecal occult blood testing or FIT,[19] to ensure that the patient would be willing to continue with a colonoscopy, should a positive result be found.

Tools to Estimate Life Expectancy

Because the benefit of screening diminishes with decreasing life expectancy, being able to estimate life expectancy is valuable in guiding the decision of whether or not to continue screening. There are existing tools to help clinicians understand probable life expectancy so that they may apply this information to the shared decision-making process.

Gait speed has been shown to correlate well with life expectancy. A gait speed of 0.8 m/s is associated with median life expectancy; as gait speed increases or decreases, life expectancy is longer or shorter, respectively (**Fig. 1**).[20]

In addition, prognostic calculators have been created and validated to estimate 9- to 10-year life expectancy in older adults. Such models take into account age, gender, comorbid conditions, and functional measures.[21,22] These and other prognostic calculators are available online at www.eprognosis.org.[23]

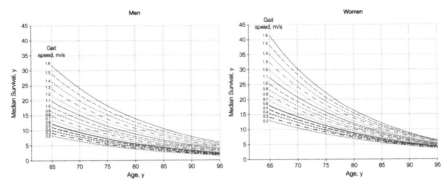

Fig. 1. Gait speed and median survival in older adults. (*From* Studenski S, Perera S, Patel K, et al. Gait speed and survival in older adults. JAMA. 2011;305(1):50–8; with permission.)

Overscreening

Despite recommendations to discontinue CRC screening in adults with less than 10 years life expectancy, many adults in this category report ongoing screening. A study from 2010 found that 51% of adults older than 75 years with life expectancies under 10 years still reported undergoing CRC screening.[24] Finding and removing premalignant lesions in this patient population is unlikely to improve quality of life or length of life. In some patients, depending on the number and severity of their comorbidities, even identifying a cancer may not alter the course of their medical treatments and clinical progression. If they are deemed too functionally debilitated to undergo treatment of the found cancer, identification of CRC does not alter their overall medical management. In fact, autopsy studies have shown that 2% to 3% of older adults have undiagnosed CRC at time of death, and 10% to 33% have colon polyps at time of death.[25] However, subjecting this population to CRC screening does put them at risk for the potential complications related to the screening procedure itself.

COLONOSCOPY IN THE ELDERLY
Sedation

Most endoscopic procedures are performed using either conscious sedation with a combination of narcotics and benzodiazepines or monitored anesthesia care with propofol. Elderly patients receiving sedation have an increased response to sedatives, and awareness of this is essential to prevent adverse sedation–related events.[15] However, chronologic age alone is not the main determinant of sedation-related complications. Age-related comorbidities and rapid or excessive dosing of sedatives are the major contributors to sedation-related complications in this group.[26] Elderly patients should be given fewer agents at a slower rate with lower initial and cumulative doses to avoid complications, such as respiratory depression, aspiration, and prolonged recovery periods.[15]

Bowel Preparation

Older patients, particularly those older than 80 years, are more likely to have inadequate bowel preparation and may have difficulty tolerating a large volume bowel preparation when undergoing colonoscopy.[15,27,28] When colonoscopy is pursued in this population, providers should strongly consider utilization of split-dose bowel preparations, which entails administering half of the preparation the evening before the colonoscopy and administering half of the preparation several hours before the colonoscopy on the day of the procedure.[15] It is the opinion of these investigators that split-dose preparation improves both tolerability and effectiveness of bowel preparation in all age groups, including the elderly. As with all patients, careful assessment of comorbid conditions and chronic medications should be part of the preprocedure evaluation in elderly patients undergoing colonoscopy. Generally, balanced-electrolyte solutions are less likely to cause fluid and electrolyte shifts in this population, especially in those with comorbid renal or cardiac issues.[15,29] In addition, blood thinners, diabetic agents, and certain antihypertensives may need to be modified or temporarily suspended in advance of bowel preparation and colonoscopy. This requires good communication between primary care providers, endoscopists, and patients in order to avoid potentially dangerous medication errors in the periprocedure period.

Procedural Considerations

In addition to issues with sedation and bowel preparation, there are specific procedural considerations to be aware of in elderly patients. In a study of 180 patients, endoscopists reported that colonoscopy was more technically difficult and time to cecal intubation was longer in patients aged 61 to 75 years compared with younger patients.[30]

It is important to understand adverse events related to colonoscopy in the elderly. In a random sample of more than 50,000 Medicare beneficiaries aged 66 to 95 years who underwent colonoscopy, adverse events were measured. Adverse events after outpatient colonoscopy increased with older age, if a polypectomy was performed, and with certain comorbid conditions, such as stroke, chronic obstructive pulmonary disease, atrial fibrillation, or congestive heart failure, all of which are more prevalent in the elderly.[31] Looking prospectively at more than 1.3 million Medicare beneficiaries aged 70 to 79 years, the excess 30-day risk for any adverse event in patients undergoing colonoscopy was 5.6 events per 1000 individuals in the 70 to 74 years age group and approximately double this at 10.3 per 1000 individuals in the 75 to 79 years age group.[17]

SHARED DECISION-MAKING IN THE ELDERLY

Once armed with information about options for screening and evidence concerning relative risks and benefits of screening based on age, comorbidities, and life-expectancy as reviewed earlier, clinicians should seek to engage in a shared decision-making process and have a collaborative, honest, open conversation with their elderly patients. It is important to begin this dialogue with an assessment of patient perceptions of CRC screening. Many patients are more likely to overestimate the benefits of screening and underestimate the harms of screening.[32] An interview study of 116 adults aged 70 years or older living in retirement communities showed that although 81% of participants believed that they would die of some disease other than cancer, only 13% thought that they would not live long enough to benefit from cancer screening tests.[33] This highlights a thought-provoking paradox in elderly patients' perceptions of the risks and benefits of cancer screening. Before exploring a patient's specific situation and making a firm recommendation about screening to that patient, it is prudent for the clinician to provide them with general information about the logistics and risks of screening.

The conversation of cessation of screening can be a delicate conversation for clinicians to approach. On what should the clinician focus? Should a patient's predicted life expectancy be directly discussed? Some clinicians may feel insensitive speaking about this in a pragmatic manner, which may lead them to avoid discussing the topic entirely, which could result in ongoing screening, even when not in the best interest of the patient. Avoiding the conversation is more likely to result in continuing CRC screening, as many older adults report that stopping screening is an active decision to be made but continuing screening is not.[34] However, elderly patients do want to discuss this topic, and there is consensus among both patients and clinicians that these are important conversations to have.[35] In one interview study, although most participants had not discussed the possibility of stopping cancer screening with their physicians, when prompted, 84% said they wanted to have these discussions.[33] In another study of 40 community dwelling adults older than 65 years who participated in semistructured interviews, participants were amenable to stopping cancer screening, especially in the context of a trusting relationship with their clinician.[36] However, in multiple studies, elderly individuals seem to be divided on whether life expectancy should be mentioned as part of the cessation of cancer screening conversation,[33,35] with 48% of patients older than 70 years preferring to not discuss life expectancy as an element in deciding about ongoing cancer screening.[33]

Some investigators recommend framing the discussion around age, health status, and helping people live longer, rather than making comments such as "you may not live long enough to benefit from this test."[36] Mentioning shifts in health priorities, and potentially avoiding an explicit discussion of life-expectancy, seems to be an acceptable communication strategy for both clinicians and older adults.[35] Overall, these interview-based studies are valuable and highlight the desire of patients to discuss screening, and cessation of screening, with their providers. They also underscore possible areas of misunderstanding that physicians can address with their elderly patients.

SUMMARY

The decision for elderly patients to continue with or forgo CRC screening is a complex and multifaceted clinical choice, which must involve an open and honest dialogue between clinicians and patients. After the age of 75 years, the risk to benefit ratio of CRC screening varies depending on prior screening status, comorbidities, predicted life expectancy, and functional capacity.[4,17,18] Once life expectancy is less than 10 years, the benefits of ongoing screening do not justify the associated risks.[4] However, predicting life expectancy in an individual patient is difficult. Gait speed and other prognostic calculators can be used to aid clinicians in assessing predicted life expectancy,[20–22] and these can be useful factors to consider when assessing if ongoing screening is justified. Once armed with accurate information about the risks and benefits of screening, the pros and cons of the multitude of screening tests, and an understanding of an individual patient's predicted life expectancy, clinicians need to engage their elderly patients in a sensitive and empathetic conversation. It is incumbent on the clinician to breach this conversation and explore patient understanding, priorities, and values as it relates to screening tests. Evidence shows that patients do want to discuss this with their doctors but may not open the conversation themselves,[33,35] further highlighting clinician responsibility for beginning this dialogue. Understanding elderly patients' hesitation to directly address life expectancy in this conversation is important. Elderly patients are split as to whether they prefer to explicitly talk about life expectancy[33,35]; therefore, focusing the conversation on patient values and health care priorities can avoid upsetting patients while still allowing them to explore the complexities of this topic with a trusted clinician.[35,36]

Engaging elderly patients in this discussion allows them the opportunity to obtain accurate information about the benefits of screening and can help dispel misconceptions about the relative risks and benefits, as many patients tend to overestimate the benefits and underestimate the risks of screening.[32,33] Furthermore, because many older adults view the decision to stop screening as an active choice and to continue screening as the default,[34] open discussion may empower patients to stop undergoing screening if that is their preference. Avoiding the conversation in this unique population could result in ongoing screening, even if not appropriate, which exposes the patients to unnecessary risk and potential harm. As the number of elderly patients continues to increase, the importance of appropriate utilization of screening tests in the elderly will become a commonly encountered clinical scenario that all clinicians will be engaging in regularly. Accurate information and empathetic shared decision-making are essential tools for clinicians and patients to successfully navigate these challenging topics.

CLINICS CARE POINTS

- Elderly patients tend to overestimate the benefits of cancer screening and underestimate the risks.
- Many elderly patients feel that the 'default' decision is to continue CRC screening, while cessation of screening requires an active decision.
- Patients want to discuss ongoing cancer screening and possible cessation of screening with their physician; however, many will not initiate this conversation. It is the responsibility of the clinician to breach this topic with patients.
- Patients have mixed preference regarding direct discussion of life expectancy as part of the CRC screening conversation. Focusing on functional status, overall health, health priorities, and quality of life is an acceptable method for framing this conversation.

DISCLOSURE

The authors have nothing to disclose.

REFERENCES

1. Siegel RL, Miller KD, Jemal A. Cancer statistics, 2020. CA Cancer J Clin 2020; 70(1):7–30.

2. Data: SRD—AT. Surveillance, Epidemiology, and End Results (SEER) Program (www.seer.cancer.gov) Research Data (1975-2016), National Cancer Institute, DCCPS, Surveillance Research Program, released April 2019, based on the November 2018 submission. 2019. Accessed.

3. Bibbins-Domingo K, Grossman DC, Curry SJ, et al. Screening for colorectal cancer: US preventive Services Task Force recommendation statement. JAMA 2016; 315(23):2564–75.

4. Rex DK, Boland CR, Dominitz JA, et al. Colorectal cancer screening: recommendations for physicians and patients from the U.S. Multi-society Task Force on colorectal cancer. Am J Gastroenterol 2017;112(7):1016–30.

5. Lansdorp-Vogelaar I, Gulati R, Mariotto AB, et al. Personalizing age of cancer screening cessation based on comorbid conditions: model estimates of harms and benefits. Ann Intern Med 2014;161(2):104–12.

6. Knudsen AB, Zauber AG, Rutter CM, et al. Estimation of benefits, burden, and harms of colorectal cancer screening strategies: modeling study for the US preventive Services Task Force. JAMA 2016;315(23):2595–609.

7. van Hees F, Habbema JD, Meester RG, et al. Should colorectal cancer screening be considered in elderly persons without previous screening? A cost-effectiveness analysis. Ann Intern Med 2014;160(11):750–9.

8. Lieberman DA, Rex DK, Winawer SJ, et al. Guidelines for colonoscopy surveillance after screening and polypectomy: a consensus update by the US Multi-Society Task Force on Colorectal Cancer. Gastroenterology 2012;143(3):844–57.

9. O'Brien MJ, Winawer SJ, Zauber AG, et al. The National Polyp Study. Patient and polyp characteristics associated with high-grade dysplasia in colorectal adenomas. Gastroenterology 1990;98(2):371–9.

10. Winawer SJ, Zauber AG, Ho MN, et al. Prevention of colorectal cancer by colonoscopic polypectomy. The National Polyp Study Workgroup. N Engl J Med 1993; 329(27):1977–81.

11. Zauber AG, Winawer SJ, O'Brien MJ, et al. Colonoscopic polypectomy and long-term prevention of colorectal-cancer deaths. N Engl J Med 2012;366(8):687–96.

12. Lee JK, Liles EG, Bent S, et al. Accuracy of fecal immunochemical tests for colorectal cancer: systematic review and meta-analysis. Ann Intern Med 2014; 160(3):171.

13. Kim HY, Kim SM, Seo JH, et al. Age-specific prevalence of serrated lesions and their subtypes by screening colonoscopy: a retrospective study. BMC Gastroenterol 2014;14:82.

14. Nosho K, Igarashi H, Ito M, et al. Clinicopathological and molecular characteristics of serrated lesions in Japanese elderly patients. Digestion 2015;91(1):57–63.

15. Chandrasekhara V, Early DS, Acosta RD, et al. Modifications in endoscopic practice for the elderly. Gastrointest Endosc 2013;78(1):1–7.

16. Sabharwal S, Wilson H, Reilly P, et al. Heterogeneity of the definition of elderly age in current orthopaedic research. Springerplus 2015;4:516.

17. Garcia-Albeniz X, Hsu J, Bretthauer M, et al. Effectiveness of screening colonoscopy to prevent colorectal cancer among Medicare beneficiaries aged 70 to 79 years: a prospective observational study. Ann Intern Med 2017;166(1):18–26.

18. Lin OS, Kozarek RA, Schembre DB, et al. Screening colonoscopy in very elderly patients: prevalence of neoplasia and estimated impact on life expectancy. JAMA 2006;295(20):2357–65.

19. Kotwal AA, Schonberg MA. Cancer screening in the elderly: a review of breast, colorectal, lung, and prostate cancer screening. Cancer J 2017;23(4):246–53.

20. Studenski S, Perera S, Patel K, et al. Gait speed and survival in older adults. JAMA 2011;305(1):50–8.

21. Cruz M, Covinsky K, Widera EW, et al. Predicting 10-year mortality for older adults. JAMA 2013;309(9):874–6.

22. Schonberg MA, Davis RB, McCarthy EP, et al. External validation of an index to predict up to 9-year mortality of community-dwelling adults aged 65 and older. J Am Geriatr Soc 2011;59(8):1444–51.

23. Soung MC. Screening for cancer: when to stop?: a practical guide and review of the evidence. Med Clin North Am 2015;99(2):249–62.

24. Schonberg MA, Breslau ES, Hamel MB, et al. Colon cancer screening in U.S. adults aged 65 and older according to life expectancy and age. J Am Geriatr Soc 2015;63(4):750–6.

25. Colon cancer screening (USPSTF recommendation). U.S. Preventive Services Task Force. J Am Geriatr Soc 2000;48(3):333–5.

26. Muravchick S. The elderly outpatient: current anesthetic implications. Curr Opin Anaesthesiol 2002;15(6):621–5.

27. Houissa F, Kchir H, Bouzaidi S, et al. Colonoscopy in elderly: feasibility, tolerance and indications: about 901 cases. Tunis Med 2011;89(11):848–52.

28. Chatrenet P, Friocourt P, Ramain JP, et al. Colonoscopy in the elderly: a study of 200 cases. Eur J Med 1993;2(7):411–3.

29. Mamula P, Adler DG, Conway JD, et al. Colonoscopy preparation. Gastrointest Endosc 2009;69(7):1201–9.

30. Ristikankare M, Hartikainen J, Heikkinen M, et al. The effects of gender and age on the colonoscopic examination. J Clin Gastroenterol 2001;32(1):69–75.

31. Warren JL, Klabunde CN, Mariotto AB, et al. Adverse events after outpatient colonoscopy in the Medicare population. Ann Intern Med 2009;150(12):849–57, w152.

32. Sutkowi-Hemstreet A, Vu M, Harris R, et al. Adult patients' perspectives on the benefits and harms of overused screening tests: a qualitative study. J Gen Intern Med 2015;30(11):1618–26.

33. Lewis CL, Kistler CE, Amick HR, et al. Older adults' attitudes about continuing cancer screening later in life: a pilot study interviewing residents of two continuing care communities. BMC Geriatr 2006;6:10.

34. Torke AM, Schwartz PH, Holtz LR, et al. Older adults and forgoing cancer screening: "I think it would be strange. JAMA Intern Med 2013;173(7):526–31.

35. Schoenborn NL, Boyd CM, Lee SJ, et al. Communicating about stopping cancer screening: comparing clinicians' and older adults' perspectives. Gerontologist 2019;59(Suppl 1):S67–76.

36. Schoenborn NL, Lee K, Pollack CE, et al. Older adults' views and communication preferences about cancer screening cessation. JAMA Intern Med 2017;177(8): 1121–8.

Inflammatory Bowel Disease in the Older Adult

Shirley Cohen-Mekelburg, MD, MS[a,b,c],*, Akbar K. Waljee, MD, MSc[a,b,c,d]

KEYWORDS

- Ulcerative colitis • Crohn's disease • Elderly-onset

KEY POINTS

- As the population continues to age, we will be seeing an increasing number of older adults with inflammatory bowel disease.
- The management of inflammatory bowel disease in the elderly comes with specific challenges, as a result of comorbidities, polypharmacy, age-related circumstances, and limited inclusion of older adults in clinical trials.
- To best care for older adults with inflammatory bowel disease, it is important to be aware of the special considerations in their treatment, with particular attention to the risk of infections, malignancy, comorbidities, and overall fitness.

Inflammatory bowel disease (IBD) is a chronic relapsing–remitting condition affecting the gastrointestinal tract. Its 2 subtypes, ulcerative colitis (UC) and Crohn's disease, lead to often disabling symptoms of diarrhea, hematochezia, and abdominal pain, in addition to multiple other clinical manifestations. UC is limited to the colon and marked by bloody diarrhea, tenesmus, and fecal urgency, in addition to more systemic symptoms such as weight loss and fevers. Crohn's disease can affect any aspect of the gastrointestinal system, including the mouth, upper gastrointestinal tract, small bowel, or colon. Crohn's disease is classified into 3 major phenotypes including nonstricturing nonfistulizing, stricturing, or fistulizing disease classifications. It most often manifests as abdominal pain and diarrhea, in addition to phenotype-specific symptoms, such as nausea and vomiting, symptomatic fistulas, and other systemic symptoms such as arthralgias, rashes, and weight loss.

[a] Inflammatory Bowel Disease Program, VA Ann Arbor Healthcare System, VA Center for Clinical Management Research, 2215 Fuller Road, Ann Arbor, MI 48105, USA; [b] Division of Gastroenterology & Hepatology, Department of Internal Medicine, Michigan Medicine, 3912 Taubman Center, 1500 East Medical Center Drive, Ann Arbor, MI 48109, USA; [c] Institute for Healthcare Policy and Innovation, University of Michigan, 2800 Plymouth Road, Ann Arbor, MI 48109, USA; [d] Michigan Integrated Center for Health Analytics and Medical Prediction (MICHAMP), University of Michigan, 2800 Plymouth Road, Ann Arbor, MI 48109, USA
* Corresponding author. Division of Gastroenterology & Hepatology, Michigan Medicine, 3912 Taubman Center SPC 5362, 1500 East Medical Center Drive, Ann Arbor, MI 48109.
E-mail address: shcohen@med.umich.edu
Twitter: @ShirleyCoMek (S.C.-M.); @AkbarWaljee (A.K.W.)

Clin Geriatr Med 37 (2021) 185–195
https://doi.org/10.1016/j.cger.2020.08.013
0749-0690/21/Published by Elsevier Inc.

geriatric.theclinics.com

The prevalence of IBD continues to increase, and spread globally. In a population-based cohort study of patients with IBD in Olmsted County, Minnesota from 1970 to 2010, age- and sex-adjusted incidence rates for Crohn's disease and UC were 8.7 and 10.7 per 100,000 person-years, respectively.[1] The age- and sex-adjusted prevalence were 246.7 and 286.3 cases per 100,000 persons, respectively.[1] Although the mean age at diagnosis for UC and Crohn's disease is 29.5 and 34.9 years, respectively, the incidence of IBD in older adults is substantial.[1] Among 60- to 69-year-old and 70- to 93-year-olds, the incidence of UC and Crohn's disease was 5.8 and 7.5 cases per 100,000 person-years, and 9.9 and 10.2 cases per 100,000 person-years, respectively.[1] This incidence compares with an incidence of 16.6 and 18.7 cases per 100,000 person-years among 20- to 29-year-olds for UC and Crohn's disease, respectively. In a similar national cohort study in Canada using the Canadian Gastrointestinal Epidemiology Consortium, the estimated prevalence of IBD among older adults was 646 per 100,000 in 2008. A primary forecasting analysis used simulation to estimate an IBD prevalence of 1370 per 100,000 by 2030 among older adults. These prevalence estimates are higher than those reported for adults 18 to 59 years of age, which were 622 and 1118 per 100,000 in 2008 and 2030, respectively.[2] The prevalence of IBD in the elderly is increasing as our population grows older.[2] In addition, more than 10% and up to 20% of new IBD diagnoses are in patients 60 years and older and defined as elderly-onset IBD.[1–4]

Although the management of IBD tends to follow a similar approach for all adults, there are certain characteristics that make IBD treatment more challenging in older patients. In the last 2 decades, the advent of novel medical treatments has changed the paradigm of IBD, with an increasing focus on the prevention of disease progression rather than symptom control alone. However, the safety of these therapies in the elderly needs to be considered. Further, the management of IBD in the elderly is confounded by comorbidities that can increase the risk of medication or surgical complications; polypharmacy and altered pharmacokinetics also increase the risk of drug–drug interactions and adverse events (**Box 1**).[5]

PRESENTATION

In older adults, IBD is more likely to be confused with other conditions, such as medication-related colitis, microscopic colitis, colonic ischemia, or diverticular disease (**Box 2**).[3] Therefore, elderly patients are more likely to have a delay in IBD diagnosis, leading to further bowel damage before treatment initiation. It is estimated that

---

Box 1
Issues important to elderly patients with IBD

- Comorbidities
- Polypharmacy
- Altered pharmacokinetics
- Competing diagnoses
- Infection risk
- Cancer risk
- Surgical complications
- Limited mobility and vision

Box 2
Differential diagnosis for IBD in older adults
• Medication-related colitis
• Microscopic colitis
• Segmental colitis associated with diverticular disease
• Colonic ischemia
• Infectious colitis
• Radiation colopathy

up to 60% of older adults with IBD are initially misdiagnosed.[6] Microscopic colitis can often be differentiated from IBD by the absence of mucosal abnormalities. Although segmental colitis associated with diverticular disease can mimic Crohn's colitis both endoscopically and histologically, the segment of inflammation is usually confined to the area involved by diverticula. Estimates of misdiagnosed segmental colitis associated with diverticular disease as Crohn's disease have been reported to be as high as 8%.[7] Colonic ischemia has been misdiagnosed as IBD in up to 50% of cases, and often can be differentiated by its acute onset of symptoms and rapid clinical improvement, in addition to differentiating characteristics on endoscopy and histology.[8]

The clinical presentation of IBD in an older adult is often similar to younger patients, but certain characteristics of elderly-onset IBD are notable. Elderly-onset IBD may be more subtle with less severe diarrhea, hematochezia, and abdominal pain.[9] In Crohn's disease, it is also more likely to present with a nonstricturing nonfistulizing phenotype.[3,9] Elderly-onset Crohn's disease is more likely to be colonic in distribution, with proctitis and left-sided colitis predominating.[3] Patient's with elderly-onset IBD are also more likely to have a stable disease course, rather than disease progression. In UC, elderly onset disease is more often left sided in distribution without proximal extension over time.[3,9] In contrast, extraintestinal manifestations are similar regardless of age.[3]

DIAGNOSIS

Following a history and physical examination, the workup for IBD in the elderly is similar to that in the general population and involves laboratory testing and an endoscopic evaluation. Laboratory testing includes blood work and stool studies may reveal results suggestive of IBD and rule out alternative diagnoses. A complete blood count may demonstrate an elevated white blood cell count, or reduced hemoglobin value consistent with anemia; this may be a result of iron deficiency and/or anemia of chronic disease. An elevated erythrocyte sedimentation rate and C-reactive protein are nonspecific markers of inflammation. An elevated fecal calprotectin, a stool test measuring a neutrophil-derived protein, is consistent intestine-specific inflammation. Stool pathogen tests, including stool culture, *Clostridium difficile* toxin testing, and gastrointestinal panels, are used to rule out an infection. An ileocolonoscopy with associated biopsies is ultimately required for luminal evaluation for inflammation. Histologic evidence of chronic inflammation in the form of lymphocytes or plasma cells, along with crypt architectural abnormalities is suggestive of IBD over alternative diagnoses. Noncaseating granulomas may also be present, and are pathognomonic for Crohn's disease. In the setting of upper gastrointestinal symptoms, an esophagogastroduodenoscopy may be indicated, to evaluate for upper gastrointestinal involvement. If suspicion for small bowel disease exists, cross-sectional imaging (in the form of computed tomography or magnetic resonance enterography) or video capsule endoscopy may also be helpful to confirm disease extent.

TREATMENT OF INFLAMMATORY BOWEL DISEASE

Medical treatment strategies for IBD are generally the same for both younger and older patients with IBD. The armamentarium of IBD targeted medications includes 5-amino-salicylates, immunomodulators, corticosteroids, and biologics. Treatment of IBD may follow a step-up or top-down approach. A step-up approach involves tiered treatment for IBD, starting with aminosalicylates and/or corticosteroids and escalating to immu-nomodulators and/or biologics as necessary. A top-down approach, in contrast, in-volves early top tier treatment, usually with biologics.

Variation in treatment is common among older adults with IBD and confounded by multiple factors including patient and provider preferences, financial barriers and payer policies, and disease severity.[10,11] In a single-center Veterans Affairs IBD cohort from 2000 to 2008, 46.5% of the study population was 60 years or older. After control-ling for disease severity, older age at IBD onset was associated with a lower likelihood of biologic use with an odds ratio of 0.97 (95% confidence interval [CI], 0.95–0.99).[12] In fact, no patients who was 70 years or older at IBD diagnosis had received a biologic.[12] However, the limited availability of biologic treatment options during the study period likely contributed to the low rates of biologic initiation among older patients in this study. In a second study using administrative data from the United States, Canada, the United Kingdom, and Denmark to examine IBD-targeted medication among older patients with IBD, variation in prescriptions was also apparent, with increasing use of infliximab toward the end of the study period in 2009.[10]

5-Aminosalicylic Acid Agents

The 5-aminosalicylic acids are used to treat mild to moderate UC.[13] Its mechanism of action is multifactorial, and is believed to work in part by inhibiting T-cell proliferation, inhibiting antibody production and mast cell release.[14] It is also thought to inhibit proinflammatory cytokines, such as IL-1 and tumor necrosis factor (TNF).[14] Cochrane systematic reviews have demonstrated the superiority of topical 5-aminosalicylic acid therapy over placebo for induction of remission in ulcerative proctitis with pooled odds ratios of 8.3 (95% CI, 4.28–16.12) and 5.3 (95% CI–3.15, 8.92) for clinical and endo-scopic remission, respectively.[15] For more extensive mild to moderate UC, combined oral and topical 5-aminosalicylic acid is the first-line therapy with a lower likelihood of failure to achieve remission (relative risk. 0.65; 95% CI, 0.47–0.91) compared with oral 5-aminosalicylic acid alone.[16] No difference in effectiveness exists between oral 5-aminosalicylic acid agents and sulfasalazine, though 5-aminosalicylic acid agents are better tolerated.[17] Similarly, no significant difference in the effectiveness of the different 5-aminosalicylic acid formulations has been demonstrated in trials, but once daily dosing is associated with improved adherence.[18] In contrast, its use in Crohn' disease is controversial, because the data suggest no difference in effective-ness as compared with placebo, but the use of 5-aminosalicylic acid–based therapy in Crohn's disease remains commonplace.[18]

An estimated 44% to 75% of elderly patients with IBD receive 5-aminosalicylic acid therapy.[19,20] Although this high rate of use is likely related to its safe side effect profile, adverse effects and the risks of inadequate IBD treatment need to be considered. The 5-aminosalicylic acids have been demonstrated to cause nephrotoxicity, pancreatitis, in addition to numerous other less severe adverse effects. They have also shown to interact with digoxin, coumadin, and thiopurines. In addition, 5-aminosalicylic acid–based enemas may be more difficult to administer in older adults in the context of limited mobility as well as decreased rectal tone or fecal incontinence. These factors all need to be considered closely in the treatment of IBD in older adults.

Systemic Corticosteroids

Systemic corticosteroids, such as prednisone or budesonide, are used for induction therapy in both Crohn's disease and UC. Although they have beneficial effects in the short term, they do not have long-term benefits and carry serious side effects, including hypertension, hyperglycemia, delirium, psychological effects, skin changes, bone loss, glaucoma, cataracts, cardiovascular complications, and an increased mortality.[13,21] They increase the risks of serious infections, and also lead to loss of bone density and fractures. Although budesonide has an extensive first-pass metabolism leading to fewer systemic effects, similar adverse events have been reported.

The use of systemic corticosteroids in elderly patients with IBD is common with prolonged corticosteroid use of over 3 months reported among 20% to 43% of older adults 65 years and older.[22,23] This frequency of use is thought to relate to the relative perceived comfort of corticosteroid prescribing and use by physicians and patients alike, as compared with immunomodulators or biologic agents. In a national cohort study of Medicare beneficiaries who were 65 years or older, only 3.7% of patients received steroid-sparing therapy with an anti-TNF agent. Additionally, 19% and 10% of these patients on anti-TNF therapy received prolonged corticosteroid courses of at least 3 or 6 months duration, respectively.[24]

Although all patients are vulnerable to the effects of systemic corticosteroids, older adults are at particularly risk of a corticosteroid-related complication.[11,25] In a population-based case-control study of patients with IBD older than 65 years using Canadian administrative health data, oral corticosteroid use was associated with a statistically significant higher likelihood of serious infection (adjusted relative risk, 2.3; 95% CI, 1.8–2.9).[26] In a second study, 40% of older adults had a corticosteroid-related adverse event, and 16% osteoporosis specifically.[27] Although this factor should be considered and discussed for all patients with IBD, a baseline bone density study and calcium and vitamin D supplementation is of particular importance in older adults especially in the setting of prolonged corticosteroid treatment.[28]

Immunomodulators

Immunomodulators, such as thiopurines or methotrexate, are used in the maintenance treatment of moderate to severe IBD.[13,29] Thiopurines (including 6-mercaptopurine and its prodrug, azathioprine) work on multiple proinflammatory pathways, ultimately inhibiting nucleic acid biosynthesis and inflammation. Methotrexate works by inhibiting various enzymes required for folic acid synthesis, ultimately inhibiting protein synthesis leading to its anti-inflammatory effects. Azathioprine has demonstrated efficacy in randomized controlled trials of patients with steroid-dependent UC as compared with oral 5-aminosalicylic acid therapy.[30] Similar studies have demonstrated the efficacy of both azathioprine and intramuscular methotrexate in maintaining remission in Crohn's disease.[29] Immunomodulators are also used in low doses in combination with biologics to decrease immunogenicity. Immunomodulators have many adverse effects, which can often limit their use. The most common adverse effects of azathioprine and 6-mercaptopurine include allergic reactions, pancreatitis, nausea, myelosuppression, infections, hepatotoxicity, and cancer. They have also been linked with a higher risk of nonmelanoma skin cancer and lymphoma.[31] Methotrexate has similar adverse effects, in addition to pneumatosis, with the exception of lymphoma.[29]

Immunomodulators tend to be used less frequently in older adults.[32] This trend may be related to concerns for adverse effects, particularly lymphoproliferative diseases or nonmelanoma skin cancer, for which increasing age is also a risk factor. In addition to these adverse effects, particular attention needs to be paid to older adults receiving an immunomodulator, given drug–drug interactions with medications that are more common in older adults, such as allopurinol or coumadin. The metabolism and excretion of these drugs needs to also be considered, because older adults tend toward higher rates of renal and hepatic impairment.

Biologics

Biologics are used for induction and maintenance of remission in both Crohn's disease and UC, and work on targeted inflammatory pathways. Current commercially available biologics include anti-TNFs such as infliximab, adalimumab, golimumab, and certolizumab; anti-integrins, such as vedolizumab; and anti-IL-12/23 inhibitors, such as ustekinumab. These medications have changed the natural history of IBD, and have demonstrated a benefit in decreasing corticosteroid use, hospitalizations, and surgeries.[33–38] These targeted therapies are increasing in their use for the treatment of moderate to severe IBD. Their more relevant adverse effects include infections, neurologic complications, dermatologic issues, and melanoma.[39]

Although biologics, especially anti-TNFs, have been increasingly common, they are less often used in the treatment of older adults with IBD.[11,12] A study using a Medicare IBD cohort from 2006 to 2009 reported 3.7% use of anti-TNF therapy among beneficiaries 65 years and older.[24] This low use may be partially related to less severe disease, but differences in use persist even when controlling for this factor. The use of anti-TNF therapy is also contraindicated in the setting of severe cardiomyopathies and heart failure, which is a more common comorbidity with increasing age. In an IBD cohort from the Netherlands, patients with elderly-onset Crohn's disease were 1.6 times less likely to use a biologic agent, and those with elderly-onset UC were 2.4 times less likely to use a biologic agent.[40] Therapy cessation rates were similar between older and younger patients, and most likely to be related to loss of response.[40] Interestingly, some observational studies have suggested lower response rates to anti-TNF therapy in older adults.[41] However, it is unclear if this finding may be related to confounding factors, such as disease duration, which are difficult to account for. A similar safety and effectiveness profile has been demonstrated for elderly patients receiving vedolizumab.[42]

SURGERY IN GERIATRIC PATIENTS

Surgery is commonly indicated for medication-refractory IBD or colonic dysplasia. Older patients with Crohn's disease are more likely to undergo a surgical resection on presentation or shortly after diagnosis, although long-term surgical rates are similar to younger patients. In a population-based IBD cohort, 14.1% of patients with elderly-onset Crohn's disease underwent a surgical resection on diagnosis as compared with 7.1% of younger Crohn's disease patients (adjusted hazard ratio, 1.88; 95% CI, 1.12–3.15).[40] Surgery at diagnosis was much less common in UC with rates of 0.5% as compared with 0.9% in elderly-onset disease as compared with a younger age of onset, respectively.[40]

Older adults are also at higher risk for surgery related complications, including postoperative infections and mortality. In UC, total proctocolectomy with end ileostomy is more common than an ileal pouch anal anastomosis as a result of concerns regarding function in older adults. However, recent studies demonstrate no difference in functional outcomes among older adults who undergo ileal pouch anal anastomosis surgery.[43,44] In a systematic review including 3 retrospective studies of pouch failure after ileal pouch anal anastomosis, there was no statistically significant difference in pouch failure by age.[43] However, given that these studies are observational in nature, they may have selected for older adults who are more likely to have favorable postsurgical outcomes.

SPECIAL CONSIDERATIONS

Older adults are less likely to be represented in clinical trials.[45] Therefore, a majority of the knowledge we have on the safety of medical and surgical therapy in the treatment of IBD, as well as IBD-related morbidity and mortality comes from observational studies.

Infections

Although patients with IBD and those receiving immune targeted therapy are at risk for certain infection, age is a major risk factor for infections. Ananthakrishnan and McGinley[46] report on the higher likelihood of infection-related hospitalizations among admitted patients with IBD older than 66 years, when controlling for comorbidities (adjusted hazard ratio, 1.20; 95% CI, 1.11–1.30). Most commonly, older age was associated with a higher risk of *C difficile* infections, bacterial pneumonia, urinary tract infections, and related sepsis.[46] Immunosuppression also places these patients at risk for opportunistic infections, such as tuberculosis, legionella, toxoplasmosis, *Pneumocystis jiroveci* pneumonia, histoplasmosis, cytomegalovirus, varicella zoster virus, and Epstein–Barr virus.[47] Elderly patients are at particularly high risk for morbidity and mortality related to these infections. In a multicenter prospectively enrolled Italian IBD cohort, patients older than 65 years were more likely to have a serious infection and a higher mortality rate than younger patients.[48] In addition, those older patients receiving an biologic therapy had higher rates of serious infections and death as compared with those on nonbiologic therapy.[48] This consideration is important in a discussion of treatment strategies for older patients with IBD. Although a top-down approach has become more commonplace, a more personalized step-up approach may be more fitting for older patients with IBD, although further studies are necessary to better understand the most effective strategies.

Given the higher risk of serious infection, infection prevention measures are particularly important in the treatment of older patients with IBD. This strategy includes an emphasis on vaccination against influenza virus and pneumococcal infections in this subgroup. Vaccination against varicella zoster virus needs to also be considered, and has become more feasible for patients on immune-targeted therapy with the recent availability of the recombinant Shingrix vaccine.

Cancer

The prevalence of cancer increases with age. This finding is particularly important to understand in the context of considering IBD treatment options in older adults with immunomodulator or biologic therapy. Thiopurines have been associated with a higher likelihood of non-Hodgkin's lymphoma and nonmelanoma skin cancer, and anti-TNF agents have been associated with a higher likelihood of melanoma. In addition, although IBD is an independent predictor of colorectal cancer, the incidence of colorectal cancer also increases with age. Therefore, cancers should be excluded before the initiation of IBD-targeted therapy in older adults, and the potential increased risk of malignancy in the setting of immunosuppressant or biologic therapy needs to be carefully weighed against the benefits in these patients. Once on immune-targeted therapy, the importance of an annual skin cancer screening should also be emphasized.

Patients with IBD of at least 8 years' duration or a comorbid diagnosis of primary sclerosis cholangitis are at higher than average risk of colorectal cancer. However, colorectal cancer surveillance in the elderly requires an individualized approach. Although colorectal cancer surveillance guidelines in IBD are the same regardless of age, life expectancy and fit for surgery need to be considered in a discussion of colorectal cancer surveillance in older patients with IBD.

Health Care Use

Overall, older patients with IBD tend to have a greater likelihood of hospitalization and are more likely to have confounding anemia, dehydration, and malnutrition.[45] In a cross-sectional study using all-payer discharge data from community hospitals, patients aged 65 years or older accounted for 25% of IBD hospitalizations.[49] A 3- to 4-fold higher in-hospital mortality has been demonstrated among older patients with IBD, with age as a strong independent predictor.[49] Infection-related admissions (especially opportunistic infections and *C difficile* infections) have been shown to particularly contribute to this morbidity and mortality.

Comorbidities and Polypharmacy

One-third of elderly patients are estimated to use 5 or more chronic medications. This predisposes patients to noncompliance, medication errors, and drug-drug interactions.[5] Specific drug–drug interaction are discussed in the Treatment of Inflammatory Bowel section. Elderly patients with mobility or vision issues may also have more difficulty with injectable medications, enemas, or suppositories, which needs to be considered when prescribing certain therapies.

SUMMARY

As the population continues to age, we will be seeing an increasing number of older adults with IBD. The management of IBD in the elderly comes with specific challenges, as a result of comorbidities, polypharmacy, age-related circumstances, and limited inclusion of older adults in clinical trials. To best care for older adults with IBD, it is important to be aware of the special considerations in their treatment, with particular attention to the risk of infections, malignancy, comorbidities, and overall fitness. Gaps in knowledge on how to best manage older patients with IBD exist. Future clinical trials should consider inclusion of older adults to gain a better understanding of treatment effectiveness and safety that may differ by age. Studies that better examine the optimal treatment strategies for older patients are also lacking.

CLINICS CARE POINTS

- Have a high index of suspicion for IBD in the presentation of an older adult with gastrointestinal complaints.
- The workup for IBD in the older adult is similar to the general population, and involves laboratory testing and an endoscopic evaluation.
- Older adults are vulnerable to the effects of systemic corticosteroids.
- Immunomodulators, biologics, and surgical interventions are all used in the management of IBD when the benefits outweigh risks.

DISCLOSURE

The authors have nothing to disclose.

REFERENCES

1. Shivashankar R, Tremaine WJ, Harmsen WS, et al. Incidence and prevalence of Crohn's disease and ulcerative colitis in Olmsted county, Minnesota from 1970 through 2010. Clin Gastroenterol Hepatol 2017;15:857–63.
2. Coward S, Clement F, Benchimol EI, et al. Past and future burden of inflammatory bowel diseases based on modeling of population-based data. Gastroenterology 2019;156:1345–1353 e4.
3. Gisbert JP, Chaparro M. Systematic review with meta-analysis: inflammatory bowel disease in the elderly. Aliment Pharmacol Ther 2014;39:459–77.
4. Norgard BM, Nielsen J, Fonager K, et al. The incidence of ulcerative colitis (1995-2011) and Crohn's disease (1995-2012) - based on nationwide Danish registry data. J Crohns Colitis 2014;8:1274–80.
5. Ahmed O, Nguyen GC. Therapeutic challenges of managing inflammatory bowel disease in the elderly patient. Expert Rev Gastroenterol Hepatol 2016;10: 1005–10.
6. Foxworthy DM, Wilson JA. Crohn's disease in the elderly. Prolonged delay in diagnosis. J Am Geriatr Soc 1985;33:492–5.
7. Hadithi M, Cazemier M, Meijer GA, et al. Retrospective analysis of old-age colitis in the Dutch inflammatory bowel disease population. World J Gastroenterol 2008; 14:3183–7.
8. Pardi DS, Loftus EV Jr, Camilleri M. Treatment of inflammatory bowel disease in the elderly: an update. Drugs Aging 2002;19:355–63.
9. Gower-Rousseau C, Vasseur F, Fumery M, et al. Epidemiology of inflammatory bowel diseases: new insights from a French population-based registry (EPIMAD). Dig Liver Dis 2013;45:89–94.
10. Benchimol EI, Cook SF, Erichsen R, et al. International variation in medication prescription rates among elderly patients with inflammatory bowel disease. J Crohns Colitis 2013;7:878–89.
11. Govani SM, Wiitala WL, Stidham RW, et al. Age disparities in the use of steroid-sparing therapy for inflammatory bowel disease. Inflamm Bowel Dis 2016;22: 1923–8.
12. Feagins LA, Spechler SJ. Biologic agent use varies inversely with age at diagnosis in Crohn's disease. Dig Dis Sci 2010;55:3164–70.
13. Harbord M, Eliakim R, Bettenworth D, et al. Third European evidence-based consensus on diagnosis and management of ulcerative colitis. part 2: current management. J Crohns Colitis 2017;11:769–84.
14. Ham M, Moss AC. Mesalamine in the treatment and maintenance of remission of ulcerative colitis. Expert Rev Clin Pharmacol 2012;5:113–23.
15. Marshall JK, Thabane M, Steinhart AH, et al. Rectal 5-aminosalicylic acid for induction of remission in ulcerative colitis. Cochrane Database Syst Rev 2010;(1):CD004115.
16. Ford AC, Khan KJ, Achkar JP, et al. Efficacy of oral vs. topical, or combined oral and topical 5-aminosalicylates, in ulcerative colitis: systematic review and meta-analysis. Am J Gastroenterol 2012;107:167–76 [author reply: 77].
17. Wang Y, Parker CE, Bhanji T, et al. Oral 5-aminosalicylic acid for induction of remission in ulcerative colitis. Cochrane Database Syst Rev 2016;(4):CD000543.

18. Ford AC, Achkar JP, Khan KJ, et al. Efficacy of 5-aminosalicylates in ulcerative colitis: systematic review and meta-analysis. Am J Gastroenterol 2011;106: 601–16.
19. Juneja M, Baidoo L, Schwartz MB, et al. Geriatric inflammatory bowel disease: phenotypic presentation, treatment patterns, nutritional status, outcomes, and comorbidity. Dig Dis Sci 2012;57:2408–15.
20. Charpentier C, Salleron J, Savoye G, et al. Natural history of elderly-onset inflammatory bowel disease: a population-based cohort study. Gut 2014;63:423–32.
21. Waljee AK, Rogers MA, Lin P, et al. Short term use of oral corticosteroids and related harms among adults in the United States: population based cohort study. BMJ 2017;357:j1415.
22. Ananthakrishnan AN, Donaldson T, Lasch K, et al. Management of inflammatory bowel disease in the elderly patient: challenges and opportunities. Inflamm Bowel Dis 2017;23:882–93.
23. Johnson SL, Palta M, Bartels CM, et al. Examining systemic steroid Use in older inflammatory bowel disease patients using hurdle models: a cohort study. BMC Pharmacol Toxicol 2015;16:34.
24. Johnson SL, Bartels CM, Palta M, et al. Biological and steroid use in relationship to quality measures in older patients with inflammatory bowel disease: a US Medicare cohort study. BMJ Open 2015;5:e008597.
25. Waljee AK, Wiitala WL, Govani S, et al. Corticosteroid use and complications in a US inflammatory bowel disease cohort. PLoS One 2016;11:e0158017.
26. Brassard P, Bitton A, Suissa A, et al. Oral corticosteroids and the risk of serious infections in patients with elderly-onset inflammatory bowel diseases. Am J Gastroenterol 2014;109:1795–802 [quiz: 803].
27. Thomas TP. The complications of systemic corticosteroid therapy in the elderly. A retrospective study. Gerontology 1984;30:60–5.
28. Lichtenstein GR, Sands BE, Pazianas M. Prevention and treatment of osteoporosis in inflammatory bowel disease. Inflamm Bowel Dis 2006;12:797–813.
29. Lichtenstein GR, Loftus EV, Isaacs KL, et al. ACG clinical guideline: management of Crohn's disease in adults. Am J Gastroenterol 2018;113:481–517.
30. Ardizzone S, Maconi G, Russo A, et al. Randomised controlled trial of azathioprine and 5-aminosalicylic acid for treatment of steroid dependent ulcerative colitis. Gut 2006;55:47–53.
31. Kappelman MD, Farkas DK, Long MD, et al. Risk of cancer in patients with inflammatory bowel diseases: a nationwide population-based cohort study with 30 years of follow-up evaluation. Clin Gastroenterol Hepatol 2014;12:265–73.e1.
32. Kariyawasam VC, Kim S, Mourad FH, et al. Comorbidities rather than age are associated with the use of immunomodulators in elderly-onset inflammatory bowel disease. Inflamm Bowel Dis 2019;25:1390–8.
33. Colombel JF, Sandborn WJ, Reinisch W, et al. Infliximab, azathioprine, or combination therapy for Crohn's disease. N Engl J Med 2010;362:1383–95.
34. Feagan BG, Rutgeerts P, Sands BE, et al. Vedolizumab as induction and maintenance therapy for ulcerative colitis. N Engl J Med 2013;369:699–710.
35. Feagan BG, Sandborn WJ, Gasink C, et al. Ustekinumab as induction and maintenance therapy for Crohn's disease. N Engl J Med 2016;375:1946–60.
36. Sandborn WJ, Feagan BG, Rutgeerts P, et al. Vedolizumab as induction and maintenance therapy for Crohn's disease. N Engl J Med 2013;369:711–21.
37. Sandborn WJ, Gasink C, Gao LL, et al. Ustekinumab induction and maintenance therapy in refractory Crohn's disease. N Engl J Med 2012;367:1519–28.

38. Panaccione R, Ghosh S, Middleton S, et al. Combination therapy with infliximab and azathioprine is superior to monotherapy with either agent in ulcerative colitis. Gastroenterology 2014;146:392–400 e3.

39. Colombel JF, Loftus EV Jr, Tremaine WJ, et al. The safety profile of infliximab in patients with Crohn's disease: the Mayo clinic experience in 500 patients. Gastroenterology 2004;126:19–31.

40. Jeuring SF, van den Heuvel TR, Zeegers MP, et al. Epidemiology and long-term outcome of inflammatory bowel disease diagnosed at elderly age-an increasing distinct entity? Inflamm Bowel Dis 2016;22:1425–34.

41. Desai A, Zator ZA, de Silva P, et al. Older age is associated with higher rate of discontinuation of anti-TNF therapy in patients with inflammatory bowel disease. Inflamm Bowel Dis 2013;19:309–15.

42. Adar T, Faleck D, Sasidharan S, et al. Comparative safety and effectiveness of tumor necrosis factor alpha antagonists and vedolizumab in elderly IBD patients: a multicentre study. Aliment Pharmacol Ther 2019;49:873–9.

43. Shung DL, Abraham B, Sellin J, et al. Medical and surgical complications of inflammatory bowel disease in the elderly: a systematic review. Dig Dis Sci 2015; 60:1132–40.

44. Longo WE, Virgo KS, Bahadursingh AN, et al. Patterns of disease and surgical treatment among United States veterans more than 50 years of age with ulcerative colitis. Am J Surg 2003;186:514–8.

45. Sturm A, Maaser C, Mendall M, et al. European Crohn's and Colitis Organisation topical review on IBD in the elderly. J Crohns Colitis 2017;11:263–73.

46. Ananthakrishnan AN, McGinley EL. Infection-related hospitalizations are associated with increased mortality in patients with inflammatory bowel diseases. J Crohns Colitis 2013;7:107–12.

47. Toruner M, Loftus EV Jr, Harmsen WS, et al. Risk factors for opportunistic infections in patients with inflammatory bowel disease. Gastroenterology 2008;134: 929–36.

48. Cottone M, Kohn A, Daperno M, et al. Advanced age is an independent risk factor for severe infections and mortality in patients given anti-tumor necrosis factor therapy for inflammatory bowel disease. Clin Gastroenterol Hepatol 2011;9:30–5.

49. Ananthakrishnan AN, McGinley EL, Binion DG. Inflammatory bowel disease in the elderly is associated with worse outcomes: a national study of hospitalizations. Inflamm Bowel Dis 2009;15:182–9.

Moving?

Make sure your subscription moves with you!

To notify us of your new address, find your **Clinics Account Number** (located on your mailing label above your name), and contact customer service at:

Email: journalscustomerservice-usa@elsevier.com

800-654-2452 (subscribers in the U.S. & Canada)
314-447-8871 (subscribers outside of the U.S. & Canada)

Fax number: 314-447-8029

Elsevier Health Sciences Division
Subscription Customer Service
3251 Riverport Lane
Maryland Heights, MO 63043

*To ensure uninterrupted delivery of your subscription, please notify us at least 4 weeks in advance of move.